Assessment Skills for Paramedics

Assessment Skills for Paramedics

Second Edition

Edited by
Amanda Y. Blaber and
Graham Harris

McGraw Hill Education · Open University Press

Open University Press
McGraw-Hill Education
McGraw-Hill House
Shoppenhangers Road
Maidenhead
Berkshire
England
SL6 2QL

email: enquiries@openup.co.uk
world wide web: www.openup.co.uk

and Two Penn Plaza, New York, NY 10121-2289, USA

First published 2011
First published in this second edition 2016

Copyright © Amanda Y. Blaber and Graham Harris (Eds), 2016

All rights reserved. Except for the quotation of short passages for the purposes of criticism and review, no part of this publication may be reproduced, stored in a retrieval system, or transmitted, in any form or by any means, electronic, mechanical, photocopying, recording or otherwise, without the prior written permission of the publisher or a licence from the Copyright Licensing Agency Limited. Details of such licences (for reprographic reproduction) may be obtained from the Copyright Licensing Agency Ltd of Saffron House, 6–10 Kirby Street, London EC1N 8TS.

A catalogue record of this book is available from the British Library

ISBN-13: 978-0-33-526216-8
ISBN-10: 0-33-526216-3
eISBN: 978-0-33-526217-5

Library of Congress Cataloging-in-Publication Data
CIP data applied for

Typeset by Aptara, Inc.

Fictitious names of companies, products, people, characters and/or data that may be used herein (in case studies or in examples) are not intended to represent any real individual, company, product or event.

Printed and bound by CPI Group (UK) Ltd, Croydon, CR0 4YY

Praise for this book

"...This book clearly sets out and balances the critical, unscheduled and urgent care assessment priorities for paramedic students and those who are looking to refresh their skills. The content, depth of discussion and signposting within the book clearly highlight and discuss critical points for the reader which are supported with appropriate supporting evidence...We recommend this book to all of our paramedic students, and it should be an 'essential' purchase for all discerning paramedic students whether they are embarking on their studies or refreshing and updating their skills..."
Mark Nevins, Programme Leader, Paramedic Practice Programme,
Teesside University, UK

"This second edition draws on additional guidelines and best practice to elegantly illustrate the fundamental knowledge and skills required to undertake a comprehensive, evidence-based approach to patient assessment. The book builds on the plethora of knowledge and understanding of patient assessment, from common presentations through to complex specialisms which require a focused and often prompt response from the out-of-hospital care provider.
This book is ideally suited to the undergraduate paramedic student, along with experienced paramedics wishing to review their assessment techniques."
John Donaghy, Principal Lecturer and Professional Lead, Paramedic Science,
University of Hertfordshire, UK

Contents

Contributors · viii

How to use this book · x

Abbreviations and acronyms · xiii

1 General principles of assessment · 1

2 Respiratory assessment · 14

3 Cardiovascular assessment · 47

4 Abdominal and gastro-intestinal assessment · 82

5 Neurological assessment · 112

6 Spinal injuries assessment · 139

7 Trauma assessment · 151

8 Musculoskeletal assessment · 176

9 Assessment of minor injuries · 205

10 Minor ailments	226
11 Child assessment	245
12 Older person assessment	273
13 Obstetric patient assessment	293
14 Assessment and care of the newborn	309
15 Mental health assessment	325
Conclusion	350
Glossary of terms	351
Index	357

Contributors

Denise Aspland RGN, RSCN, DipHE Child Health, BSc (Hons) Health & Social Care Professional Practice. APLS Instructor, Senior Sister/Practice Development Sister, Darent Valley Hospital NHS Trust.

Chris Baker MSc, BSc (Hons) with Emergency Care Practice, CertEd. Clinical Tutor/Link Tutor, University Team (Saint George's University of London Honorary contract), London Ambulance Service.

Amanda Blaber PG (Dip)Ed, MSc Sociology of Health and Welfare, BSc (Hons) Health and Community Studies, Dip HE (Accident & Emergency), RGN. Honorary FCPara. Senior Lecturer, University of Brighton.

Vince Clarke BSc (Hons), PGCE, MA, MCPara. Principal Paramedic Tutor, Higher Education Team, London Ambulance Service NHS Trust.

Kevin Dark BSc (Hons), PGCE, MCPara. Paramedic Clinical Tutor, Higher Education Team. London Ambulance Service NHS Trust.

Stuart Elms Dip HE, MCPara. Clinical Director, East of England Air Ambulance Service.

Graham Harris MSc, BSc, PGCE, Advanced BTEC, Chartered MCIPD, FCPara. Director of Professional Standards, The College of Paramedics.

David Kerr MA, BSc (Hons), CertEd, MCPara. Senior Lecturer/Programme Leader Paramedic Science, Department of Adult Nursing & Paramedic Science, University of Greenwich.

Rehan Khan BSc (Clinical Sciences), MBBS, MRCOG. Consultant in Obstetrics and Gynaecology (Specialist in Maternal Medicine and Medical Education), RCOG tutor, Barts and the London NHS Trust.

Jaqualine Lindridge BA (Hons) DipHE, MA, PGCert, MCPara. Consultant Paramedic, London Ambulance Service NHS Trust.

Tracy Nicholls PGC (TLHE) (Open), FHEA, MCPara. Council Member for the East of England, The College of Paramedics.

Nandiran Ratnavel MBBS, MRCPCH. Consultant Neonatologist, Barts Health NHS Trust; Director, London Neonatal Transfer Service; Lead Clinician, Royal London Hospital Neonatal Services; Joint Clinical Lead, North East North Central London Neonatal Network.

Ursula Rolfe PhD student, MPhil media management, PG Cert Ed (Higher education), BSc, (Hons) Urgent and emergency care, BA (Hons) English and Psychology, MCPara. Programme Lead MSc Trauma Sciences, Southampton University.

Rob Slee BSc (Hons), PGCE, MCPara. Lecturer, Department of Adult Nursing & Paramedic Science, University of Greenwich.

Marlon Stiell MSc, BSc, Dip HE, MBPS (Member of the British Psychological Society). Senior Lecturer, Department of Adult Nursing and Paramedic Science, University of Greenwich.

Paul Townsend BSc (Hons), PGCE, MCPara. Paramedic Clinical Tutor. Higher Education Team. London Ambulance Service NHS Trust.

Nigel Ward Dip HE (Paramedic Science), MCPara. Paramedic Team Leader, London Ambulance Service NHS Trust.

How to use this book

This book is about *the process and skills of assessment*. Primarily the text is aimed at undergraduate student paramedics, and registered paramedics who may wish to revisit their knowledge of assessment. It does not explain how to obtain vital signs or demonstrate anatomy and physiology of systems, as these elements would be covered in other modules of learning in the curricula. Each chapter covers a particular system (e.g. respiratory) or subject (e.g. minor illness). Where applicable the chapters are written using the **primary** and **secondary** survey format, however, the content of Chapters 9, 10 and 14 cover assessment and care of the specialism instead.

Patient assessment does not necessarily incorporate or require the use of all the techniques discussed and described within the text. However, you may wish to use the text as an aide-mémoire, or if you feel that your subject knowledge and/ or relevant skills of assessing a particular area require updating or refreshing, then turn to the appropriate chapter. Here you will be able to review the evidence provided and, where applicable, appraise the subject knowledge and practise the skills/techniques identified. Following this, you will be able to implement these into your practice through your future patient assessments.

Each chapter commences with a brief description of the content, and where applicable a **Scene Assessment** appropriate to the particular chapter.

The **Primary Survey** configuration covers the **DR ABCDE** framework where appropriate and incorporates:

    D – Danger
    R – Response
    A – Airway
    B – Breathing
    C – Circulation
    D – Disability
    E – Expose, Examine and Evaluate

This presents a structured systematic format for the paramedic to follow.

The **Trauma** Chapter 7 includes the additional **'C'** for **Catastrophic Haemorrhage** element, DR 'C' ABCDE.

The **Obstetrics** Chapter 13 includes the additional **'F'** and **'G'** elements, **Fundus** and **Get to the point quickly**.

The **Child Assessment** Chapter 11 relates to the use of the 'ABC **'DEFG'** format, the latter specifically relating to **'Don't Ever Forget Glucose'**.

If, on completing the primary survey elements of your assessment, you identify that the patient does have a **time critical** condition, then you will need to manage the respective element/s accordingly and convey the patient to the appropriate place of care. Throughout the text **red flags** are represented by this symbol and advise the reader of areas of concern that may require immediate attention and/or action.

However; if your assessment has clearly identified that the patient **DOES NOT** have a time critical or a **red flag** condition, then your assessment of the patient should continue by implementing and conducting a **Secondary Survey**.

The chapter continues with a description of the assessment/examination for that particular area or speciality of the secondary survey, followed by information on conditions specific to that system or area of speciality, which where appropriate adheres to the following structure:

Presenting Complaint	**(PC)**
History of Presenting Complaint	**(HPC)**
Past Medical History	**(PMH)**
Drug/Medication History	**(DMH)**
Social/Family History	**(SFH)**
Review of Systems	**(ROS)**

This affords a continuation of the structured arrangement which provides a systematic format of obtaining the **History** of the patient in relation to their presenting complaint and the area or systems affected. Following this structure while performing the secondary survey will enable the paramedic to obtain all of the elements of a focused history, which include:

- History
- Vital signs
- Physical assessment.

These elements enable the paramedic to identify illnesses or injuries not ascertained during the primary survey. They simultaneously provide the opportunity

How to use this book

of detecting less obvious illnesses/injuries and/or signs and symptoms of underlying medical conditions.

Throughout the chapter there are action boxes. These include a summary of the key points of the **Possible actions to be taken** for the respective element of the survey. Depending on your findings from the assessment you will decide whether or not the action or actions are appropriate to the respective patient, and therefore whether these actions need to be addressed. As stated if the patient has a **time critical** and/or **red flag** condition identified in the **Primary Survey**, then the paramedic will need to manage this accordingly.

The end of chapter contains the reference list. There is a comprehensive glossary of terms at the back of the text and the terms are given in ***bold italic*** on their first occurrence.

Throughout the book the reader may come across repetition of certain conditions, and this is due to these being relevant to each particular chapter. For example, in Chapter 2 Respiratory assessment, the authors describe injuries to the respiratory system, including tension pneumothorax, and in Chapter 7 Trauma assessment, the authors describe various life-threatening injuries caused by trauma that affect the patient's breathing, one of which includes tension pneumothorax.

Remember that with many patients and their presenting conditions you may be assessing several systems, and in certain instances two or more patients simultaneously. Paramedics, as Health and Care Professions Council (HCPC) registrants, are required to maintain their knowledge and competency of skills. Whether you are a student or experienced paramedic, the information provided in this text will assist you in obtaining a structured assessment of your patients, and will be a useful aid in maintaining your knowledge and competency of assessment skills.

Abbreviations and acronyms

AAA	Abdominal Aortic Aneurysm
AACE	Association of Ambulance Chief Executives
ACCP	American College of Chest Physicians
ACJ	Acromioclavicular Joint
ACS	Acute Coronary Syndrome
ACT	Assess the scene, Communicate, Triage, treat and transport
ADL	Activity of Daily Living
AF	Atrial Fibrillation
ALS	Advanced Life Support
ALSG	Advanced Life Support Group
AMHP	Approved Mental Health Professional
AMI	Acute Myocardial Infarction
AMT	Abbreviated Mental Test
APH	Ante-Partum Haemorrhage
APR	Active, Passive, Resisted
AR	Aortic Regurgitation
ARVC	Arrhythmogenic Right Ventricular Cardiomyopathy
AS	Aortic Stenosis
ASD	Atrial Septal Defect
ATMIST	Age, Time of incident, Mechanism, Injuries, Signs and Symptoms, Treatment given/immediate needs
AVNRT	Atrioventricular Nodal Re-entry Tachycardia
AVPU	A – alert, V – responds to verbal stimuli, P – responds to painful stimuli, U – unresponsive.
BASICS	British Association of Immediate Care Schemes
BECHS	Bradycardia, Exhaustion, Central Cyanosis, Hypotension and a Silent chest
BGL	Blood Glucose Level
BLS	Basic Life Support
BNF	British National Formulary

Abbreviations and acronyms

BP	Blood Pressure
BPM	Beats Per Minute
BTS	British Thoracic Society
BVM	Bag Valve Mask
CABG	Coronary Artery Bypass Grafting
CAD	Coronary Artery Disease
CAP	Community Acquired Pneumonia
CBR	Capillary Bed Refill
CBRNE	Chemical, Biological, Radiological, Nuclear, and Explosive Incidents
CCF	Congestive Cardiac Failure
CHD	Coronary Heart Disease
CHL	Conductive Hearing Loss
CIMAH	Control of Industrial Major Accident Hazards
CMACE	Centre for Maternal and Child Enquiries
CN	Cranial Nerve
CoP	College of Paramedics
COPD	Chronic Obstructive Pulmonary Disease
CPAP	Continuous Positive Airway Pressure
CRT	Capillary Refill Time
CSF	Cerebral Spinal Fluid
CVD	Cardiovascular Disease
CVS	Cardiovascular System
DCM	Dilated Cardiomyopathy
DELIRIUMS	Drugs or toxins, Emotional (psychiatric), Low pO_2, Infection, Retention (stool/urine), Ictal (seizures), Under nutrition/dehydration, Metabolism, Subdural haematoma
DH	Department of Health
DIB	Difficulty In Breathing
DKA	Diabetic Ketoacidosis
DMH	Drug/Medication History
DNAR	Do Not Attempt Resuscitation
DOB	Date of Birth
DR 'C' ABCDE	Danger, Response, Catastrophic Haemorrhage, Airway, Breathing, Circulation, Danger, Expose-Examine-Evaluate
DSH	Deliberate Self-Harm
DVT	Deep Vein Thrombosis
ECG	Electrocardiogram

Abbreviations and acronyms

ED	Emergency Department
EDD	Estimated Date of Delivery
ENT	Ear, Nose & Throat
ETA	Estimated Time of Arrival
EtCO$_2$	End Tidal Carbon Dioxide
ETI	Endotracheal Intubation
ETT	Endotracheal Tube
FAST	Face, Arms, Speech, Test
FEV	Forced Expiratory Volume
FGAs	First Generation Anti-psychotics
FLACC	Face, Legs, Activity, Cry, Consolability
FLAPS	Feel the chest, Look at the chest, Listen to the chest (auscultate), Percuss the chest, Sides under the sides of the chest and shoulders
FOOSH	Fall Onto Out Stretched Hand
GAD	General Anxiety Disorder
GCS	Glasgow Coma Score/Scale
GI	Gastro-intestinal
GMC	General Medical Council
GP	General Practitioner
GSW	Gunshot Wound
GU	Genito-urinary
HART	Hazardous Area Response Team
HASU	Hyper Acute Stroke Unit
HCl	Hydrochloric Acid
HCM	Hypertrophic Cardiomyopathy
HCPC	Health and Care Professions Council
HEMS	Helicopter Emergency Medical Service
HF	Heart Failure
HOCM	Hypertrophic Obstructive Cardiomyopathy
HPC	History of Presenting Complaint
HR	Heart Rate
HSE	Health and Safety Executive
IAPP	Inspection, Auscultation, Percussion, Auscultation
ICC	Inherited Cardiac Conditions
ICD	Implantable Cardioverter Defibrillator
ICP	Intracranial Pressure
ICS	Intercostal Space

Abbreviations and acronyms

IHD	Ischaemic Heart Disease
IPPA	Inspection, Palpation, Percussion, Auscultation
ISS	Injury Severity Score
ITU	Intensive Therapy Unit
JACCOL	Jaundice, Anaemia, Clubbing, Cyanosis, Oedema, Lymphadenopathy
JVP	Jugular Venous Pressure
LBBB	Left Bundle Branch Block
LLQ	Left Lower Quadrant
LMP	Last Menstrual Period
LOC	Level of Consciousness
LOC	Loss of Consciousness
LQTS	Long QT Syndrome
LSSA	Local Social Services Authority
LVF	Left Ventricular Failure
LVH	Left Ventricular Hypertrophy
LUQ	Left Upper Quadrant
MAOIs	Mono-Amine Oxidase Inhibitors
MCP	Metacarpo-Phalangeal Joints
MDT	Mobile Data Terminal
METHANE	Major incident standby or declared, Exact location of incident, Type of incident, Hazards (present and potential), Access and egress routes, Number, severity and type of casualties, Emergency services present on scene and further resources required.
MHL	Mixed Hearing Loss
MHRA	Medicines and Healthcare Products Regulatory Agency
MI	Myocardial Infarction
MILS	Manual Inline Stabilization
MIU	Minor Injury Unit
MOI	Mechanism of Injury
MSC	Motor, Sensory, Circulation
MSD	Musculoskeletal Disorder
MSI	Musculoskeletal Injury
MSU	Mid-Stream Urine
NAEMT	National Association of Emergency Medical Technicians
NAI	Non-Accidental Injury
NAO	National Audit Office
NARU	National Ambulance Resilience Units

NASSAs	Nor-Adrenaline and Specific Serotonergic Antidepressants
NCCfMH	National Collaborating Centre for Mental Health
NCEPOD	National Confidential Enquiry into Patient Outcome and Death
NCGC	National Clinical Guideline Centre
NHS	National Health Service
NICE	National Institute for Health and Care Excellence
NLS	Newborn Life Support
NOF	Neck of Femur
NP	Nasal Pharyngeal
NSAID	Non-Steroidal Anti-Inflammatory Drugs
NSPCC	The National Society for Prevention of Cruelty to Children
OCD	Obsessive Compulsive Disorders
ONS	Office for National Statistics
OPA	Oral Pharyngeal Airway
OTC	Over the Counter
PALS	Paediatric Advanced Life Support
PC	Presenting Complaint
PCI	Percutaneous Coronary Intervention
PE	Pulmonary Embolism
PEF	Peak Expiratory Flow
PERRLA	Pupils Equal and Round; React to Light and Accommodation
PGDs	Patient Group Directives
PIH	Pregnancy-Induced Hypertension
PIP	Proximal Inter-Phalangeal Joint
PMH	Past Medical History
PND	Paroxsymal Nocturnal Dyspnoea
PND	Postnatal Depression
PPCI	Primary Percutaneous Coronary Intervention
PPE	Personal Protective Equipment
PR	Per Rectum
PRICE	Protection, Rest, Ice, Compression, Elevation
PTCA	Percutaneous Transluminal Coronary Angioplasty
PTSD	Posttraumatic Stress Disorder
PV	Per Vagina
RAD	Right Axis Deviation
RBBB	Right Bundle Branch Block
RFS	Red Flag Sepsis

RICE	Rest, Ice, Compression, Elevation
RLQ	Right Lower Quadrant
ROLE	Recognition of Life Extinct
ROM	Range of Movement
ROS	Review of Systems
ROSC	Return of Spontaneous Circulation
RR	Respiratory Rate
RTC	Road Traffic Collision
RUQ	Right Upper Quadrant
RVF	Right Ventricular Failure
RVP	RendezVous Points
SAH	Sub-Arachnoid Haemorrhage
SAMPLE	Signs & Symptoms, Allergies, Medications, Past medical history, Last meal, Events leading up to the incident
SCCM	Society of Critical Care Medicine
SCENE	Safety, Cause including (MOI), Environment, Number of patients, Extra resources needed
SCI	Spinal Cord Injury
SCJ	Sternoclavicular Joint
SFH	Social/Family History
S/FMH	Social/Family Medical History
SGA	Supra-Glottic Airway
SGAs	Second Generation Anti-psychotics
SGD	Supraglottic Airway Device
SHL	Sensorineural Hearing Loss
SIRS	Systemic Inflammatory Response Syndrome
SLIPDUCT	Swelling, Loss of function, Irregularity, Pain, Deformity, Unnatural movement, Crepitus, Tenderness
SNRIs	Serotonin and Noradrenaline Reuptake Inhibitors
SOB	Shortness of Breath
SOCRATES	Site, Onset, Character, Radiates, Associated symptoms, Time/duration, Exacerbating factors, Severity
SORT	Special Operations Response Team
SpO$_2$	Oxygen saturation monitor
SROM	Spontaneous Rupture Of Membranes
SSRIs	Selective Serotonin Reuptake Inhibitors
STEMI	ST-segment Elevated Myocardial Infarction
TARN	Trauma Audit and Research Network

Abbreviations and acronyms

TIA	Transient Ischaemic Attack
TMJ	Temporomandibular Joint
TWELVE	Tracheal deviation, Wounds, Emphysema (surgical), Laryngeal crepitus, Venous distension, Expose the thorax and Exclude injuries.
UECC	Urgent & Emergency Care Centre
UK	United Kingdom
URTI	Upper Respiratory Tract Infection
UTI	Urinary Tract Infection
VA	Visual Acuity
VF	Ventricular Fibrillation
VSD	Ventricular Septal Defect
VT	Ventricular Tachycardia
WBC	White Blood Cell
WHO	World Health Organization
WIC	Walk-In Centre

1 General principles of assessment
Graham Harris

This chapter will provide a brief overview of the general principles of assessment. It will include how to undertake an *assessment* of the scene, conducting a primary and secondary survey, and the evidence that the paramedic needs to obtain while performing the assessment.

SCENE ASSESSMENT

As with any situation, the attending paramedic can obtain a wealth of information and details from assessing the scene of the incident: these can be divided into sections on safety and the situation itself.

Safety

When approaching any scene or incident, consideration should be given to the following:

- Safety for self, colleague(s), patient(s) and other persons on the scene
- Are other emergency services present on the scene; are they required?
- Can the scene be secured? Rescue attempts should only be undertaken by trained personnel (*besides Fire and Rescue Services, this includes Hazardous Area Response Team (HART) and/or Special Operations Response Team (SORT) trained personnel*) (College of Paramedics (CoP), 2015a)
- If the situation is hazardous, can the patients be moved to safe area?
- Consider the possibility of further threat to self, colleague(s) or patient(s) from:
  - fire
  - blood or other body fluids
  - weapons
  - traffic
  - environmental conditions (e.g. *flash floods*).

SITUATION

While the situation itself is assessed following the safety assessment, in essence, these features tend to have significant overlap, as certain situations pose differing safety hazards:

- What has taken place at the scene?
- What is the nature of the incident/illness (e.g. *trauma due to a road traffic collision (RTC), or the onset of an acute or exacerbation of a chronic medical condition*)?
- What is the **mechanism of injury (MOI)** (e.g. *fall, blunt or penetrating trauma*)?
- How many patients are there, and what are their ages?
- Do you require further paramedic assistance (e.g. *specialist, advanced or consultant paramedic*), or supportive areas of practice (e.g. *HART or SORT team, or helicopter emergency medical services (HEMS)*)?

PRIMARY SURVEY

The purpose of conducting a **primary survey** is to identify if there are any life-threatening problems, and to manage them accordingly while determining if early transportation is required. Depending upon the nature of the incident/situation, the paramedic conducts a primary survey using the **DR ABCDE** framework (Resuscitation Council (UK), 2011), however; in certain trauma incidents because of '**catastrophic haemorrhage**', there may be a requirement to use the **DR 'C' ABCDE** framework (Hodgetts et al., 2006). In essence, the primary survey is undertaken with an instantaneous overview of all elements in relation to the patient's respective system conditions.

Element	System
D – Danger	
R – Response	(Neurological system)
A – Airway/including 'C' spine immobilization	(Respiratory system)
B – Breathing/severe illness/chest injuries	(Respiratory system)
C – Circulation/**haemorrhage**/shock	(Cardiovascular system)
D – Disability	(Neurological system)
E – Expose/Examine/Environment	

DANGER

This element covers the safety of the paramedic, colleagues and the patient(s). It is simultaneously ascertained as part of the scene assessment. The reasoning for this is that if the paramedic is overcome by the circumstances of the incident (*inhalation of smoke, gases, flash-flooding*), they will be of no benefit to the patient.

General principles of assessment

The paramedic needs to differentiate between the actual and potential aspects of danger of any incident they attend. This could incorporate anything from:

- positioning of the vehicle (*fend off*) to provide protection at the scene of a road traffic collision
- approaching chemical, biological, radiological, nuclear and explosive, (CBRNE) incidents (AACE, 2013a)
- approaching fires and hazardous material (*hazmat*) incidents safely
- requesting that pets are secured in another room
- requesting the attendance of police at a possible crime scene
- ensuring that appropriate personal protective equipment (PPE) is worn in relation to the incident, for example, hi-visibility jackets when attending a road traffic incident.

Possible actions to be taken:

- Ensure **personal protective equipment (PPE)** is worn
- Request fire/police service assistance
- Request a (*HART* and/or *SORT*) team as appropriate
- Request the assistance of an appropriate specialist, advanced or consultant paramedic (College of Paramedics, 2015b).

RESPONSE

This provides the paramedic with the opportunity to introduce themselves and obtain an initial assessment of the patient's ability to respond to verbal communication. The paramedic introduces themselves and asks the patient what has happened. How the patient responds (or does not respond) will provide significant information as to their level of consciousness. In the primary survey the **AVPU** framework is used:

> **A** – The patient is **A**lert, conscious and responds directly and appropriately to the paramedic's question/introduction.
> **V** – The patient responds to the **V**erbal command, which may be a grunt or groan.
> **P** – The patient responds only to **P**ainful stimuli.
> **U** – The patient is **U**nresponsive.

Possible actions to be taken:

- Record the patient's level of consciousness (LOC)
- Record any period of **unconsciousness** (*it may be part of the patient's **lucid interval***).

AIRWAY

- Does the patient have a patent airway? If so, are they able to maintain it for themselves?
- The patient who responds **A** on the **A**VPU scale is described above as Alert. This can be considered to be the case if the patient is talking, therefore the airway is open. However, the patient may be making unusual sounds such as snoring or making gurgling sounds, a **stridor** or wheezing may be heard, all of which could indicate there is some form of airway obstruction.
- Gurgling indicates that there is fluid in the airway and there is a need for suction (Resuscitation Council (UK), 2011).
- Snoring may indicate a soft tissue problem either with the tongue, swelling or foreign body obstruction.
- Stridor indicates a problem above the vocal cords in the upper airway, whereas wheezing indicates the problem is below the vocal cords in the lower airways.
- If the patient is unresponsive, ascertain if there is an obstruction due to fluids or foreign bodies in the airway and manage accordingly. Open the airway, depending on the MOI, consider a 'C' spine manoeuvre (*jaw-thrust technique*), alternatively if there is no 'C' spine problem, then consider using the (*head-tilt-chin-lift technique*) (see *Spinal Injuries Assessment, Chapter 6*).
- If appropriate, consider the use of an adjunct (*oral (OP) and nasal (NP) pharyngeal airways*) in maintaining the airway (Resuscitation Council (UK), 2011).

Possible actions to be taken:

- Consider 'C' spine problems and use the appropriate technique
- Ensure airway is patent and secure before proceeding to next element.

BREATHING

- Look to see that the patient is breathing. Look, listen and feel for no more than 10 seconds to determine if the victim is breathing normally (Resuscitation Council (UK), 2010).
- If *apnoeic*, then commence immediate **ventilations** using bag-valve-mask (BVM) and supplemental oxygen before continuing with the next element of the assessment.
- Look to see if the patient is using **accessory muscles**, supraclavicular retraction (*suprasternal retractions are the inward movement of the*

General principles of assessment

muscles above the sternum), or intercostals retraction (***intercostal retractions*** *occur when the muscles between the ribs pull inward*).
- Is there any **flaring of nostrils**, or **pursed lips**?
- Look for **flail segments**, **paradoxical breathing**, bruising and deformities of the thorax.
- Listen for **sucking chest wounds**, audible wheezes.
- If the patient is breathing, assess their respiratory rate and effort and ensure that this is adequate enough to ensure oxygenation. If available, measure the oxygen saturation (SpO_2) and ensure an inspired oxygen concentration of 94% or more. Oxygen therapy should be administered in accordance with current guidelines (British Thoracic Society, 2015).
- Listen to the patient talking and assess if they are able to complete a sentence in one breath.
- **Auscultate** the chest and listen for normal and abnormal breath sounds over a minimum of five positions on each lung (Bickley, 2013). A wheeze indicates **bronchospasm**, whereas coarse sounds indicate pulmonary oedema.
- Feel the patient's chest for expansion, irregularity and tenderness.
- A patient with a respiratory rate of <10 or >29 breaths per minute may potentially require ventilatory support, as both rates are indicative of inadequate minute volumes and respiratory failure.

Possible actions to be taken:

- If patient is not responding: look, listen and feel for breathing for 10 seconds
- Ensure that the patient is not hypoxic (*diminished levels of oxygen to tissues*)
- Manage breathing/**hypoxia** effectively before moving to the next element.

CIRCULATION

- Look to see if the patient has any form of haemorrhage, internal or external. Manage the haemorrhage accordingly (*see Trauma Assessment, Chapter 7*).
- Assessment of the patient's circulatory system includes palpating and recording the radial pulse, note the rate and volume/character:
  - Is it tachycardic or **bradycardic**? Is it full and bounding or weak, regular or irregular? If the radial pulse cannot be palpated, can the femoral or carotid pulses be palpated? A palpable peripheral pulse can provide the paramedic with a rough estimate of blood

pressure: radial = a systolic of 80 mmHg, femoral = a systolic of 70 mmHg and carotid = a systolic of 60 mmHg (Salomone and Pons, 2014). However, Deakin and Low (2000) state that these rough estimates generally overestimate a patient's systolic blood pressure and therefore underestimate the degree of hypovolaemia. The paramedic needs to be aware of these varying schools of thought and research findings, when only using the presence of pulses as a guide to the patient's systolic blood pressure.
- Assess the colour of the skin. Is it pale, indicating poor **perfusion**? This indicates partial oxygenation. Assess the temperature and the moisture of the skin: normal skin temperature is warm to touch, whereas cool skin indicates poor perfusion. Is the patient cyanosed? Are they **jaundiced**? (Longmore et al., 2014). The paramedic should also assess and examine the patient's skin **turgor** to ensure the patient is hydrated (Rushforth, 2009). Check turgor by lightly pinching the skin of the patient's forearm between the paramedic's thumb and forefinger. Normal turgor is a return to normal contour <3 seconds; if the skin remains elevated (tented) >3 seconds, turgor is decreased.
- Check the capillary bed refill (CBR) by pressing over the nail bed for 5 seconds and then releasing: normal refill should occur within 2 seconds, an alternative location is the patient's sternum or forehead.

Possible actions to be taken:
- Control external haemorrhage
- Manage shock accordingly (see *Trauma Assessment, Chapter 7*)
- Palpate, assess and record pulse rate and rhythm.

DISABILITY

- Assess the patient's level of consciousness (LOC). The **Glasgow Coma Scale (GCS)** provides an assessment of three specific key areas, Best Eye (4), Best Motor (5), and Best Verbal (6), with a respective maximum score of 15, and minimum score of 3.
- Record **T** if an **endotracheal tube (ETT)** is inserted when scoring Best Verbal (Smith et al., 2011).
- A GCS score of 3–8 may indicate that the patient has sustained either a severe head injury or a major **cerebral insult**.
- A GCS score of 14–15 is mild.
- A GCS score of 15 is normal.
- A GCS score of 8 defines coma (Kaplan and Roesler, 2013).
- In the UK, the majority of fatal head injury outcomes are in the moderate (GCS 9–12) or severe (GCS 8 or less) groups (NICE, 2014).

General principles of assessment

- Remember to assess both the patient's posture and pupillary response. In patients who are comatose (GCS 8), note any **decerebrate** or **decorticate posture** and pupillary responses to light (*normal response is constriction*).
- Remember that the AVPU scale used in the response element is accepted as a quicker tool for use within the primary survey.
- Assess the patient's pupils for size, reaction and accommodation (*occurs when the patient converges their eyes and constricts their pupils to a near object*). The use of the following framework will assist the paramedic: **P**upils **E**qual and **R**ound; **R**eact to **L**ight and **A**ccommodation (**PERRLA**) (*see Neurological Assessment, Chapter 5*).
- Assess blood glucose levels (***hypo/hyperglycaemia** may be the cause of altered levels of consciousness*).

Possible actions to be taken:

- Assess and document LOC
- Note abnormal postures (*decerebrate/decorticate*) (*see Neurological Assessment, Chapter 5*)
- Assess and document size, equality and accommodation of pupils
- Assess blood glucose levels.

EXPOSE/EXAMINE/EVALUATE

- Expose the patient's injury/injuries, e.g. on a trauma patient completely remove all clothing but remember to consider the environment and ensure that the patient is covered to prevent **hypothermia** and maintain dignity, as far as possible. Look for medical alert tag; this will often reveal information about the patient's past medical history or supply a telephone number where this information can be obtained (*see Neurological Assessment, Chapter 5*).
- Consent: Obtain valid consent. Remember, not every patient is unconscious (Department of Health, 2009).
- Crime scene: Paramedics attend incidents involving violent crime, and need to be aware of maintaining the integrity of the crime scene, including any physical evidence (*body materials, objects and impressions*) (Pilbery, 2014).
- Evaluate the findings within the primary survey that you have just completed and if you have identified any **time critical** problems within any of the elements, then consider the need to transport and transfer immediately to an appropriate treatment centre, or remain on scene and conduct a **secondary survey**.

> **Possible actions to be taken:**
> - Obtain valid consent
> - Expose the patient's affected area(s) and examine
> - Ascertain if the patient has medical alert tag/bracelet
> - Remember the patient's dignity and possible hypothermia
> - Evaluate – transfer or move onto secondary survey?

SECONDARY SURVEY

This is a focused history and physical examination to identify injuries or problems not identified during the primary survey. It provides the paramedic with the opportunity of detecting less obvious injuries and/or signs and symptoms of underlying medical conditions. There are three key elements to the secondary survey:

- history
- **vital signs**
- the physical assessment.

History

The key elements of obtaining a patient history are described in this section, and an example of how the elements could be recorded is provided below:

- PC: 48 ♀ C/O difficulty in breathing (DIB) (**dyspnoea**)
- HPC: History of feeling unwell for several days, developing a **productive cough** for 3/7, yellowish green in colour, according to the patient, and today they feel unable to cope with the dyspnoea.

Presenting complaint (PC)

The following are examples of questions you might ask yourself. See the appropriate chapter for specific questions related to each area of assessment.
- What is the presenting complaint? (*This may be due to an illness (abdominal pain), or a specific injury (fell over and hurt my ankle).*)
- Is it because:
  - the patient has difficulty in breathing?
  - they were involved in a motor vehicle collision?
  - or they have severe abdominal pain?
- The paramedic should clearly identify the reason(s) why the patient or caller has requested their attendance; this includes ascertaining the mechanism of injury (MOI) in patients who have suffered trauma (Bledsoe et al., 2014).

General principles of assessment

History of presenting complaint (HPC)

- What is the history of the presenting complaint? Through a process of questions, further history may become available. For example, a patient is complaining of difficulty in breathing (DIB) (dyspnoea). On questioning, it becomes apparent that they have a history of feeling unwell for several days, developing a productive cough over the past three days and today find it extremely difficult to breathe.
- The above example explains why the history leading up to the presenting complaint is extremely important and can assist the paramedic in making a provisional diagnosis, and instigating appropriate, timely treatment and management of the patient's problems (Limmer et al., 2014).

Past medical history (PMH)

- What is the patient's past medical history?
- Have they had similar episodes previously?
- Do they have any other medical conditions? Consider the following mnemonic:
    - **MR C. J. THEADS** to ascertain if they have, or have had any of the following: **M**yocardial Infarction (Heart Attack); **R**heumatic Fever/ **R**heumatoid Arthritis; **C**ancer(s); **J**aundice; **T**uberculosis (TB); **H**ypertension; **E**pilepsy; **A**sthma; **D**iabetes; **S**trokes
- If they are diabetic, what type: I or II?
- Do they suffer from other respiratory diseases and/or conditions such as **chronic obstructive pulmonary disease (COPD)**, **emphysema** or **chronic bronchitis**?
- Do they have a cardiac condition, such as **angina**, **left ventricular failure (LVF)**, or right ventricular failure (RVF)?
- Consider patients presenting with DIB who have an inhaler, or chest pain who have a GTN spray, or those with an allergic reaction who have an **epipen**. These patients have been prescribed these for an existing medical condition (Limmer et al., 2014).
- Have they ever been hospitalized or had any operations? If so, what for?

Drug/medication history (DMH) (to include prescribed, or recreational drugs, over the counter (OTC) and other health products), and allergies

- Is the patient currently prescribed medications for any pre-existing condition(s)? If so, what medications are they?
- Using the patient's medications, ask the patient to explain to you why they take each medication. This will help you to explore the patient's knowledge and understanding of their prescribed medications.

- Are they compliant with their medications?
- Have they purchased any OTC medications to relieve their symptoms?
- Has the patient taken any analgesics for any pain they may be suffering? If so, at what time did they take the medicines?
- Are they taking or undergoing any courses of **complementary therapy medicines**?
- Do they have any known allergies (*food, medication, latex*)? Have they ever previously had an anaphylactic reaction? (*anaphylaxis is extreme sensitivity to a protein or drug*). If so, do they have medication(s); Epipen (adrenaline)?

Possible actions to be taken:

- If transporting the patient, best practice dictates taking their medications with them, as the receiving unit may not stock particular medicines
- This also enables the receiving unit to record medicines, dosages and establish patient compliance.

Social/family medical history (S/FMH)

- Depending upon the age of the patient, ascertain if they live alone or have relatives/carers or external agency input (social service input, meal deliveries, etc.).
- Consider the activities of daily living (ADL), what can the patient do or not do for themselves? Has this changed?
- Remember to differentiate between *physical* activities such as bathing, dressing and feeding, and *instrumental* activities, such as shopping, housekeeping and taking medications (Bickley, 2013).
- Depending on the presenting medical condition, do other members of the patient's family also suffer from the condition/illness? Familial history is often a factor in patients presenting with many conditions, for example, cardiac, diabetes and strokes.

Review of systems (ROS)

- The signs and symptoms are ascertained as part of the physical assessment, as the paramedic conducts a review of the patient's major systems: respiratory, cardiovascular, neurological, gastro-intestinal (GI), etc.
- Modify questions to the system: Respiratory – Are you asthmatic? Is it normally well controlled? What medications/inhalers do you use? Have you tried them today? When was your last attack?

General principles of assessment

- On auscultation, are there **adventitious sounds** (*abnormal lung sounds, e.g. wheeze, crackles (rales) or stridor*)? Is there pain on inspiration?
- When assessing a patient's pain, use the **SOCRATES** framework (AACE, 2013b):

    S – Site, where exactly is the pain?
    O – Onset, what were they doing when the pain started?
    C – Character, what does the pain feel like? Is it constant, colicky, sharp or heavy?
    R – Radiate, does the pain go anywhere else?
    A – Associated symptoms, is it associated with any other symptoms? E.g nausea and/or vomiting?
    T – Time/duration, how long have they had the pain?
    E – Exacerbating/relieving factors, does anything make the pain better or worse?
    S – Severity, obtain an initial pain score (0 = no pain, 10 = worst pain ever).

Record the vital signs which should include the following evidence regarding the patient:

- Respiratory rate (RR), character and work of breathing
- Heart rate (HR), character, volume and rhythm
- Blood pressure (BP)
- **Electrocardiogram (ECG)**, including 3-lead monitoring and 12-lead ECG acquisition
- Blood glucose levels
- GCS neurological status
- Pupils
- **Peak expiratory flow (PEF)** (best of three readings)
- Temperature
- Oxygen saturations (SpO_2)
- Pain score
- Signs and symptoms of each system obtained during the secondary survey.

The use of the following **SAMPLE** framework may assist the paramedic (see *Respiratory Assessment, Chapter 2*):

    S – Signs and symptoms
    A – Allergies
    M – Medications
    P – Past medical history
    L – Last meal
    E – Events leading up to the incident

IMPRESSIONS (OVERALL OF THE PATIENT/ SITUATION) (IMP)

- What is your overall impression of the patient and the situation? Remember someone who is not dressed and/or unwashed, without their hair being groomed, halfway through the day may be like this due to the effects of their illness/condition.
- If the scene is the patient's home, what is the condition of their surroundings?
- All of this information is useful to **handover**, if the patient is being **conveyed**. Any information you have about the patient's home surroundings is lost once you leave the patient, if you do not mention any concerns/observations. If not provided as part of your patient handover, then this may mean that the patient is discharged without appropriate support or investigation.
- Is their accommodation safe for them to return to?

OTHER CONSIDERATIONS

Towards the end of each chapter the following considerations will be discussed where applicable to either the system and/or the patient's age/gender/religion:

- *Communication* – How the paramedic deals with the problem of communicating with someone whose first language is not English, or patients who may be deaf or have a learning disability.
- *Destination/receiving specialist units/non-conveyance* – How does the paramedic decide on the destination if the patient needs to be transported? What specialist units are available 24/7 for **primary angioplasty**? Are specialist hyper acute stroke units (HASU), burns or regional trauma units available? What primary care agencies/facilities are available for the patient if the decision by the paramedic is not to convey the patient?
- *Social/family/carer/guardian* – What social implications are there when patients are transported for care, either for the patient or the family/carer/guardian? If a full-time carer was taken ill and required hospitalization, what problems would this cause the attending paramedic?
- *Ethical and legal* – What are the **ethical** and legal dilemmas of obtaining **consent** in every emergency situation? What happens when a patient does not have **capacity** to provide consent?

REFERENCES

Association of Ambulance Chief Executives (2013a) *UK Ambulance Services Clinical Practice Guidelines 2013 Pocket Book: Chemical, Biological, Radiological, Nuclear and Explosive Incidents*. Bridgwater: Class Professional Publishing.

Association of Ambulance Chief Executives (2013b) *UK Ambulance Services Clinical Practice Guidelines 2013 Pocket Book: Pain Assessment Model*. Bridgwater: Class Professional Publishing.

Bickley, L.S. (2013) *BATES' Pocket Guide to Physical Examination and History Taking* (7th edn). Philadelphia, PA: Lippincott Williams & Wilkins.

Bledsoe, B.E., Porter, R.S. and Cherry, R.A. (2014) *Paramedic Care: Principles and Practice*, vol. 5, *Trauma* (4th edn). Harlow: Pearson Education Limited.

British Thoracic Society (2015) *Emergency Oxygen Use in Adult Patients: Guideline*. Available at: https://www.brit-thoracic.org.uk/searchresults/?txtSearch=2015+Oxygen+Guidelines&search= (accessed 14 February 2015).

College of Paramedics (2015a) *Paramedic Curriculum Guidance* (3rd edn, revised). Bridgwater: College of Paramedics.

College of Paramedics (2015b) *Paramedic Post Registration: Career and Competency Framework* (3rd edn). Bridgwater: College of Paramedics.

Deakin, C.D. and Low J.L. (2000) Accuracy of the advanced trauma life support guidelines for predicting systolic blood pressure using carotid, femoral, and radial pulses: observational study. *British Medical Journal* 321: 673–74.

Department of Health (2009) *Reference Guide to Consent for Examination or Treatment* (2nd edn). London: Department of Health.

Hodgetts, T., Mahoney, P., Russell, M. and Byers, M. (2006) ABC to [C]ABC: redefining the military trauma paradigm. *Emergency Medical Journal* 23: 745–6.

Kaplan, L.J. and Roesler, D.M. (2013) *Critical Care Considerations in Trauma: Neurologic Injury*. Available at: http://emedicine.medscape.com/article/434445-overview (accessed 25 November 2014).

Limmer, D.J., O'Keefe, M.F., Grant, H.T., Murray, B., Bergeron, J.D. and Dickinson, E.V. (2014) *Emergency Care* (12th edn). Harlow: Pearson Education Limited.

Longmore, M., Wilkinson, I.B., Baldwin, A. and Wallin, E. (2014) *Oxford Handbook of Clinical Medicine* (9th edn). Oxford: Oxford University Press.

NICE (National Institute for Health and Care Excellence) (2014) *Head Injury: Triage, Assessment, Investigation and Early Management of Head Injury in Children, Young People and Adults*. NICE clinical guideline 176. Available at: http://www.nice.org.uk/guidance/cg176 (accessed 25 November 2014).

Pilbery, R. (2014) *Nancy Caroline's Emergency Care in the Streets: United Kingdom* (7th edn). Burlington: Jones & Bartlett Learning.

Resuscitation Council (UK) (2010) *2010 Resuscitation Guidelines*. London: Resuscitation Council (UK).

Resuscitation Council (UK) (2011) *Advanced Life Support* (6th edn). London: Resuscitation Council. Reprinted in 2012 (with corrections).

Rushforth, H. (2009) *Assessment Made Incredibly Easy* (UK edn). Philadelphia, PA: Lippincott Williams & Wilkins.

Salomone, J.P. and Pons, P.T. (2014) *Pre-Hospital Trauma Life Support (PHTLS)* (8th edn). Maryland Heights, MO: Mosby Elsevier.

Smith, S.F., Duell, D.J. and Martin, B.C. (2011) *Clinical Nursing Skills: Basic to Advanced Skills* (8th edn). London. Pearson Education Ltd.

2 Respiratory assessment
Vince Clarke and Paul Townsend

In the out-of-hospital environment, patients often present with a wide range of acute and chronic respiratory emergencies. For safe practice, the paramedic should rely on thorough and effective assessment skills in order to provide timely intervention. The aim of this chapter is to provide an overview of the clinical skills required for an effective respiratory system assessment to be conducted in the pre- and out-of-hospital environment. It will identify areas of key importance and discuss the equipment available to aid in the assessment process.

SCENE ASSESSMENT

Information provided by the caller is often displayed on the mobile data terminal (MDT) and can alert you to the patient's condition as well as providing clues as to the likely respiratory assessments and treatments the patient may require. Respiratory emergencies could result from medical conditions, such as **asthma**, or from trauma.

Use the time while en route to the scene to prepare yourself. Ask yourself:

- How am I going to approach the scene?
- What equipment will I need to perform a respiratory assessment?
- What primary survey **A**irway and **B**reathing problems are time critical?

Equipment available for respiratory assessment:

- **Stethoscope**
- Peak flow meter, to assess peak expiratory flow (PEF)
- Oxygen saturation monitor (SpO_2), to measure peripheral capillary oxygen saturation
- End tidal carbon dioxide monitor ($EtCO_2$), to measure levels of exhaled carbon dioxide.

Respiratory assessment

Global overview

This is the paramedic's immediate impression of the patient's condition from the scene that is presented to them and should not take more than a few seconds. This skill will develop with both experience and clinical knowledge and can perhaps begin to explain how experienced paramedics can rapidly recognize the degree to which a patient is unwell. An abundance of information from both the environment and patient can be obtained prior to verbal questioning or physical assessment and should not be overlooked by the paramedic, as it will aid them in their differential diagnosis, ideally leading to a preferred diagnosis.

Look for signs of respiratory distress in the patient:

- Reduced level of consciousness
- Unable to complete a sentence in one breath
- Patient positioning, such as sitting forward in the tripod position (see Figure 2.1)
- Use of accessory muscles around the neck and shoulders
- **Intercostal recession**, where the tissue between the ribs is drawn inwards
- **Flared nostrils/pursed lips**
- Abnormal or additional sounds such as wheezing
- **Cyanosis**, blue-tinged lips and/or buccal mucosa.

Consider, where appropriate, information within the environment:

- Immediate surroundings – industrial (*chemicals*), agricultural, fire calls, water and/or explosive/flammable products
- Home oxygen
- Cigarettes
- Medication – inhalers
- Smells – gases, damp.

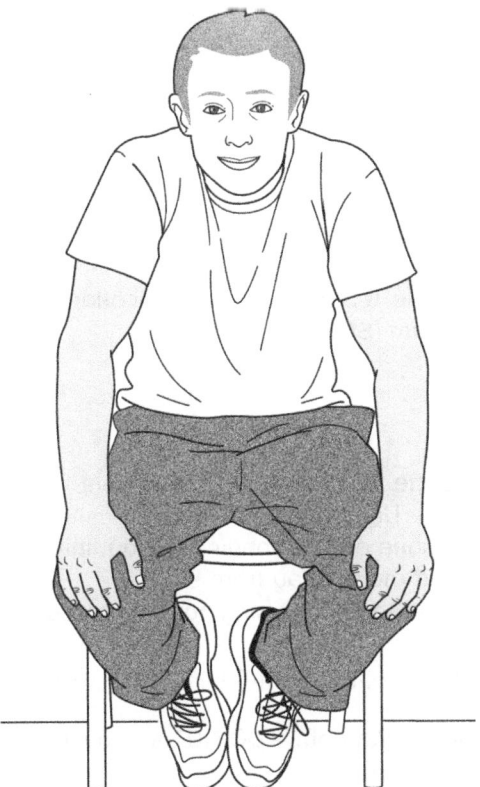

Figure 2.1 Tripod position

PRIMARY SURVEY

The primary survey is fundamental in the early identification of time critical patients. It should take between one and two minutes and includes Danger, Response, (Catastrophic Haemorrhage), Airway, Breathing, Circulation, Disability and Exposure. Any patient that fails an element of the primary survey should be treated as time critical. Treatment should be commenced at the earliest opportunity and continued en route to hospital. Remember do not move on to the next element of the primary survey until the element you are dealing with has been managed.

DANGER

- Although the majority of patients presenting with respiratory distress are experiencing an exacerbation of a chronic respiratory illness, environmental factors may sometimes be the cause.
- Consideration, therefore, needs to be given to the environment as being potentially dangerous. Environmental risks that may affect the respiratory system can occur from toxic agents, e.g. smoke/gas/carbon monoxide.

Possible actions to be taken:

- Remove patients into an open space and fresh air
- Request fire brigade/police assistance
- Request Hazardous Area Response Team (HART), or in Scotland, Special Operations Response Team (SORT), if available.

RESPONSE

- Initial response is obtained using the AVPU scale: is the patient A – Alert, V – Verbal, P – Pain or U – Unresponsive?
- If there are multiple patients and none are responding to you, initiate the Step 1, 2, and 3 procedure and move away from scene.
  - *Step 1* – One Collapsed Patient – Approach using normal procedures (*CBRN contamination unlikely*)
  - *Step 2* – Two Collapsed Patients – Approach with caution – (*CBRNE contamination possible*)
  - *Step 3* – Three or More Collapsed Patients – DO NOT approach the scene – (*CBRN contamination likely*)
  - If possible: Withdraw, Contain and Report. DO NOT compromise your safety or that of your colleagues or the public (AACE, 2013a).

Respiratory assessment

Possible actions to be taken:

- Major incident – provide an appropriate report (METHANE)
- Withdraw; Contain; Management; Refer to Triage SIEVE CBRNE, and Re-Assess.

AIRWAY

- Is the airway patent? Is the patient able to maintain their own airway?
- Correct any airway deficits immediately by using stepwise airway management.
- Are there any abnormal sounds? If so, the airway may be obstructed.
  - Gurgling: fluid in the airway and there is need for suction.
  - Snoring: soft tissue problem due to the tongue occluding the airway.
  - Stridor: upper airway problem (*partial obstruction of the larynx or trachea*).
  - Wheezing: lower airway problem (*below the vocal cords*).

Possible actions to be taken:

(Consider cervical spine)

- Head tilt, chin lift if no risk to C-spine; or, Jaw thrust if C-spine injury is suspected
- Recovery position (*injury permitting*)
- Suction
- Oralpharyngeal (OP)/nasopharyngeal (NP) airway adjuncts
- Supraglottic airway device (SGD)
- Endotracheal intubation (ETI)
- Needle cricothyroidotomy.

BREATHING

- Look, listen and feel for the presence of breathing for no more than 10 seconds.
- If the patient is not breathing, commence Basic Life Support (BLS) as per current guidelines.
- If the patient is breathing, obtain a preliminary respiratory rate and determine the pattern and work of breathing. A patient with a respiratory rate of less than (<)10 or greater than (>)29 breaths per minute may potentially require ventilatory support, as both rates are indicative of inadequate minute volumes and respiratory failure (*carpopedal spasm of the patient's hands may be due to hyperventilation*).

- If the respiratory rate is outside normal parameters, expose and assess the patient's chest for the use of accessory muscles and any chest trauma (*sucking chest wounds or flail segments, if so, manage appropriately*).
- Auscultate the chest for breath sounds (*ascertain if there are any abnormal sounds*) and feel the patient's chest for equal expansion, crepitus and tenderness.
- Feel for and ascertain if the trachea is central (*tracheal deviation is a late sign of a tension **pneumothorax***).
- If resources allow, consider measuring SpO_2 and $EtCO_2$.

Possible actions to be taken:

- Commence BLS if the patient is not breathing
- Seal sucking chest wounds, stabilize flail segments, decompress tension pneumothoraces accordingly (see *Trauma Assessment, Chapter 7*)
- Reverse hypoxia
- Administer oxygen appropriately to patient's illness/injury in accordance with current guidelines (British Thoracic Society, 2015).

CIRCULATION

Circulatory problems, such as heart failure, may produce symptoms which manifest during assessment of the respiratory system, e.g. pulmonary oedema. Basic circulatory checks within the primary survey are therefore vital in providing an insight to underlying respiratory problems.

- Palpate and assess the patient's radial pulse and ascertain the rate.
- Assess the colour of the skin: pallor, or pale skin, is indicative of poor tissue **perfusion**. Cyanosis is indicative of **hypoxaemia**.
- Assess the skin temperature. Moist clammy skin suggests decreased tissue perfusion.
- Assess the patient's capillary refill. Delayed refill, greater than (>) 2 seconds also suggests poor perfusion.
- All of these findings are potentially indicative of respiratory problems manifesting in the circulatory system.

Possible actions to be taken:

- Ascertain if there is internal haemorrhage
- Arrest external haemorrhage
- Manage shock accordingly (see *Trauma Assessment, Chapter 7*).

DISABILITY

Underlying respiratory problems such as hypoxia may result in cerebral deficit and reducing levels of consciousness.

- AVPU scoring is an adequate measure of a patient's disability within the primary survey.
- The Glasgow Coma Scale (GCS) requires accurate recording and may not be an appropriate measure in the immediately life-threatening situations.
- Assess the patient's pupils for both size and reaction. Check to see if the pupils are equal, round, react to light and accommodate. The use of the following framework will assist the paramedic: **P**upils **E**qual and **R**ound; **R**eact to **L**ight and **A**ccommodation (PERRLA) (see *Neurological Assessment, Chapter 5*).

Possible actions to be taken:

- Document AVPU score
- Document size and equality and accommodation of pupils.

EXPOSE/EXAMINE/EVALUATE

Appropriate exposure of a patient is important in order to make an accurate assessment of their presenting condition.

Possible actions to be taken:

- Expose and examine the patient
- Remember patient dignity and possible hypothermia
- Evaluate – transfer immediately or move onto secondary survey.

SECONDARY SURVEY

History

History taking is an important skill for the paramedic to master in order to provide timely interventions and treatment. Below are a series of questions that you should be asking your patient in order to gather an accurate history:

Presenting complaint
- Do you have any pre-existing medical conditions related to your breathing?

- Are you short of breath (SOB)?
- Do you have any difficulty in breathing (DIB)?
- Is this level of DIB/SOB normal for you?
- Do you have any other symptoms?
- Are these new or old?

History of presenting complaint
- When did the SOB/DIB start?
- What were you doing when it started?
- Have you experienced previous episodes of this before?
  - If so, when?
- Do you have a cough?
  - Is it productive?
  - Does it produce phlegm? If so, what colour is the phlegm? (*Yellow/green sputum may suggest infection, possible* **bronchiectasis** *or pneumonia. Pink frothy sputum may suggest pulmonary oedema.*)
  - Have you coughed up any blood? (**Haemoptysis** *(blood in sputum) may suggest malignancy, TB, infection or trauma*).
  - Clear sputum (*probably saliva*).
- The paramedic should consider that a cough can be a relatively non-specific symptom which can occur due to irritation of the air passages from the pharynx to the lungs. The character of the cough may, however, give these clues:
  - Loud brassy cough – *suggests pressure on trachea, e.g. tumour*
  - Hollow 'bovine' cough – *suggests recurrent laryngeal nerve palsy*
  - Barking (**croup**) cough – *suggests acute epiglottitis*
  - Chronic cough – *suggests pertussis, TB, foreign body, asthma (e.g. nocturnal)*
  - Dry, chronic cough – *suggests either acid irritation of the lungs, oesophageal reflux, or due to the side effects of ACE inhibitors.*
- DO NOT ignore the change in chronic coughs as it may indicate a new problem such as infection.
- Have you taken any of your prescribed medicine?
  - If so, when?
- Has it relieved the symptoms?
- Do you have any pain?
  - If so, where, exactly, is the pain?
  - Is it worse on inspiration? Remember that pleuritic pain is exacerbated by inspiration, whereas musculoskeletal pain, such as a fractured rib, is exacerbated by pressure on the affected area.

See Box 2.1 for an outline of a pain assessment framework.

> **Box 2.1** Pain Assessment Framework
>
> When assessing a patient's pain, use the SOCRATES framework (AACE, 2013b):
>
> **S** – Site. Where exactly is the pain?
> **O** – Onset. What were they doing when the pain started?
> **C** – Character. What does the pain feel like? Is it constant, colicky, sharp or heavy?
> **R** – Radiate. Does the pain go anywhere else?
> **A** – Associated symptoms. Is it associated with any other symptoms? For example, nausea and/or vomiting
> **T** – Time/duration. How long have they had the pain?
> **E** – Exacerbating/relieving factors. Does anything make the pain better or worse?
> **S** – Severity. Obtain an initial pain score (*0 = no pain, 10 = worst pain ever*).
>
> The pain framework can also be adapted to assess the severity of a patient's SOB/DIB.

The use of the following framework (SAMPLE) will assist the paramedic in gaining a full and thorough history:

>   **S** – Signs and symptoms
>   **A** – Allergies
>   **M** – Medications
>   **P** – Past medical history
>   **L** – Last meal, what time did they last eat?
>   **E** – Events leading up to the incident

Allergies, drug/medication history
- Do you have a history of allergies?
  - If you have an allergy, can you describe the symptoms you presented with?
- Do you take any prescribed medications?
  - If so, what are they? (*The paramedic should note the type and dosage of each drug, the time of day the drug is administered and whether the patient is compliant with their medication. In addition, the paramedic should take time to check if the drug is in date.*)
- Have you purchased any over-the-counter medications?
- Have you taken any pain relief (analgesics)?
  - If so, what time did you take the medicines?

- Are you undergoing any courses of complementary therapy?
- Do you take any recreational drugs?
  - If so, what did you take and when?

Past medical history
- Do you have a history of a chronic respiratory illness?
  - If so, what is the condition?
- Do you suffer with asthma, emphysema or bronchitis?
- Have you ever been hospitalized with the condition?
- Have you spent time in intensive care with this condition?
- Have you ever had a pulmonary embolism?
- Have you ever had any surgery?
  - If so, what for?
- Do you have any other medical conditions?

Social/family medical history
- Do you smoke?
  - If so, how many cigarettes do you smoke a day?
- How long have you been smoking? (*Record appropriate pack years, e.g. 20 cigarettes a day = 1 pack, × length of period smoking, e.g. 5 years, so that would be written as 1 pack × 5 years.*)
- Have you been in contact with any external agents that could cause respiratory agitation? For example, industrial chemicals, building site materials such as cement or asbestos, farming chemicals or prolonged exposure to a damp environment.
- Do you have a family history of asthma or any other respiratory illness?
- Is there a family history of any other medical conditions? For example, ischaemic heart disease or cancer.

REVIEW OF SYSTEMS RELATED TO THE RESPIRATORY SYSTEM

Cardiovascular
- Do you experience SOB on exercise?
- Are you experiencing any chest pain or palpitations?
- Do you have any DIB when lying flat? **Orthopnoea** is the sensation of breathlessness in the recumbent position, relieved by sitting or standing.
- Have you been using more pillows to help you sleep at night?
- Paroxysmal nocturnal dyspnoea (PND) is a sensation of shortness of breath that awakens the patient, often after 1 or 2 hours of sleep, and is usually relieved in the upright position. It is often seen in patients with left ventricular failure (LVF).

- Do you have any oedema/swelling of lower limbs?
- Do you suffer from anaemia? (see Cardiovascular Assessment, Chapter 3)

Neurological

- Have you experienced any dizziness recently?
- Have you experienced any fits, faints or 'funny turns' recently?
- Have you experienced a headache, lethargy or SOB?
- Is there a history of any head trauma recently?
- Was there any loss of consciousness (LOC)?
- Have you vomited? (see Neurological Assessment, Chapter 5)

Musculoskeletal

- Do you have any muscular pain surrounding your chest?
- Does this pain get worse on inspiration, palpation or coughing?
- Have you experienced any recent trauma to the chest? (see Musculoskeletal Assessment, Chapter 8)

VITAL SIGNS

Vital signs are essential to all patient assessments. They should be used in conjunction with the information found within the history taking and physical examination process to differentiate between time critical and non-time critical patients.

The paramedic must remember continual reassessment of the vital signs is an essential part of patient assessment.

Respiratory rate

The respiratory rate is a highly sensitive physiological indicator in determining if there is deterioration in a patient's condition. The following will help accurate measurement:

- Record the rate, depth and rhythm over one minute. Do not tell the patient you are recording their respiratory rate as they may alter their breathing rate as a result. The paramedic could record the respiratory, rate immediately after taking a pulse rate without the patient's knowledge. A patient with a respiratory rate of <10 or >29 breaths per minute may potentially require ventilatory support, as both rates are indicative of inadequate minute volumes and respiratory failure.
- Other methods for obtaining an accurate respiratory rate from the patient are observing oxygen mask misting, abdominal breathing or chest rise where appropriate.

Pulse oximetry

Oxygen is expressed as a percentage. Supplemental oxygen should be administered in accordance with current guidelines (British Thoracic Society, 2015).

- Advantages of pulse **oximetry** are:
  - Simple, quick and non-invasive measurement.
- Limitations of pulse oximetry are:
  - Inaccurate measurements when exposed to movement, bright light, metallic nail varnish or cold environments.

The paramedic should be aware that haemoglobin has a greater affinity to carbon monoxide compared to oxygen. This may result in a dangerously false pulse oximetry reading, as the pulse oximetry sensor cannot differentiate between oxyhaemoglobin and carboxyhaemoglobin. In cases of suspected carbon monoxide poisoning, consider the use of HART/SORT teams who may have access to carboxyhaemoglobin saturation monitoring.

Peak expiratory flow

Peak expiratory flow (PEF) provides a measure of adequacy of the ventilation within the lungs in the form of the forced expiratory volume (FEV). This is an essential assessment tool for any asthmatic patient, however, the paramedic should recognize that the patient may not be able to perform the task due to the severity of their dyspnoea.

- A peak flow meter with a disposable mouthpiece is required. Be careful to warn the patient not to obstruct the movement of the measurement gauge.
- PEF should be recorded as the best of three forced expiratory volumes. This should be compared to the patient's estimated value from a peak expiratory flow chart or known normal value (AACE, 2013c).
- Readings should be taken both pre- and post-treatment so a comparison can be made on the effectiveness of the treatment provided.

Special attention should be given to asthmatic patients with peak flows of 33–50% (acute severe asthma) or <33% (life-threatening asthma) of their normal expected value.

Capnometry (end tidal carbon dioxide, $EtCO_2$)

End tidal carbon dioxide (tCO_2) is a non-invasive measurement of carbon dioxide at the end of expiration and provides an accurate insight into the ventilation and circulation of a patient, i.e. the effectiveness of the cardiorespiratory system.

Respiratory assessment

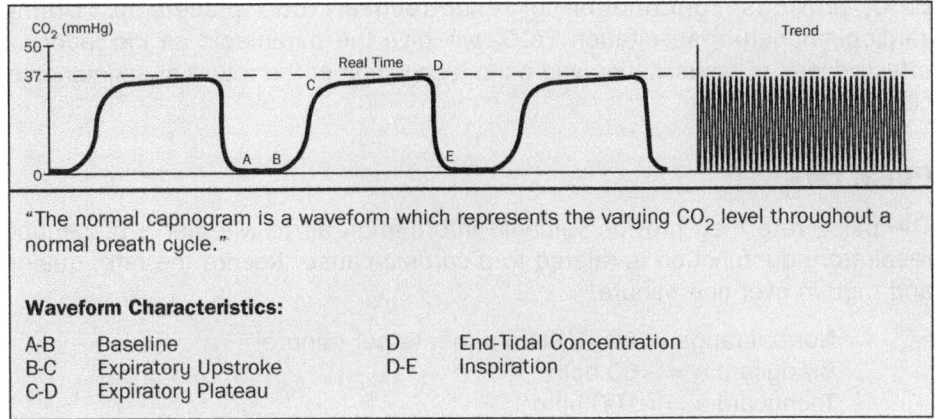

"The normal capnogram is a waveform which represents the varying CO_2 level throughout a normal breath cycle."

Waveform Characteristics:

A-B	Baseline	D	End-Tidal Concentration
B-C	Expiratory Upstroke	D-E	Inspiration
C-D	Expiratory Plateau		

Figure 2.2 Normal capnogram waveform. Normal $EtCO_2$ 35–45 mmHg.

Capnography displays the $EtCO_2$ as a waveform with the normal physiological range of 35 mmHg–45 mmHg or 4.6 kPa–6 kPa forming a 'box' waveform (see Figure 2.2).

For patients whose cardiorespiratory system is not functioning properly, these values will change, for example, severe asthmatics may present with a slightly elevated $EtCO_2$ reading although the shape of the waveform may be of greater diagnostic value. with the asthmatic patient generally being characterized by a 'shark fin'-shaped waveform (see Figure 2.3). However, during cardiac arrest, these values typically decrease due to a reduction in gaseous exchange (see Figure 2.4).

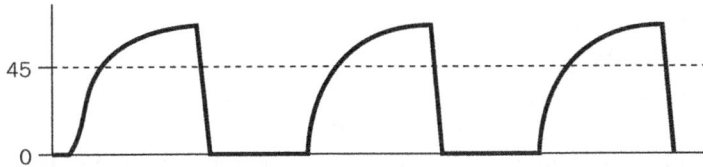

Figure 2.3 Shark-fin appearance waveform (seen in asthmatic and COPD patients)

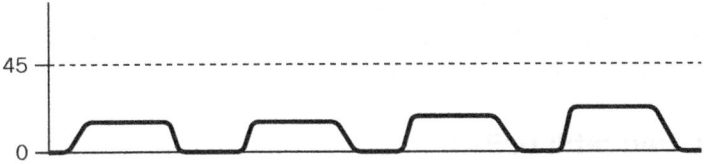

Figure 2.4 CPR intubated patient waveform (attempt to maintain a minimum of 10 mmHg)

EtCO$_2$ provides confirmation of endotracheal tube placement. During cardiopulmonary resuscitation EtCO$_2$ will give the paramedic an indication of effectiveness of resuscitation and early recognition of the return of spontaneous circulation (ROSC).

Pulse rate

The pulse rate may provide valuable information as to whether a presenting respiratory dysfunction is related to a cardiac cause. Record the rate, quality and rhythm over one minute:

>Normal range = 60–100 bpm (beats per minute)
>Bradycardia = <60 bpm
>Tachycardia = >100 bpm

Blood pressure

Blood pressure is a primary vital sign and gives an important indication of the patient's cardiovascular status.

- Normal adult blood pressure is defined as a systolic blood pressure of 120 mmHg and a diastolic blood pressure of 80 mmHg.
- **Hypertension** is defined as a systolic blood pressure equal to or above 140 mmHg and/or diastolic blood pressure equal to or above 90 mmHg.

Electrocardiogram (ECG)

When appropriate, it is important to obtain a 12-lead ECG to identify any underlying cardiovascular causes of respiratory dysfunction.

- Sinus arrhythmia can occur in a patient presenting with a normal respiratory rate, rhythm and depth.
- A patient presenting with a respiratory illness and **tachypnoea** may produce large amounts of artefact on the ECG, making it difficult to accurately interpret.
- Approximately 75% of patients with COPD have ECG abnormalities. P – pulmonale is often but not invariably present. There may also be low amplitude of QRS complexes as hyperinflated lungs are poor electrical conductors (Morris et al., 2008).

Capillary bed refill (CBR)

A CBR assessment can be recorded peripherally or centrally, although cold temperatures and dirt may hinder peripheral recording.

- For peripheral CBR assessment, use the fingernail beds.
- For central CBR assessment, use the sternum or forehead.
- Pressure should be applied for 5 seconds and capillary refill should return in less than 2 seconds.
- >2 seconds suggests poor tissue perfusion.

Glasgow Coma Score (GCS)

The GCS evaluates three areas of behaviour: eye opening, verbal response and motor response to give a cumulative score out of 15. Due to the complexity of GCS and the time required to measure it effectively, the AVPU scale may be a more appropriate measurement in the immediate out-of-hospital environment (see *Neurological Assessment, Chapter 5*).

Blood glucose level (BGL)

Recording the patient's glucose level gives the paramedic an indication of the systemic blood sugar levels in mmols/l.

- Normal range for non-diabetic patient 3.0–5.6 mmols/l (AACE, 2013d).
- A patient that is hyperglycaemic may present with Kussmaul's breathing, which is a deep sighing respiratory pattern and is associated with diabetic ketoacidosis. Such patients may have an acetone odour to their breath, often likened to 'pear-drops'.

Temperature

The paramedic should be aware that extremes of temperature can affect the patient's respiratory rate, rhythm and depth. You should:

- Record using a tympanic thermometer.
- Monitor the temperature for a possible underlying infection.

   Hypothermia = <35°C
   Severe hypothermia = <30°C, may cause **bradypnoea**
   Hyperthermia = >40°C, may cause tachypnoea/hyperventilation syndrome

PHYSICAL ASSESSMENT

As the paramedic enters the room, it is appropriate practice to introduce yourself and your colleagues and ask for the patient's name. This helps to foster the trust of the patient and will provide a good environment for gaining the consent required to perform the respiratory assessment.

Creating a suitable environment

Patients value their privacy and dignity and a paramedic should promote and protect the patient's modesty at all times. This could be facilitated in an office environment by asking colleagues to leave the room or by using the private setting of the ambulance.

Consent

Paramedics must ensure that they gain appropriate informed consent for any treatment that they carry out. In emergencies it may not be possible to gain consent, in which case the paramedic must act in the best interests of the patient by adopting the common law doctrine of necessity. In cases where a patient does not consent to examination or treatment, they must be fully informed of the possible consequences of their refusal. If consent is still withheld, the reasons must be fully and accurately documented (Department of Health, 2009).

RESPIRATORY ASSESSMENT

Respiratory assessment is carried out by using IPPA (Inspection, Palpation, Percussion, Auscultation).

Inspection

Appropriately expose the patient's chest while maintaining their privacy and dignity at all times. The paramedic should inspect the whole chest including the posterior, anterior and axilla surfaces for:

- Respiratory rate, depth and rhythm (note abnormal, Kussmaul's, Cheyne-Stokes)
- Normal chest shape and equal chest rise
- Accessory muscle use – sternocleidomastoid, scalene muscles
- Chest wall markings – wounds, bruising, bleeding, swelling
- Scars – with credible history
- Implantable devices – pacemaker, implantable cardioverter-defibrillator (ICD)
- Medication patches – **glyceryl trinitrate (GTN)**, nicotine, analgesia
- Rashes – hives that are indicative of allergy or petechial haemorrhage indicative of meningococcal septicaemia.

Palpation

The paramedic is required to use both their hands and fingers to palpate the anterior, posterior and axilla chest walls. Palpation should start above each clavicle and systematically progress down the anterior chest wall followed by the posterior chest wall, then the axilla. The paramedic should note any of the following findings:

- Tenderness – bruising, muscle damage
- Crepitus – fractures
- Surgical emphysema – popping under the skin caused by trapped air.

Equal and bilateral air entry of the lungs can be palpated through visualizing respiratory expansion. The paramedic can enhance this movement by appropriately placing their hands on either the posterior chest wall with their thumbs meeting over the spine or the anterior chest wall with their thumbs meeting over the sternum. Equal and symmetrical hand movement, associated with normal inspiration, can be seen when thumbs separate on inspiration and return to original position on expiration. A lack of symmetry could indicate problems on either or both sides of the thorax.

Tactile fremitus is the palpable vibration created by the spoken word and indicates areas of consolidation within the lungs. Consolidation, also known as exudate, is a solid mass containing a mixture of white blood cells, red blood cells and fibrin, which are leaked through capillary walls as a result of inflammation. The paramedic should use the ulnar edge of their hands and systematically move over the anterior and posterior aspects of the chest wall asking the patient to repeat '99' at each point. Areas of consolidation, from pneumonia, for example, produce increased fremitus, whereas conditions where there is reduced air entry, such as emphysema, produce decreased fremitus.

Percussion

The paramedic should recognize that percussion is best performed in a quiet and calm environment in order to hear the resonance of the lungs. This environment is hard to create in the pre-hospital setting and therefore its application may be limited.

The percussing finger is the middle finger of one hand. This is placed on the chest wall with the remaining fingers spread. See Figure 2.5. The middle finger of the opposing hand should be used to strike the planted finger on the chest wall. Percussion should start above the clavicles and systematically progress down the chest wall at 3–4 cm intervals. Go from right to left chest comparing the percussion notes between the two sides (including the clavicles and axillae). The left side of the chest wall should be compared to the right side of the chest wall at each percussion point. (See Figure 2.5.) Percussion should be performed over intercostal spaces, moving down the chest at intervals of 3–4 cm comparing both sides. Remember to percuss laterally. Do not

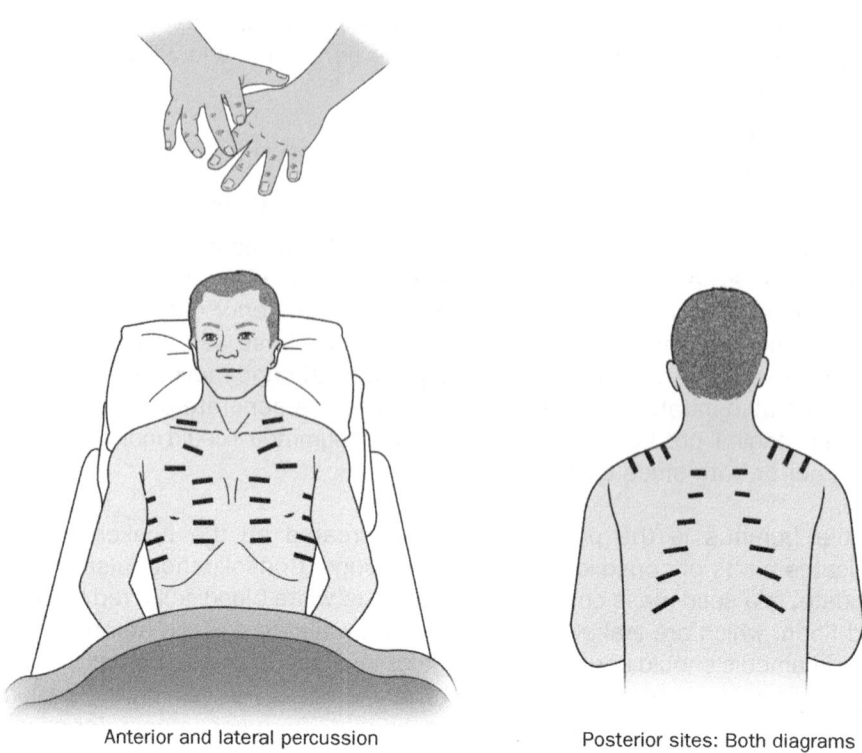

Anterior and lateral percussion

Posterior sites: Both diagrams scanned from Macleod, Clinical Examination

Figure 2.5 The finger positions and percussion sites

percuss over the scapula. Percuss down to the 6th rib anteriorly, the 8th rib in the axilla and the 10th rib posteriorly.

Table 2.1 provides examples of conditions and percussion notes.

Table 2.1 Percussion note examples

Condition	Percussion note
Pneumothorax	Hyper-resonant
Normal lung	Resonant
Collapse or consolidation	Dull
Emphysema or pneumothorax	
Pleural effusion	'Stony' or very dull

Auscultation

Auscultation (see Figures 2.6, 2.7 and 2.8) is the process of listening to the lungs using a stethoscope. Prior to commencing the assessment, the paramedic should ensure that the earpiece of the stethoscope is pointing forward into the external ear. In addition, they should check that the diaphragm, as opposed to the 'bell', is engaged and used for the auscultation process.

Anterior chest: Auscultate at least six areas on the anterior chest in order to listen to all lobes. Compare the left side of the lung to the right side moving systematically down the anterior wall (see Figure 2.6).

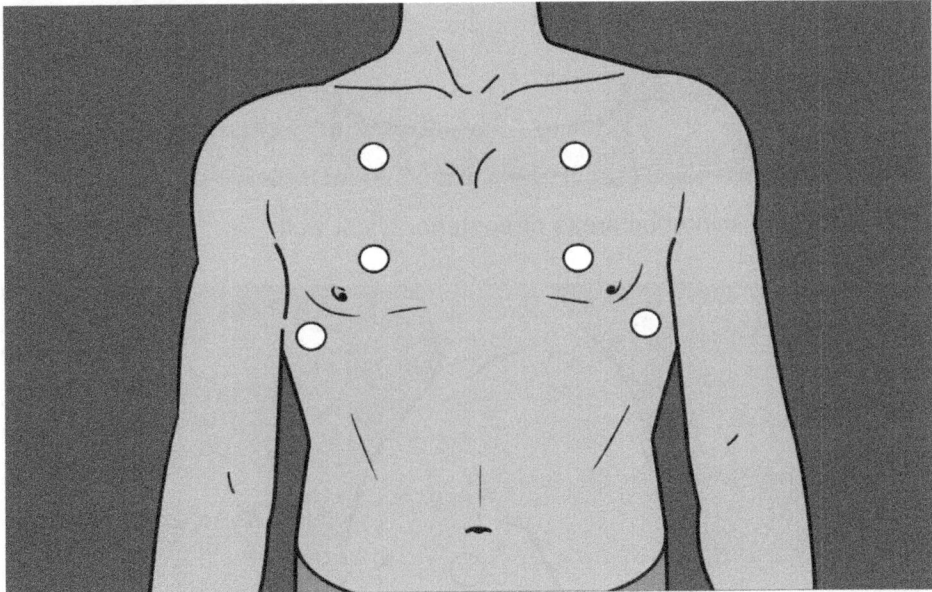

Figure 2.6 Auscultation areas of anterior chest wall

Posterior chest: Auscultate at least eight areas on the posterior chest in order to listen to all lobes (see Figure 2.7). To enhance auscultation, ask the patient to cross their arms, which will remove the scapula from the auscultation field. Compare the left side of the lung to the right side moving systematically down the posterior wall.

Axilla: Auscultate at least three areas on each axilla in order to listen to all lobes (see Figure 2.8). Move systematically over each axilla separately.

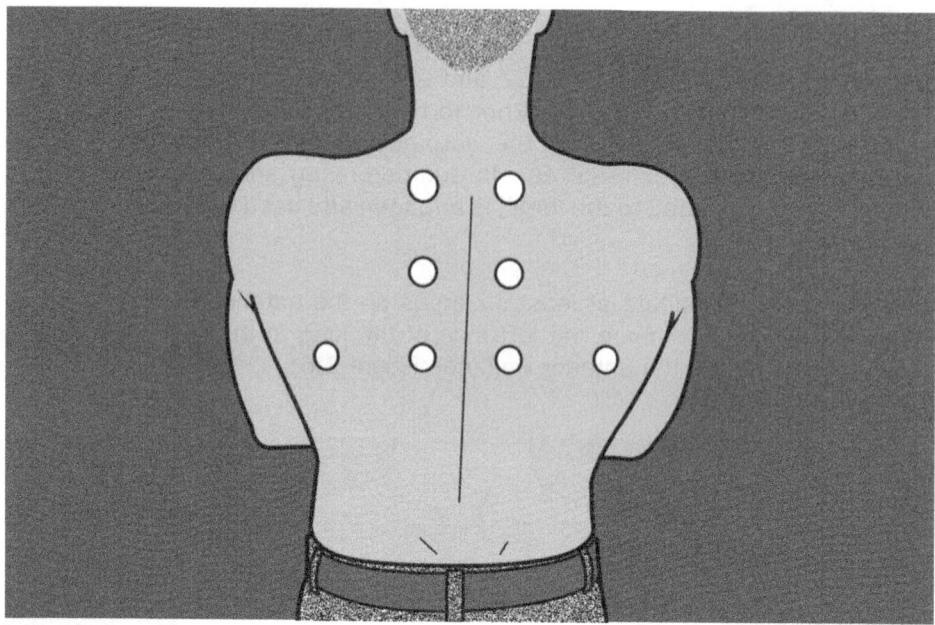

Figure 2.7 Auscultation areas of posterior chest wall

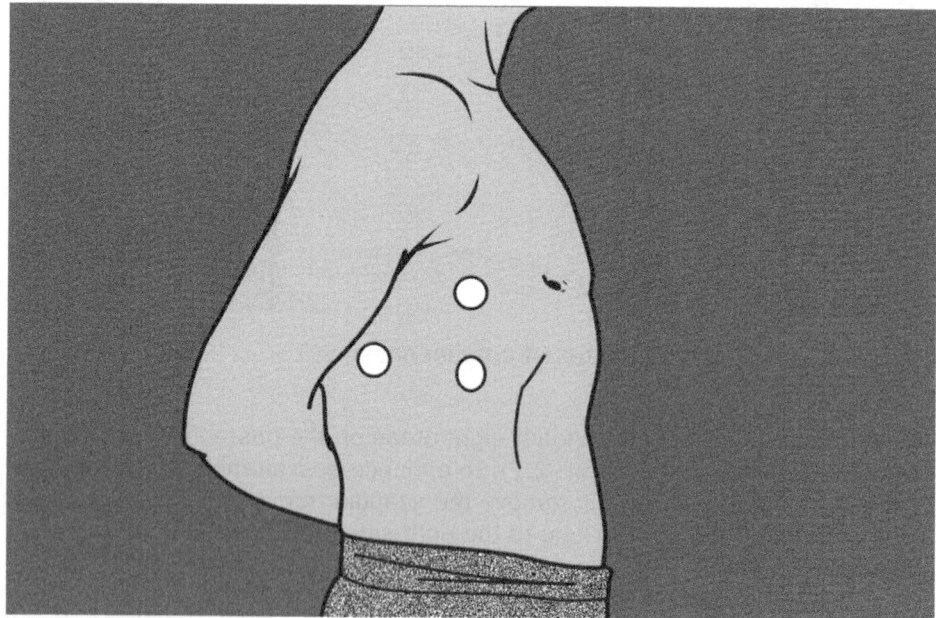

Figure 2.8 Auscultation areas of axillary region

Sounds found on auscultation:

- Expiratory wheeze – the sound created by air passing through narrowed airways on expiration (asthma, COPD).
- Inspiratory wheeze – high-pitched sound heard on inspiration (foreign body obstruction).
- Fine crackles – sound created at the end of expiration by the reopening of the small airways or air passing through intra-alveolar fluid. This is normally heard in the basal lung fields (pulmonary oedema).
- Coarse crackles – sound created on both inspiration and expiration due to fluid or sputum in the larger airways (pneumonia).
- Pleural rub – creaking sound heard on deep inspiration and expiration (pleurisy).
- Absent breath sounds – could indicate a severe life-threatening condition (tension pneumothorax, life-threatening asthma).

COMMON RESPIRATORY CONDITIONS

Asthma

Asthma is a common and chronic inflammatory condition of the airways.

Epidemiology
Currently 5.4 million people in the UK are receiving treatment for asthma. This equates to 4.3 million adults (1 in 12) and 1.1 million children (1 in 11). In Europe the UK still has some of the highest rates for asthma, and on average three people a day die from asthma. In 2011, there were 1,167 deaths from asthma in the UK, and an estimated 75% of hospital admissions for asthma are avoidable and as many as 90% of the deaths from asthma are preventable.

Asthma across the UK
- In Northern Ireland, 182,000 people (1 in 10) are currently receiving treatment for asthma. This includes 146,000 adults and 36,000 children.
- In Scotland, 368,000 people (1 in 14) are currently receiving treatment for asthma. This includes 296,000 adults and 72,000 children.
- In Wales, 314,000 people (1 in 10) are currently receiving treatment for asthma. This consists of 256,000 adults and 59,000 children (Asthma UK, 2015).

Pathophysiology
Asthma is often triggered by an inhaled irritant that causes the muscles of the airway walls to constrict. In addition, it is often characterized by an increased

inflammation of the lining of the airways, which causes swelling. The narrowing of the airways is occasionally exacerbated by the production of excessive sticky mucus.

Signs and symptoms
An asthmatic patient presents with a variable airway obstruction and more than one of the following symptoms:

- Wheeze
- Breathlessness
- Tight chest
- Cough
- Moderate exacerbation of asthma
- PEF >50%–75% best or predicted
- No features of acute severe asthma.

Acute severe asthma

- PEF 33%–50% best or predicted
- Respiratory rate ≥25/min
- SpO_2 ≥92%
- Heart rate ≥110/min
- Inability to complete a sentence in one breath.

Life-threatening asthma

- PEF <33% best or predicted
- SpO_2 <92%
- Altered consciousness level
- Exhaustion
- Arrhythmia
- Hypotension
- Cyanosis
- Silent chest
- Poor respiratory effort.

Patient-specific questions
- Is there a family history of asthma?
- How regularly do you have asthma attacks?
- Have you ever been admitted into intensive care due to your asthma? This is an important indicator of the likelihood of a patient deteriorating rapidly – consideration of previous hospital admissions should be taken very seriously when implementing a treatment plan for these patients.

Possible actions to be taken:
- Auscultate all lung fields to confirm an expiratory wheeze and to exclude evidence of a pneumothorax
- Provide supplementary oxygen to maintain saturations of 94%–98%
- Regular PEFR measurement and reassessment
- Administer drug therapy for asthma as per current local guidelines
- Pre-alert hospital depending on the severity of the attack.

Chronic obstructive pulmonary disease (COPD)

COPD is the preferred term for patients suffering with airway obstruction associated with **emphysema** and bronchitis, although pathological changes associated with chronic asthma can lead to the disease too. It is a chronic progressive disease process which is not fully reversible and is predominantly caused by smoking. Exacerbations often occur, where there is a rapid and sustained worsening of symptoms beyond normal day-to-day variations (NICE, 2010).

Epidemiology
An estimated 3 million people are affected by COPD in the UK, of which 2 million remain undiagnosed. It accounts for approximately 30,000 deaths within the UK, of which 90% occur in the over-65-year-old age group. By the year 2020, COPD is set to become the third leading cause of death worldwide, surpassed only by heart disease and stroke (NICE, 2010).

Pathophysiology
Emphysema is characterized by the destruction of alveolar walls and reduction in the elasticity of the lungs, which reduces the effective surface area for gas exchange. As a result, large spaces remain filled with air during expiration. Smoking is thought to reduce the effectiveness of the body's defence mechanism against this process, allowing sustained alveolar destruction to occur.

Bronchitis is characterized by excessive secretion of bronchial mucus and a productive cough for at least three months a year for two successive years (NICE, 2010). Chronic mucus production affects both large and small airways as a result of an increased number and size of mucous glands and goblet cells. This process causes a narrowing of the airways, increasing airway resistance.

Signs and symptoms of exacerbation of COPD
- Dyspnoea
- Tachypnoea

- Increased sputum production
- Increased wheeze on auscultation
- Chest tightness
- Reduced exercise tolerance
- Fatigue
- Acute confusion
- Cyanosis
- **Tachycardia**
- SpO_2 markedly reduced.

Patient-specific questions
- Does your difficulty in breathing increase with exercise?
- How far can you walk without stopping on a normal day? How does this compare to today?
- Do you have a productive cough? What colour is the sputum?
- What is your normal SpO_2 level?
- Do you use home oxygen? How many litres are you on and for how long in the day?
- Have you been admitted to intensive care with the condition before? If so, when? As with asthma (above), this is an important indicator of the likelihood of a patient deteriorating rapidly – consideration of previous hospital admissions should be taken very seriously when implementing a treatment plan for these patients.

Possible actions to be taken:
- Early respiratory assessment including SpO_2 reading
- Provide supplementary oxygen for a target saturation of 88%–92%
- Administer drug therapy for COPD as per local guidelines (AACE, 2013e)
- Pre-alert hospital depending on the severity of the attack.

Pulmonary embolism (PE)

Emboli can also be caused by air and amniotic fluid in pregnant females. Paramedics should be aware that changes in ECG features associated with pulmonary artery obstruction can occur and may cause acute right ventricular dilation. This can produce an S wave in lead I, a Q wave in lead III, and T wave inversion in lead III, producing the well-known S1, Q3, T3 pattern. The S1, Q3, T3 pattern is seen in approximately 12% of patients presenting with a massive pulmonary embolus.

Epidemiology
In the UK, a pulmonary embolism (PE) following deep vein thrombosis (DVT) causes between 25,000 and 32,000 deaths each year in the hospitalized patient. DVT often occurs post-surgery in patients with reduced mobility. PE is the immediate cause of death in 10% of all patients who die in hospital.

Pathophysiology
A PE is a thrombus, commonly formed in the lower limb or pelvic veins, which becomes dislodged and is carried in the blood to the lungs where it occludes the pulmonary artery or one of its branches. An acute massive pulmonary embolism often kills immediately.

Signs and symptoms
- DIB or SOB
- Tachypnoea
- Acute onset of chest or upper back pain, often sharp or stabbing, worse on inspiration
- Confusion/apprehension
- Tachycardia
- Coughing, usually dry but may cough up blood, mucus or blood-stained mucus
- Feeling light-headed or dizzy
- Leg pain/clinical deep vein thrombosis (DVT).

Patient-specific questions
Does the patient present with any of the following pre-disposing risk factors?
- Recent surgery
- Prolonged period of recent immobility
- Pregnancy and recent childbirth
- Malignancy
- Recent myocardial infarction (MI)
- Oral contraceptive pill
- Age >40 years old
- Family history of DVT/PE.

Possible actions to be taken:
- Provide supplementary oxygen to maintain saturations of 94%–98%
- Thorough history taking with high index of suspicion
- Be prepared for a cardiorespiratory arrest
- Pre-alert hospital (AACE, 2013f).

Anaphylaxis

Anaphylaxis is a severe, life-threatening systemic hypersensitivity reaction.

Epidemiology
One in 1333 patients in the English population has experienced anaphylaxis at one point in their lives. There are approximately 20 anaphylaxis-related deaths per year, although this figure is believed to be an underestimate due to a lack of clinical recognition.

Pathophysiology
Anaphylaxis is a form of shock that affects both the respiratory and circulatory system. An initial exposure to an allergen stimulates the production of antibodies, such as immunoglobulin E (IgE), which attach to mast cells. Secondary exposure to the same allergen triggers IgE that stimulate the mast cells, causing them to degranulate and produce large quantities of histamine. The subsequent release of histamine causes vasodilation, increased permeability of the blood vessels and constriction of the smooth muscle in the airways.

Signs and symptoms
Anaphylaxis is likely when all of the following three criteria are met:

- Sudden onset and rapid progression of symptoms
- Life-threatening airway and/or breathing and/or circulation problems
- Skin and/or mucosal changes.

Sudden onset of symptoms
- Airway swelling
- Dyspnoea/dysphagia
- Stridor/hoarse voice
- Shortness of breath
- Tachypnoea
- Lethargy and confusion
- Cyanosis
- Respiratory arrest
- Signs of shock – pale/clammy
- Tachycardia
- Hypotension
- Decreasing levels of consciousness
- ECG changes (ischaemia and arrhythmias)
- Cardiac arrest
- Sense of 'impending doom'
- Urticaria (hives)
- Pruritus (itching).

Patient-specific questions
- Have you experienced an anaphylactic reaction before?
  - If so, when?
- Describe the symptoms you experienced?
- Do you have an epipen?
- Have you used it today?
- Do you know what triggered this reaction?
- Have you been admitted to an intensive therapy unit (ITU) with this condition? This is an important indicator of the likelihood of a patient deteriorating rapidly – consideration of previous hospital admissions should be taken very seriously when implementing a treatment plan for these patients.

Possible actions to be taken:
- Early adrenaline therapy if indicated, as per local guidelines
- Provide supplementary oxygen to maintain saturations of 94%–98%
- Administer drug therapy for anaphylaxis as per local guidelines
- If time critical, pre-alert the hospital with information of the attack (AACE, 2013g).

Pneumonia

Pneumonia is an infection causing the inflammation and oedema of the alveoli and small airways of the lungs.

Epidemiology
The incidence of community-acquired pneumonia (CAP) varies with age and is commonly found in the elderly or very young. Between 22% and 42% of adults with CAP are hospitalized.

Pathophysiology
Pneumonia reduces the viable surface area for external respiration, resulting in less oxygen reaching the pulmonary circulation.

Signs and symptoms
- Dyspnoea
- Tachypnoea
- Productive cough
- Reduced breath sounds
- Tachycardia
- Pyrexia.

Patient-specific questions
- Have you had a recent chest infection?
- Do you suffer with recurrent chest infections?
- Are you a smoker?

> **Possible actions to be taken:**
> - Provide supplementary oxygen to maintain saturations of 94%–98%
> - If possible, collect sputum sample for culture analysis at hospital
> - Beware of sepsis in the critically ill patient
> - If time critical, pre-alert the hospital.

Pulmonary oedema

Pulmonary oedema is an accumulation of fluid in the lungs which inhibits gas exchange across the alveoli and capillary membranes.

Epidemiology
Pulmonary oedema presenting to the UK ambulance service is predominantly caused by acute and heart failure (NICE, 2015). The condition is associated with significant morbidity levels within the pre-hospital arena, with an in-hospital short-term mortality figure varying between 20% and 30% and a five-year mortality figure nearing 50%.

Pathophysiology
Pulmonary oedema is caused by left ventricular failure (LVF) as a result of the myocardium becoming damaged. This damage results in the left ventricle becoming an ineffective pump, creating an accumulation of blood in the left atrium. Over time, this results in the back-up and accumulation of blood in the pulmonary veins, increasing the pressure at the pulmonary capillaries, leading to pulmonary oedema.

Signs and symptoms
- Dyspnoea
- Pink-stained frothy white sputum
- Orthopnoea
- Anxiousness/restlessness
- Associated with angina.

Patient-specific questions
- Have you been waking at night with shortness of breath?
- Have you been sleeping 'sitting up' or with more pillows recently?

Respiratory assessment

- Have you noticed any swelling in your legs recently?
- Do you suffer from heart failure? Have you had a previous MI, angina attack, angioplasty or coronary artery bypass?

Possible actions to be taken:
- Provide supplementary oxygen if SpO_2 <93%
- Upright patient positioning
- Consider early sublingual glyceryl trinitrate (GTN) if systolic blood pressure >90 mmHg
- Consider continuous positive airway pressure (CPAP) therapy if available and trained
- If time critical, pre-alert the hospital.

Hyperventilation syndrome

Hyperventilation syndrome is an anxiety disorder defined by a tachypnoea exceeding normal physiological requirements. The cause may be related to a stressful event, pain, excitement or an idiopathic reason.

Epidemiology
There is limited statistical data as to the occurrence of hyperventilation syndrome. Experience has shown that this syndrome can occur at any age after infancy but the onset is usually between the ages of 15 and 55 years, affecting a greater proportion of females.

Pathophysiology
The underlying mechanism of how some patients develop hyperventilation is unknown, however, once initiated, it can become a vicious cycle. During episodes of tachypnoea the patient expires excessive carbon dioxide (CO_2), resulting in *hypocapnia*. This leads to respiratory alkalosis causing the common symptoms of tetany, paraesthesia and carpopedal spasms. The experience of these symptoms exacerbates the patient's anxiety which fuels further hyperventilation.

Signs and symptoms
- Acute anxiety
- Tachypnoea
- Tetany
- Paraesthesia (mouth, lips and fingers)
- Carpopedal spasms
- Palpitations
- Dizziness.

Patient-specific questions
- Do you suffer from anxiety attacks?
- What has happened to cause your anxiety today?

Possible actions to be taken:
- Take a thorough history and examination of patient to identify life-threatening causes, (manage A and B problems)
- Consider differential diagnosis (i.e. PE, acute asthma, acute myocardial infarction)
- Maintain a calm and sympathetic approach to the patient's condition
- Provide an explanation as to the symptoms the patient is experiencing and reduce their respiration through effective coaching (AACE, 2013h).

INJURIES TO THE RESPIRATORY SYSTEM

Chest trauma

Chest trauma is a major contributor to mortality in the pre-hospital environment and can involve injuries such as flail segments, massive haemothoraces, open pneumothoraces and tension pneumothoraces.

Epidemiology

Thoracic injuries account for 25% of all deaths in trauma. The primary cause of death is due to hypoxia caused by ventilatory failure or secondary to hypovolaemia from a massive **haemothorax**.

Flail segment

A flail segment occurs when two or more adjacent ribs are broken in two or more places. A paradoxical movement of the lungs occurs due to the free floating flail segment that moves independently of the remainder of the ribs. The flail segment moves in with inhalation and out with exhalation, opposing the normal movement of ribs in respiration, causing inadequate ventilation.

Signs and symptoms
- Significant blunt trauma to the chest
- Paradoxical breathing
- Reduced chest expansion on affected side
- Pain
- Dyspnoea.

Possible actions to be taken:

- 15 l/min O_2 for trauma patients
- Appropriate positioning of patient and stabilization/splinting of the flail segment
- Analgesia as per local guidelines
- Pre-alert the nearest trauma centre.

Tension pneumothorax

A tension pneumothorax occurs when an opening is created within the pleural lining of the lung. If a one-way valve is created, air will enter the pleural space on inhalation but will not leave on exhalation. This creates an increased intra-pleural pressure, leading to the collapse of the lung. As the tension pneumothorax increases in size, the pressure pushes the contents of the mediastinum to the opposite side of the body, obstructing the blood flow of the heart, thus reducing cardiac output. In addition, the tension may compress the diaphragm and the opposing lung. Without immediate intervention the tension pneumothorax will initially result in respiratory arrest, and if interventions are still not undertaken, this condition will result in the patient suffering a cardiac arrest.

Signs and symptoms
- Mechanism of illness or injury
- Dyspnoea often severe RR >30 breaths per minute
- Reduced air entry on injured side
- Reduced SpO_2
- Surgical emphysema
- Hyper-resonance on percussion.

Possible actions to be taken:

- 15 l/min O_2 for trauma patients
- Needle decompression as per local guidelines
- Constant reassessment of presenting condition
- Pre-alert the nearest trauma centre.

Open pneumothorax

An open pneumothorax is caused by a penetrating injury to the chest wall causing air to enter the pleural space. The negative pressure created in the thoracic cavity can draw air through the hole in the chest wall. This may present as a 'sucking chest wound'.

Signs and symptoms
- Penetrating trauma to the chest
- Dyspnoea
- Sucking chest wound
- Reduced air entry on affected side
- Surgical emphysema
- Hyper-resonance on percussion.

Possible actions to be taken:
- 15 l/min O_2 for trauma patients
- Three-sided dressing applied to the wound with opening on inferior side, such as the application of a specific chest dressing, for example the 'Russell Chest Seal'
- Constant reassessment with high suspicion of tension pneumothorax
- Pre-alert the nearest trauma centre.

Haemothorax

A haemothorax occurs when blood enters the pleural space within the lungs. The pleural space of the lungs can hold up to 3 litres of blood and therefore can represent a significant source of blood loss.

Signs and symptoms
- Mechanism of injury – blunt or penetrating trauma to the chest
- Dyspnoea
- Reduced chest expansion on side of injury
- Reduced air entry on side of injury
- Signs of hypovolaemic shock
- Dull sound on percussion.

Possible actions to be taken:
- 15 l/min O_2 for trauma patients
- IV access and intravenous fluids en route as per local guidelines
- Pre-alert the nearest trauma centre.

MECHANICAL FACTORS THAT AFFECT THE RESPIRATORY SYSTEM

The paramedic should be aware that the following mechanical factors might have an influence on the efficacy of undertaking a respiratory assessment and could impact on the normal measurements and therefore distort a paramedic's assessment of the respiratory system:

- Pregnancy – a gravid female may not be able to fully expand her lungs due to the splinting of the diaphragm by the in-situ foetus.
- Obesity – these patients may have an increased weight on their chest and therefore will require a greater mechanical effort to breathe normally. In addition, their increased abdominal mass will impede on lung expansion.
- Abdominal distension – this could be due to either: *fluid* from ascites, impacted *faeces*, *fat*, *foetus* and *flatus*.

CHAPTER KEY POINTS

- In your initial assessment of the respiratory system the **DR 'C'ABCDE** framework should be used to identify life-threatening conditions and the time critical patient, conveyed to the appropriate treatment/management unit.
- If the patient does not have a time critical condition, a thorough secondary survey should be performed.
- The paramedic should endeavour to maintain a professional approach to all patients and treat them with the dignity and respect that they deserve.

REFERENCES

Association of Ambulance Chief Executives (2013a) *UK Ambulance Services Clinical Practice Guidelines 2013 Pocket Book: Chemical, Biological, Radiological, Nuclear and Explosive Incidents*. Bridgwater: Class Professional Publishing.

Association of Ambulance Chief Executives (2013b) *UK Ambulance Services Clinical Practice Guidelines 2013 Pocket Book: Pain Assessment Model*. Bridgwater: Class Professional Publishing.

Association of Ambulance Chief Executives (2013c) *UK Ambulance Services Clinical Practice Guidelines 2013 Pocket Book: Asthma Peak Flow Charts*. Bridgwater: Class Professional Publishing.

Association of Ambulance Chief Executives (2013d) *UK Ambulance Services Clinical Practice Guidelines 2013 Pocket Book: Glycaemic Emergencies (Adults)*. Bridgwater: Class Professional Publishing.

Association of Ambulance Chief Executives (2013e) *UK Ambulance Services Clinical Practice Guidelines 2013 Pocket Book: Chronic Obstructive Pulmonary Disease*. Bridgwater: Class Professional Publishing.

Association of Ambulance Chief Executives (2013f) *UK Ambulance Services Clinical Practice Guidelines 2013 Pocket Book: Pulmonary Embolism*. Bridgwater: Class Professional Publishing.

Association of Ambulance Chief Executives (2013g) *UK Ambulance Services Clinical Practice Guidelines 2013 Pocket Book: Allergic Reactions Including Anaphylaxis (Adults)*. Bridgwater: Class Professional Publishing.

Association of Ambulance Chief Executives (2013h) *UK Ambulance Services Clinical Practice Guidelines 2013 Pocket Book: Hyperventilation Syndrome*. Bridgwater: Class Professional Publishing.

Asthma UK (2015) *Asthma Facts and Frequently Asked Questions (FAQs)*. Available at: http://www.asthma.org.uk/asthma-facts-and-statistics (accessed 14 February 2015).

British Thoracic Society (2015) *Emergency Oxygen Use in Adult Patients Guideline*. Available at: https://www.brit-thoracic.org.uk/searchresults/?txtSearch=2015+Oxygen+Guidelines&search= (accessed 14 February 2015).

Department of Health (2009) *Reference Guide to Consent for Examination or Treatment* (2nd edn). London: Department of Health.

Morris, F., Brady, W.J. and Camm, J. (2008) *ABC of Clinical Electrocardiography* (2nd edn). Malden, MA: Blackwell Publishing Ltd.

NICE (National Institute for Health and Care Excellence) (2010) *Chronic Obstructive Pulmonary Disease. Management of Chronic Obstructive Pulmonary Disease in Adults in Primary and Secondary Care (Partial Update)* (CG101). London: National Institute for Health and Care Excellence.

NICE (National Institute for Health and Care Excellence) (2015) *Acute Heart Failure: Diagnosis and Management in Adults* (CG108). London. National Institute for Health and Care Excellence.

3 Cardiovascular assessment
Graham Harris and Tracy Nicholls

Cardiovascular disease (CVD) is a significant cause of mortality and morbidity in the UK, and accounts for almost one third of all deaths. According to the National Institute for Health and Clinical Excellence (NICE), in 2010 (NICE 2010b), cardiovascular disease accounted for 24% of premature deaths. NICE has implemented a health check programme for everyone between the ages of 40 and 74 who has not yet been diagnosed with cardiovascular disease, chronic kidney disease or diabetes to receive a free health check every five years which includes a CVD risk assessment (NICE, 2014a).

Cardiovascular assessment is an appraisal of the cardiovascular system (CVS) which is in essence the *transport* system of the body, comprising the pump (the *heart*), a control centre and miles of various blood vessels, the heart being the central component. It is connected to all the other body systems, supplying oxygen and nutrients and removing waste products, to help maintain homeostasis.

The aim of this chapter is to provide the paramedic with a systematic approach to the assessment of the cardiovascular system to enable them to undertake an evaluation of the condition and function, and identify abnormalities of the heart and circulatory system, whether they are of a non-serious, serious or life-threatening nature. For further evidence of individual cardiovascular conditions, NICE has published guidelines (NICE, 2015a).

SCENE ASSESSMENT

Information received regarding the incident may provide the paramedic with potential expectations prior to arriving at the scene. A call given as: 'Male, 55 years of age, collapsed? Heart attack?' indicates a potential medical emergency, whereas a call given as: 'Male, 55 years of age, massive blood loss' indicates a potential trauma emergency (see *Trauma Assessment, Chapter 7 for cardiothoracic injuries*).

Initial questions to ask are:

- Is the patient in a collapsed condition?
- If so, is this because the patient has suffered a cardiac arrest, or is it due to shock?

A cardiovascular assessment commences as you approach the patient: these observations may provide evidence of cardiovascular compromise:

- Do they appear to be in obvious distress?
- Do they have obvious dyspnoea?
- Do they appear ill or time critical?
- Are they holding their chest?
- Do they look pale?
- Are they diaphoretic?
- Are they cyanosed?
- Are they sitting upright with legs dependent?

PRIMARY SURVEY

The patient may present and appear well to the paramedic, however, remember that as with other systems, deterioration of the cardiovascular system (CVS) can be both rapid and potentially fatal.

DANGER

- Ensure the safety of yourself, your colleagues, the patient, relatives/bystanders.
- Patients with existing cardiac conditions may have an implanted cardioverter defibrillator (ICD) fitted, or be administered glyceryl trinitrate (GTN) via patches; the latter may present a potential safety issue.
- External defibrillators may be used in cardiac resuscitation and the paramedic has a responsibility to ensure the safety of all persons present prior to delivering shocks as part of advanced cardiac life support (Resuscitation Council (UK) ALS, 2011).

RESPONSE

- Assess the patient's response using the AVPU scale and record appropriately.
- Remember that alterations in the patient's level of consciousness (LOC) may be cardiac in origin; a patient's cerebral hypoxia may be due to the inability of the heart to pump effectively.
- Remember that brain malfunction such as LOC may be the first symptom of hypoxia (British Thoracic Society (BTS), 2015).

Cardiovascular assessment

AIRWAY

- Ascertain if the patient has a patent airway, and is able to maintain it.
- A patient who has collapsed and may have had a heart attack may also have vomited.
- The mouth and/or oropharynx may require immediate management.

Possible actions to be taken:

- Ensure airway is patent and secure before proceeding to next element.

BREATHING

- Ascertain the patient's oxygen saturation levels (SpO_2) as oxygen desaturation occurs in over 50% of cardiac patients.
- Does the patient have shortness of breath, dyspnoea?
- Is the dyspnoea exacerbated by exertion?
- Does the dyspnoea wake them up? (*paroxysmal nocturnal dyspnoea (PND)*)
- Is the dyspnoea due to an existing cardiac condition such as **left ventricular failure (LVF)** or mitral stenosis?
- If so, is the LVF associated with **orthopnoea**? Ask the patient about changes to their sleep patterns; how many pillows they sleep with?
- Does the patient have a dry, chronic cough? This could be an imminent sign of PND.
- Ask the patient if they have been prescribed ACE inhibitors, beta-blockers or amiodarone. Coughing may occur as a side-effect of the drugs (Longmore et al., 2014).

Possible actions to be taken:

- Ensure that the patient is not hypoxic, administer O_2 if required to overcome any hypoxia
- Manage breathing problems and associated hypoxia effectively before moving to the next element.

CIRCULATION

Is the patient complaining of central chest pain? Ascertain if cardiac in origin, obtain electrocardiogram (ECG) trace and manage accordingly (Camm and Bunce, 2012).

Patients presenting with a ruptured abdominal aortic aneurysm (AAA) may present with signs and symptoms of hypovolaemic shock.

If the patient presents with chest trauma or shock, manage accordingly (Salomone and Pons, 2014) (see *Trauma Assessment, Chapter 7*).

- Assess the patient's radial pulse to ascertain the *rate* and *rhythm*.
- Assess the patient's brachial or carotid pulses to ascertain the *character* and *volume*.
- Is the rate tachycardic (>100 beats per minute)?
- If so, identify the cause and manage accordingly if appropriately qualified.

For initial termination of atrioventricular nodal re-entry tachycardia (AVNRT), try vagal manoeuvres (e.g., *carotid sinus massage, exposure of the face to ice water,* or *Valsalva manoeuvre*) before initiating drug treatment.

Drugs used to terminate an acute episode of atrioventricular nodal re-entry tachycardia (AVNRT) include: adenosine (first-line), calcium channel blockers, beta-blockers and digitalis (Olshansky, 2015).

- Is the rate bradycardic (<60 beats per minute)? If so, ask the patient if they take any of the following medications:
- calcium channel blockers, such as diltiazem, amlodipine, nifedipine, verapamil
- alpha- (α) or beta- (β) adrenergic blockers, such as atenolol, propranolol, metoprolol
- glycosides, such as digoxin.

These can all cause pathological sinus bradycardia (Tidy, 2011).

- Check the *rhythm* of the pulse; an irregularly irregular pulse may occur in either atrial fibrillation (AF) or multiple ectopics. However, a regular irregular pulse can occur in a second degree (2°) heart block.

The patient's blood pressure (BP) can provide the paramedic with important information concerning the assessment of their CVS. Remember that hypotension (<90 mmHg) is a significant clinical observation of the patient's cardiac output.

Ascertain if they have a radial pulse.

Possible actions to be taken:

- Administer O_2 and gain IV access
- Obtain an ECG trace and manage accordingly
- Control external haemorrhage (see *Trauma Assessment, Chapter 7*)
- Manage shock accordingly (see *Trauma Assessment, Chapter 7*).

DISABILITY

- Assess the patient's LOC, record the AVPU level (*see Neurological Assessment, Chapter 5*). Consider the younger patient who presents with a transient loss of consciousness may have an undiagnosed cardiac arrhythmia (Department of Health, 2005; Fisher et al. 2013).
- Assess the patient's blood glucose levels.
- Assess the patient's pupils for size and reaction (PERRLA).

Possible actions to be taken:
- Assess and document LOC
- Assess and document blood glucose levels
- Assess and document size and equality of pupils.

EXPOSE/EXAMINE/EVALUATE

Expose and examine the patient, look for scars over sternum (*cardiac surgery*), check for pacemakers and or an implantable cardioverter defibrillator (ICD) (AACE, 2013a) (*normally found just below the patient's left clavicle*) (Figure 3.1),

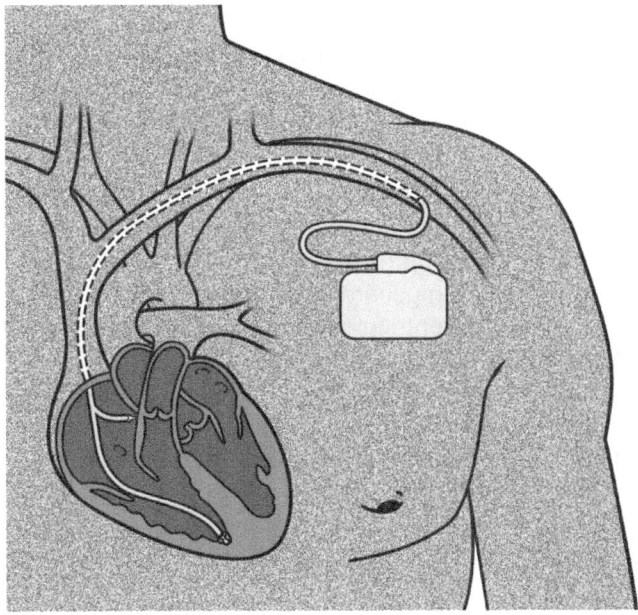

Figure 3.1 Position of implantable cardioverter defibrillator (ICD) or pacemaker

or if the patient has GTN patches on their thoracic wall. Remember: consider the environment and maintain dignity, as far as possible. Consider consent, especially in emergency situations (DH, 2009).

Evaluate the findings from the primary survey. If any time critical problems have been identified within any of the elements, then transport and transfer immediately to an appropriate treatment centre (NICE, 2013); if not, then remain on scene and conduct a secondary survey.

Actions to be taken:
- Expose patient and examine
- Remember consent and patient dignity
- Evaluate – transfer to an appropriate treatment centre (*primary percutaneous coronary intervention – PPCI*), or move on to the secondary survey.

SECONDARY SURVEY

The focused history and assessment conducted as part of this survey can assist the paramedic to establish illnesses and problems that may not have been identified within the primary survey. These may be due to either new or pre-existing cardiac conditions. The paramedic should remember that patients presenting with cardiac conditions can and will be from across the lifespan. However, the types of cardiac conditions that patients typically present with are likely to be from either one or more of the following:

- Angina
- Atrial fibrillation (AF) (*the commonest arrhythmia*)
- Ischaemic heart disease (IHD)
- Heart attack – acute myocardial infarction (AMI)
- Heart failure – right ventricular failure (RVF), left ventricular failure (LVF), and congestive cardiac failure (CCF)
- Cardiac arrythmias
- Congenital heart disease
- Inherited cardiac conditions (ICC)
- Valvular heart disease.

HISTORY

The history of the presenting complaint is a short story about how the patient has come to be unwell, and how their problem is progressing. The key elements

Cardiovascular assessment

of obtaining a patient history are described and an example of how the elements could be recorded is described:

- PC: 52 ♂ C/O central chest pain
- HPC: History of angina, at home watching TV and developed sudden onset of central chest pain. Self-administered GTN with no relief of symptoms, and wife dialled 999. Extremely pale and diaphoretic.

Presenting complaint (PC)

Asking the patient to state what the problem is and to explain their symptoms will assist the paramedic. The most common symptoms that patients with cardiac conditions present with are:

- chest pain
- dyspnoea
- palpitations
- dizziness and syncope
- nausea (and potentially vomiting)
- oedema
- transient loss of consciousness (Swanton and Banarjee, 2008; NICE, 2010a; Bickley and Szilagyi, 2012; Longmore et al., 2014).

Patients may present with one or more symptoms simultaneously, or in certain cases be asymptomatic. The symptoms may be related to specific cardiac conditions. Acute central chest pain is a common presenting symptom of cardiovascular disease. The site, character and related symptoms can assist in identifying the cause. It can be associated with *stable angina* which starts in the retrosternal region and may or may not radiate to the jaw, teeth or arms.

Patients complain of either tightness or heaviness which is associated with exercise and is normally relieved by rest. (*ECG recordings of angina patients often show ST segment depression, and either flattening of or inversion of the 'T' wave.*) However, patients with *unstable angina* may have similar symptoms but explain that the pain occurred at rest, which is potentially more serious as it may progress to a myocardial infarction (MI). Patients who have other forms of chest pain such as *pericardial pain* often present with sharp pain, either retrosternal or epigastric. It is exacerbated by movement and respiration, but relieved by sitting forward. ECG recordings in patients with pericarditis may show saddle-shaped ST elevation (Longmore et al., 2014).

Some patients may experience no chest pain, and experience *silent myocardial ischemia* (Porth, 2014). The factors causing this appear to be the same as for angina: impaired blood flow from the effects of atherosclerosis or vasospasm. There are three main groups of people who seem to experience silent myocardial ischemia: (1) people who are asymptomatic without other evidence of CHD; (2) people who have had myocardial infarct and continue to have episodes of silent ischemia; and (3) people with angina who have episodes of silent ischemia. The reason for these painless episodes is unclear (Porth, 2014). Possible reasons may be that these episodes are shorter and do not involve as much myocardial tissue, so they produce less pain, autonomic neuropathy with sensory denervation, or a defect in pain threshold or pain transmission. There is increased incidence of silent myocardial ischemia in people who have diabetes mellitus, probably as a result of autonomic neuropathy, a common complication of diabetes (Porth, 2014). One point the paramedic needs to remember is that a person with diabetes presenting with unexplained nausea and vomiting needs to be fully assessed and this includes a 12-lead ECG. You never know what you may find.

Aortic pain due to acute thoracic aortic dissection presents as a sudden severe tearing retrosternal pain which radiates to the back; the degree of the radiation will depend on the blood vessels involved. If branch arteries are affected, the patient can present with neurological signs, the absence of pulses and unequal blood pressure in their arms. *Non-cardiac pain* can be oesophageal (*reflux oesophagitis*) or mediastinal with similar dissemination to cardiac pain but is not triggered by effort (Swanton and Banarjee, 2008).

Patients with cardiac conditions commonly present with dyspnoea; the commonest cardiac cause of exertion dyspnoea is left ventricular heart failure. Dyspnoea can also occur at rest; patients present with breathlessness when they lie flat (*orthopnoea*). Alternatively the patient may present or complain of waking suddenly at night because of paroxysmal nocturnal dyspnoea (PND) due to pulmonary oedema caused by the accumulation of fluid in the lungs. (*An imminent sign of PND is a dry nocturnal cough.*) However, in acute pulmonary oedema, the patient may cough up pink frothy sputum or it may be streaked with **haemoptysis** (Swanton and Bannarjee, 2008).

Palpitations are an awareness of the heartbeat. There are times, such as during exercise, or if when anxious, that we become aware of our normal heartbeat. However, if the patient presents with palpitations in other circumstances, they may indicate a cardiac arrhythmia, notably ectopic beats or a paroxysmal tachycardia.

Assessment: ask the patient to tap out the rate and regularity of the palpitations. Irregular, fast palpitations are likely to be atrial fibrillation, whereas slow palpitations are likely to be due to beta-blocker drugs (Longmore et al., 2014). Ascertain from the patient when the symptom occurs, and if it is associated with other symptoms, such as dyspnoea or syncope, which may indicate haemodynamic compromise.

Patients presenting with dizziness or syncope (*faint*), may classically explain that they had one of their 'funny turns'. Cardiac causes of syncope can be due to either a ventricular tachycardia (VT) or complete heart block, both of which are unable to maintain cardiac output in the acute setting. Ask the patient or eye-witness what they were doing when the syncope occurred. It can occur in men at night after micturition, whereas effort syncope commonly occurs secondary to aortic valve or sub-valve stenosis in adult patients and children with Fallot's tetralogy (Swanton and Bannarjee, 2008).

Patients with deep vein thrombosis (DVT) or right heart failure (RHF) may present with oedema caused by increased venous pressure. Dependent oedema appears predominantly in the feet and ankles when sitting; however, in patients who are bedridden, the oedema will transfer and occur in the sacrum (Bickley and Szilagyi, 2012).

History of presenting complaint (HPC)

The following questions can assist the paramedic in obtaining the appropriate history surrounding the presenting complaint:

- What were you doing before the problem started?
- When did the symptoms start?
- What was the first thing that you noticed?
- Have you ever had this problem before?

Use the SOCRATES framework to structure your pain assessment questions; the SOCRATES framework is described below:

- **S** – Site. Where exactly is the pain? Is it retrosternal? Acute central chest pain is normally cardiac in origin.
- **O** – Onset. Did it commence gradually (*heart attack, myocardial infarction MI*) or suddenly (*aortic dissection*)?
- **C** – Character. Do they explain it as a tightness, heaviness or crushing?
- **R** – Radiation. To the jaw or arms (*angina*) or to the back (*aortic dissection*)?
- **A** – Associated symptoms. Are they nauseous, or diaphoretic (*myocardial infarction MI*)?
- **T** – Time/duration. When did the pain commence, and its duration?
- **E** – Exacerbating/relieving factors. Does the pain increase with movement? Or is it relieved by sitting forward (*pericarditis*)?
- **S** – Severity. How does the patient score the pain on a scale of 0–10? (*0 = no pain, 10 = worst pain ever*) (AACE, 2013b; Longmore et al., 2014).

Past medical history (PMH)

When asking patients about their medical history the paramedic should use the appropriate terminology. If you ask them if they have hypertension, they may answer no, but if you ask if they have any problems with their blood pressure, their answer is yes. The purpose of this element is to ascertain the patient's past medical history, which can provide important information concerning their condition.

- Have you had this problem before? If so, when?
- Do you have angina?
- Have you ever had a heart attack?
- Do you have a problem with your heart?
- Can you tell me what this is?
- Do you have a problem with your blood?
- Can you tell me what this is?
- Do you have a problem with your blood pressure?
- Have you ever had a 12-lead ECG recorded before? If yes, why?
- Have you ever had an ultrasound of your heart? If yes, why?
- Have you ever had a stroke?
- Do you have any other medical problems that you see your doctor about, or take tablets for? (*Patients with comorbidities have increased risk of developing cardiovascular disease, including, diabetes, hypertension, dyslipidaemia, chronic kidney disease, influenza, rheumatoid arthritis, serious mental health problems and periodontitis (NICE, 2014a).*)
- Have you had rheumatic fever? (*Patients may develop right heart failure/mitral stenosis.*)
- Have you ever been admitted to hospital or had any operations?
- If so, what was it for? Consider that cardiac operations/surgery may include:
  - heart transplant
  - coronary artery bypass grafting (CABG)
  - percutaneous transluminal coronary angioplasty (PTCA) (*balloon dilation*)
  - percutaneous coronary intervention (PCI) (*stent*)
  - valve replacement
  - pacemaker or implantable cardioverter defibrillator (ICD).

Drug/medication history (DMH)

Ask the patient general questions about any tablets or injections that they have to take or administer, remember to ask if they have purchased and or taken any over-the-ounter (OTC) medicines, or if they are taking any herbal remedies.

- Is the patient currently prescribed or taking medications for any existing medical problem?

Cardiovascular assessment

- If so, what for? Use the medications to confirm this by asking the patient what they take each medication for.
- Medications for cardiac conditions may include: beta-blockers, cardiac glycosides, ACE inhibitors, angiotensin II receptor antagonists, diuretics, anti-coagulants, statins, calcium channel blockers, potassium channel blockers and nitrates.
- Have they been compliant with their medications?
- Ask patients who present with angina and prescribed GTN spray, if they have used it.
- If yes, has it relieved the pain? If not, ask if they have a headache. If not, check that the drug is in-date.
- Have they recently started a new, or stopped a previous, medication?

Social/family medical history (S/FMH)

Consider that patients who present with cardiac conditions may be from across the lifespan; a young person presenting with syncope during exercise requires a detailed assessment of the family history to ascertain if there are risk factors. Alternatively, the older person who presents with symptoms of heart failure may have had recurrent scarlet fever as a child.

- Remember to use probing as opposed to prying questions, such as, who else is there at home?
- Depending upon the age of the patient, ascertain if they live alone or have relatives who visit, carers, nurses or other external agency input.
- Consider mobility, does the person use any walking aids?
- Are there stairs in the property? If so, can the patient climb them unaided?
- What can the patient not do for themselves because of the illness or symptoms, which normally they could?
- Depending on the presenting medical condition, ask if other members of the patient's family also suffer from the condition or illness.
- Ask about congenital conditions; long QT syndrome and hypertrophic cardiomyopathy (HCM).
- Ask about the patient's parents and siblings; specifically their age, health and if known, cause of death.
- To identify if there is a significant family history of coronary heart disease (CHD), ask the patient about the health of their grandparents and any male siblings, if they smoked, had hypertension or hyperlipidaemia before their 60th birthday, and where applicable, ascertain the cause of death.
- Ascertain and identify if the patient has any of the following risk factors: family history of CHD, hypertension, diabetes mellitus, sedentary lifestyle, diet, recreational drugs, alcohol and smoking status.

- Regular use of cocaine increases coronary atherosclerosis and the risk of a myocardial infarction (Burnett, 2015).
- Regarding alcohol and smoking, ascertain how much, how long, and if appropriate when ceased.
- Smoking is quantified in pack years (20 cigarettes smoked per day for 1 year = 1 pack year) (Longmore et al., 2014).

EXAMINATION

While this commenced with the primary survey, the examination itself comprises various components, some of which may be new to the paramedic. The component tests are simple to perform and to the experienced paramedic, their results will be objective.

The following systematic format will assist the paramedic. Appearance, hands, pulses, blood pressure, praecordium, jugular venous pressure (JVP), auscultation (*heart and lungs*), oedema, abdomen and peripheral pulses.

Appearance

- Does the patient look ill?
- Are they pale, cold, clammy (*signs of shock and cardiovascular compromise*)?
- Check their eyelids for evidence of xanthelasma (*sharply demarcated yellowish collection of cholesterol underneath the skin, around the eyelids, common in people of Asian and Mediterranean origin, and associated with hyperlipidaemia*).
- Do they have corneal arcus (*greyish-white ring, or part of a ring*) opacity occurring in the periphery of the cornea due to a lipid infiltration of the corneal stroma?
- Does the patient have proptosis (*bulging eyes*)? Graves' disease (*associated with atrial fibrillation*)?
- Does the patient have a Malar flush (*redness around the cheeks and is indicative of mitral stenosis*)?

Possible actions to be taken:

- Assess the patient's appearance, including face
- Assess the eyelids and cornea for evidence of hyperlipidaemia
- Record findings appropriately.

Hands

- Are the patients hands warm, and well perfused, or sweaty, or cold and moist?
- Veins that are dilated may be due to carbon dioxide (CO_2) retention.
- Are any rings on the patient's fingers tight because of oedema?
- Are there splinter haemorrhages under the patient's nail beds?
- Do they have Janeway lesions (*red macules*) on the palm of the hand?
- Osler's nodes (*tender lumps in the pulp of the fingertips*)?
- Are there nicotine stains?
- Does the patient have finger clubbing (see Figure 3.2) (*associated with endocarditis, atrial myxoma and cyanotic congenital heart disease*)?

Possible actions to be taken:

- Assess the patient's hands, including fingers and nails
- Assess for finger clubbing (*ask the patient to place the fingernails of the same finger on opposite hands against each other, nail to nail, a small kite/diamond shape is normally apparent between the nail beds*) (see Figure 3.2)
- If this window is obliterated, the test is positive and clubbing is present.

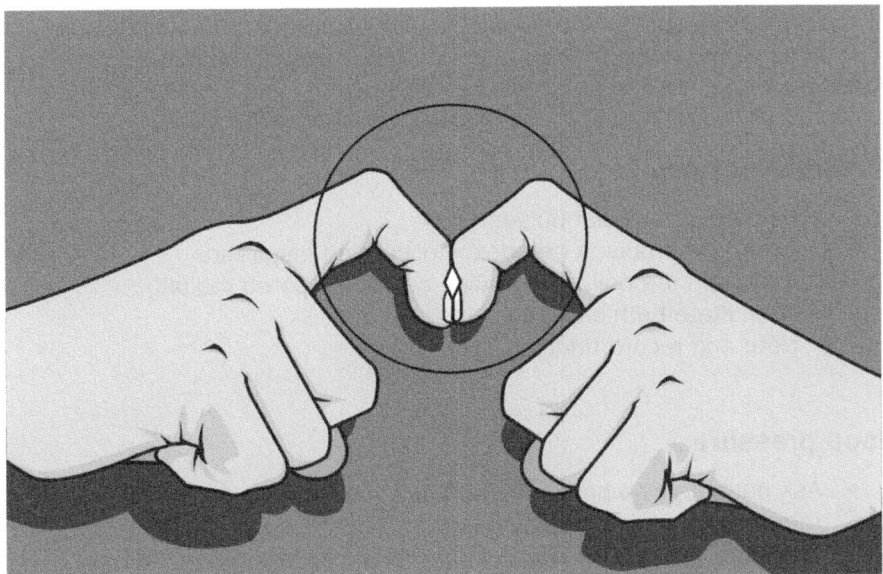

Figure 3.2 Finger clubbing assessment

Pulses

- Assess radial pulses for *rate* and *rhythm* and the carotid pulse for *character* and *volume*.
- Assess both radial pulses simultaneously and check that they are equal (*unequal pulses can indicate atherosclerosis or aortic dissection*).
- Is the pulse irregularly irregular (*indicative of atrial fibrillation (AF) or multiple ectopics*)?
- Is the pulse regularly irregular (*indicative of second degree heart block and ventricular bigeminy*)?
- Auscultate lightly and listen for carotid artery bruits (*indicative of artherosclerotic narrowing*) – (ask the patient to briefly hold their breath as you auscultate each artery in turn).
- A small volume pulse (*indicative of shock, aortic stenosis and pericardial effusion*).
- A jerky pulse (*indicative in hypertrophic obstructive cardiomyopathy, HOCM*).
- Ascertain if *pulsus paradoxus* occurs when the patient inspires (*systolic pressure reducing >10 mmHg*), this may be due to pericardial constriction or cardiac tamponade (Longmore et al., 2014).
- A *collapsing pulse* can be felt radially.

Assessment

Lift the patient's right arm up above the height of their shoulder, and let their radial pulse beat against the flat of your hand. If present, a slapping sensation caused by the collapsing pulse will be noted.

Possible actions to be taken:

- Palpate both radial pulses
- Ascertain if pulsus paradoxus occurs on inspiration
- Ascertain if a collapsing pulse can be palpated radially
- Auscultate both carotid pulses
- Note and record findings.

Blood pressure

- Ask patients who have a history of hypertension if they know what their blood pressure reading is normally.
- The blood pressure may be either raised or lowered in patients presenting with unstable angina, myocardial infarction or a serious underlying arrhythmia.

- A narrow *pulse pressure* is indicative of aortic stenosis.
- A wide *pulse pressure* is indicative of aortic regurgitation.
- A fall in systolic pressure >10 mmHg on inspiration indicates *pulsus paradoxus* and may be due to pericardial constriction or cardiac tamponade.
- Postural hypotension occurs with a fall of (*systolic >15 mmHg or diastolic >10 mmHg*) on standing, and may be due to hypovolaemia, idiopathic orthostatic hypotension or vasodilator and diuretic drugs.

Praecordium

- Inspect for scars (*median stenotomy*).
- Inspect for any deformity.
- Inspect for pulsations.
- Inspect for an ICD and or pacemaker (see Figure 3.1).
- Palpate the *apex beat* (see Figure 3.3).
- An apex beat that is *tapping* (*quick and light*) indicates mitral stenosis.
- An apex beat that is *thrusting* (*diffuse and long*) indicates aortic stenosis.
- An apex beat that is *heaving* (*sharp and firm*) indicates mitral or aortic regurgitation.

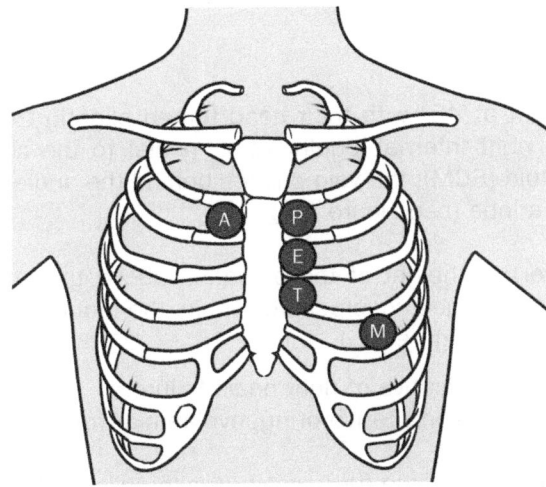

(A) **Aortic Valve** — 2nd right intercostal space (ICS), right sternal border
(P) **Pulmonary Valve** — 2nd left intercostal space (ICS), left sternal border
(E) **Erb's Point** — 3rd left intercostal space (ICS), left sternal border
(T) **Tricuspid Valve** — 4th left intercostal space (ICS), left sternal border
(M) **Mitral Valve** — 5th intercostal space (ICS), mid-clavicular line

Figure 3.3 Auscultation positions

Assessment

Ask the patient to turn on their left side and hold their breath after exhalation.

The normal apex beat is found in the left 5th intercostal space, in the mid-clavicular line (see Figure 3.3). It is palpable but does not lift the finger off the chest wall.

Jugular venous pressure (JVP)

As part of the assessment of the right side of the patient's heart, the paramedic will need to evaluate the JVP. The JVP of the internal jugular vein correlates with the pressure in the right atrium, and an elevation of the JVP may be indicative of right heart failure (RHF). There are two features requiring observation:

1. Visual assessment of the height JVP
2. The waveform of the pulse.

While not every paramedic may be fortunate to have the expertise and ability to evaluate the waveform, you can, with practice, perfect the skill of assessing the height-JVP.

Assessment

Position the patient at 45° with their head turned slightly to the left. Locate and observe the right internal jugular vein, medial to the clavicular head of sternocleidomastoid (SCM); the vein passes behind the angle of the jaw in the direction of the earlobe (see Figure 3.4).

The JVP is the vertical height of the pulsation above the sternal angle. The pulsation reflects changes in pressure within the right atrium. The JVP is elevated if >4 cm (see Figure 3.5).

- Raised JVP is indicative of right heart failure.
- Decreased JVP is indicative of hypovolaemia from GI bleeding or dehydration.
- Inspiratory filling of the neck veins (Kussmaul's sign) is indicative of constrictive pericarditis (Longmore et al., 2014).

Auscultation (heart and lungs)

Normal heart sounds are produced by the closing of the heart's valves, which cause changes to the flow of blood. The first heart sound (S_1) generates the 'lub' of the 'lub–dub' and is formed by the closure of the mitral (M_1) and tricuspid (T_1) valves at the start of ventricular systole. The second heart sound

Cardiovascular assessment

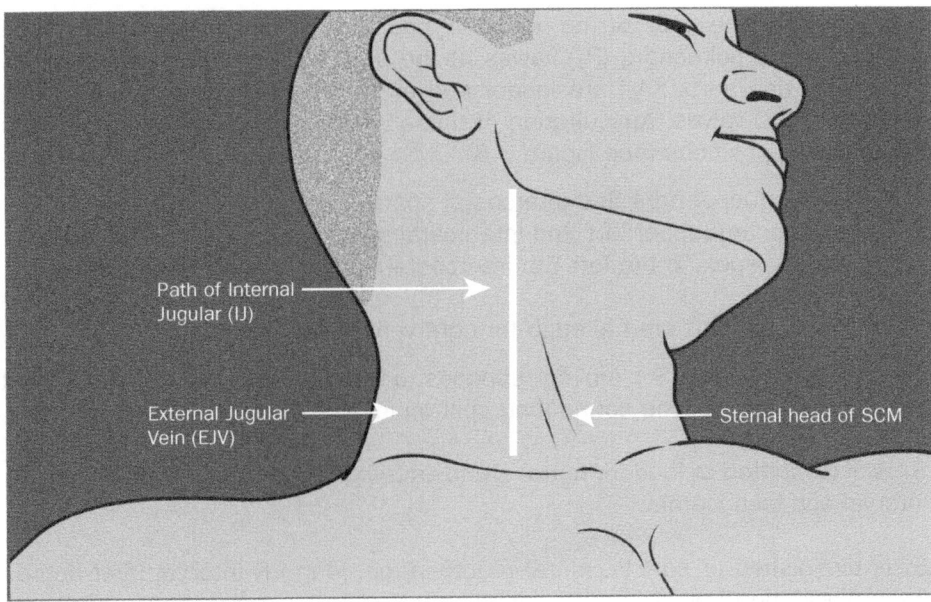

Figure 3.4 Landmarks required for jugular venous pressure measurement (JVP)

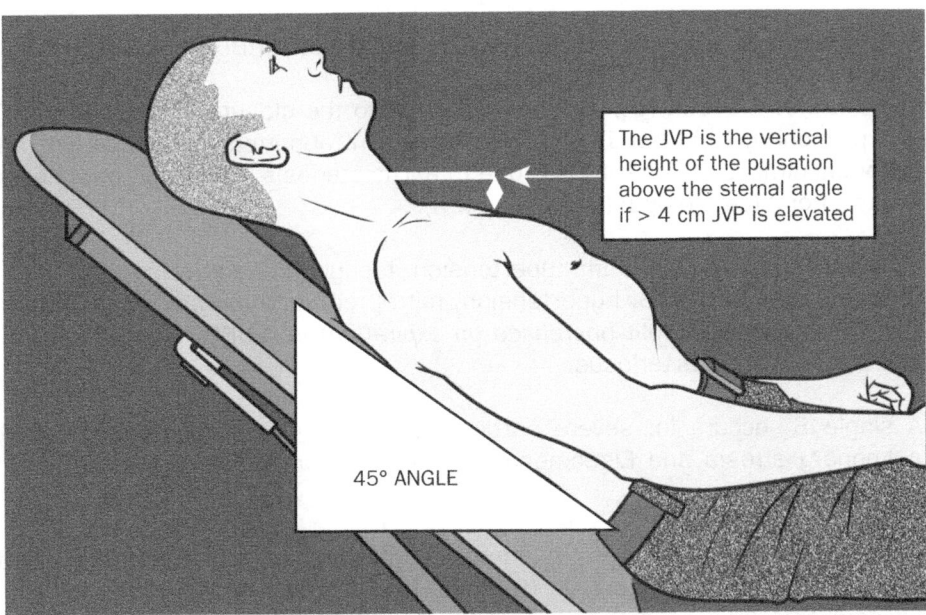

Figure 3.5 Position for measuring jugular venous pressure measurement (JVP)

(S_2) generates the 'dub' of the 'lub–dub' and is formed by the closure of the aortic (A_2) and pulmonary (P_2) valves at the start of ventricular diastole. The mitral (M_1) and aortic (A_2) are louder and occur before the tricuspid (T_1) and pulmonary (P_2) valves. Auscultation of these areas of the heart is obtained in the following positions (see Figure 3.3).

- Aortic (upper right 2nd intercostal space)
- Pulmonary (upper left 2nd intercostal space)
- Mitral (apex, in the left 5th intercostal space, in the mid-clavicular line)
- Tricuspid (left sternal edge for right ventricular area).

The first heart sound (S_1) 'lub' corresponds to the closure of the mitral (M_1) and tricuspid (T_1) valves. The sound may split on inspiration and is normal.

S_1 is accentuated or loud in: mitral stenosis (*tapping apex beat*), shortened PR interval and tachycardia.

S_1 is diminished or soft in: mitral regurgitation, long PR interval (*first degree heart block*), heart block and diminished left ventricular contraction – infarction.

S_1 is variable in: third degree heart block, AF, nodal tachycardia and ventricular tachycardia (VT).

S_1 is widely split in: right and left bundle branch block (RBBB and LBBB).

The 2nd heart sound (S_2) 'dub' corresponds to the closure of the aortic (A_2) and pulmonary (P_2) valves. The most significant abnormality of A_2 is when it becomes diminished or softened due to aortic stenosis. S_2 can be best heard at Erb's Point (cardiology) (see Figure 3.3).

A_2 is accentuated or loud in: hypertension, tachycardia and transposition. A_2 is widely split in: RBBB, hypertension, mitral regurgitation and deep inspiration. A_2 is reversed split (*increased on expiration*) in: LBBB, aortic stenosis, and patent ductus arteriosus.

A single S_2 occurs in: severe aortic or pulmonary stenosis, hypertension, pulmonary atresia and Eisenmenger syndrome (*congenital ventricular septal defect*).

P_2 is accentuated or loud in: pulmonary hypertension, and P_2 is diminished or soft in: pulmonary stenosis (Swanton and Bannarjee, 2008; Bickley and Szilagyi, 2012; Longmore et al., 2014).

Cardiovascular assessment

A third heart sound (S_3) can occur just after the second heart sound (S_2). It is pathological in patients over 30 years of age, however:

- It can occur normally in fit young adults (*athletes*).
- It occurs abnormally in patients with heart failure.
- In patients with left heart failure – S_3 is best heard in the mitral area.
- In patients with right heart failure – S_3 is best heard in the tricuspid area.

A fourth heart sound (S_4), if produced, occurs just before S_1 and is always abnormal. It signifies the atrial contraction against a stiffened ventricle which can be caused by aortic stenosis or hypertensive heart disease. It can also occur in heart failure.

There are several websites on the internet where you can practise listening to heart sounds and murmurs, the following provides an online course, but you will require headphones: http://auscultation.education/heart-sounds

Possible actions to be taken:

- Use the diaphragm of the stethoscope to auscultate for the high pitched sounds of S_1 'lub' and S_2 'dub'
- Auscultate and listen to all areas: M_1, T_1, and A_2, P_2
- Remember to listen on inspiration and on held expiration
- Listen at the apex, with the patient in the left lateral position, for low-pitched sounds of left-sided S_3, S_4 and mitral stenosis, with the bell of the stethoscope
- Listen at the apex with the patient sitting up, leaning forward holding their breath after expiration for possible aortic regurgitation
- Lungs – auscultate the base of the lungs and listen for evidence of cardiac failure crepitations and pleural effusion.

Oedema

Oedema occurs due to the accumulation of excessive fluid in the interstitial tissue spaces and in patients with cardiac conditions should include both peripheral and pulmonary assessment.

- Bilateral oedema of the legs implies systemic disease, is dependent and the ankles and legs will be affected.
- In bed-bound patients, the fluid moves to new areas and the sacrum will be affected.
- Patients with LVF can present with severe pulmonary oedema.

Abdomen

- Patients presenting with a ruptured abdominal aortic aneurysm (AAA) may present with signs and symptoms of hypovolaemic shock and intermittent or continuous abdominal pain that radiates to the back, iliac fossae or groins.
- A pulsatile mass may or may not be present.
- Ascites (*free fluid in the peritoneal cavity*) may occur in right heart failure.
- Check for bruits over the aorta and renal arteries (*indicative of artherosclerotic vascular disease*) (see *Figure 4.4, Abdominal Assessment, Chapter 4*).

Peripheral pulses

- Palpate the patient's radial, brachial, carotid and dorsalis pedis pulses.
- Feel for radio-radial delay (*indicative of aortic arch thoracic aneurysm*).
- Auscultate for bruits over the carotid, aorta and renal arteries, particularly if there is inequality or absence of the pulses (*this may be due to artherosclerosis in the older patient or vasculitis in the younger*).

Vital signs

Record the findings of each element of the assessment, which should, where appropriate, provide the following evidence regarding the patient:

- Respiratory rate, character and work of breathing
- Heart rate, character, volume and rhythm
- Blood pressure (BP)
- Electrocardiogram (*a 12-lead ECG should be recorded when undertaking a CVS assessment, specifically when the patient presents with acute central chest pain*)
- Blood glucose levels
- GCS neurological status
- Pupils
- Peak expiratory flow (PEF) (*best of three readings*)
- Temperature
- Oxygen saturations (SpO_2)
- Pain score
- Signs and symptoms of each system obtained during the secondary survey.

COMMON CARDIAC CONDITIONS

Angina

Angina pectoris is the name for the chest pain that arises from the heart due to myocardial ischaemia. The types of angina are **stable** (*due to effort and relieved with rest and or medication*), **unstable** (*occurs at rest; has an increased risk of myocardial infarction*), **decubitus** (*caused by lying flat*) and **Prinzmetal's** (*caused by coronary artery spasm*).

Signs and symptoms/presentations

- Central chest pain expressed as either tightness, heaviness or a crushing sensation.
- The pain may radiate to the neck, jaw, teeth and to either one or both arms.
- It can be exacerbated by cold weather, emotion (*anger and excitement*) and heavy meals.
- Diaphoresis, dyspnoea, nausea and faintness.
- ECG findings – ST segment depression, inverted or flattened 'T' waves.

Atrial fibrillation (AF)

Atrial fibrillation is an extremely common arrhythmia with over 835,000 people in England alone with the condition. Due to its effects on both the heart rate and rhythm, it is a major cause of morbidity and mortality owing to the increased susceptibility of suffering a stroke (NICE, 2014b).

Signs and symptoms/presentations
- Palpitations
- An irregularly irregular pulse
- Acute pulmonary oedema
- ECG findings – absent 'P' waves and irregular ventricular response (*fine oscillation/fibrillation*).

Ischaemic heart disease (IHD)

Ischaemia of the heart muscle arises from the imbalance between the supply and demand of oxygen to the myocardium. Atheroma of the coronary arteries due to coronary artery disease (CAD) is the leading cause of ischaemic heart disease due to obstruction of blood flow. It is the highest rated cause of death in the world with a total of 7.6 million, followed by stroke with 6.7 million (World Health Organization, 2014).

Signs and symptoms/presentations
- Patients with myocardial ischaemia caused by CAD can present with a variety of clinical presentations. These range from those presenting with stable angina, to the patient who may have an acute coronary syndrome (ACS), such as unstable angina and myocardial infarction.
- ECG findings – may include either ST segment depression, or ACS with or without ST elevation.

Acute myocardial infarction: heart attack

A myocardial infarction (MI) is caused by a rupture of an atherosclerotic plaque, resulting in thrombosis and occlusion of the coronary artery. Diagnosis is based upon presentation or assessment of two out of three of the following: (1) history (*central chest pain*); (2) ECG changes; and (3) cardiac markers (*enzymes*) rise. In the out-of-hospital arena, the paramedic is called to the first (*acute central chest pain*) and should be proficient in obtaining and interpreting the second (ECG changes) (College of Paramedics, 2015).

Signs and symptoms/presentations
- Acute central chest pain >15 minutes duration.
- Patients may also present with no pain (*silent MIs*), this can occur in elderly, hypertensive or diabetic patients.
- Diaphoresis, dyspnoea, nausea, emesis, and appear pale and grey.
- ECG findings – ST elevation in two or more leads in the following views:
  - Inferior infarct – in leads II, III, and AVF
  - Lateral infarct – in leads I, II, and AVL
  - Anterior infarct – in leads V_2–V_6
- Complications (cardiac arrest).

Possible actions to be taken:
- Undertake a cardiovascular assessment and obtain a 12-lead ECG recording
- If complicated, establish cardiac arrest (VF)
- Manage in accordance with UK Resuscitation Council and NICE Guidelines (Resuscitation Council (UK), 2011; NICE, 2013).

Heart failure (left ventricular failure – LVF, right ventricular failure – RVF and congestive cardiac failure – CCF)

Heart failure (HF) is the term used to describe the inability of the heart to pump effectively to meet the demands of the body, mainly due to inadequate cardiac output and blood pressure. In England and Wales, acute heart failure is one

Cardiovascular assessment

of the commonest causes of admission to hospital (over 67,000 per annum), and in the UK is the leading cause of hospital admission in people 65 years or older (NICE, 2014c).

Chronic heart failure is a complex clinical syndrome of signs and symptoms which suggest impairment of the heart as a pump supporting physiological circulation. It is caused by structural or functional abnormalities of the heart. The incidence of heart failure and chronic heart failure increases with age, with approximately 1 in 35 people aged 65–74 years having heart failure. This increases to about 1 in 15 for those aged 75–84 years, and to just over 1 in 7 in those aged 85 years and above (NICE, 2010b).

Signs and symptoms (LVF)
- Dyspnoea (*associated with exertion*)
- Tachycardia
- Tachypnoea
- Orthopnoea
- Dry nocturnal cough (*associated with paroxysmal nocturnal dyspnoea*)
- Coughing up pink frothy sputum streaked with haemoptysis (*associated with acute pulmonary oedema*)
- Wheeze
- Cold peripheries
- Muscle wasting and weight loss
- Basal lung crepitations
- Decreased systolic BP.

Signs and symptoms (RVF)
- Peripheral oedema (*ankles and calves in ambulant patients*)
- Sacral oedema (*in bed-bound patients*)
- Abdominal distension (*associated with ascites*)
- Engorgement (*puffiness*) of the face
- Pulsation in the neck and face (*associated with tricuspid regurgitation*)
- Epistaxis
- Distended varicose veins
- Nausea
- Anorexia.

Signs and symptoms (CCF)
- Typically these present as a combination of RVF and LVF signs and symptoms.
- Consider that patients may also present with depression or the side effects of drug-related treatment.
- Paramedics should remember that the ECG itself is a poor indicator of heart size, however, depending on the cause, the ECG may show: ST

depression – ischaemia, ST elevation – myocardial infarction (STEMI), or left ventricular hypertrophy (LVH) – hypertension. Suspect LVH:
- if the R wave in V6 >25 mm;
- or if the sum of S wave in V1 and the R wave in V6 is >35 mm.
• Suspect RVH if there is:
- dominant R wave in V1, T wave inversion in V1–V3 or V4, deep S wave in V6, right axis deviation (RAD) (Longmore et al., 2014).

Cardiac arrhythmias

Some cardiac arrhythmias are common; these are often benign and intermittent. Occasionally, however, cardiac arrhythmias cause cardiac compromise. Depending on the arrhythmia, it may be classified as bradycardic or tachycardic in origin; remember that the patient may be asymptomatic.

Signs and symptoms
- Palpitations
- Chest pain
- Dyspnoea
- Collapse
- Hypotension
- Syncope
- Pulmonary oedema.

Possible actions to be taken:

- Obtain a 12-lead ECG recording and diagnose arrhythmia (*bradycardia – tachycardia*)
- Bradycardia – if <40 bpm or patient is symptomatic, manage appropriately
- Tachycardia – ascertain from the ECG recording if it is broad complex (*rate >100 bpm and QRS complex >120 ms*) or narrow complex (*rate >100 bpm and QRS <120 ms*) and manage appropriately (Resuscitation Council (UK) ALS, 2011).

Congenital heart disease

The diversity of congenital heart disease in adults is different from that of children due to adults being unlikely to have complex lesions. The commonest in order of occurrence are:

- Bicuspid aortic valve – In adulthood, this is likely to develop aortic stenosis (AS) or aortic regurgitation (AR).

Cardiovascular assessment

- Atrial septal defect (ASD) – A hole connecting the atria, the commonest of which (*ostium secondum*) occurs high in the septum. This type of ASD is often asymptomatic until adulthood. As the compliance of the ventricles diminishes with age, the patient develops left-to-right shunting.

Signs and symptoms
- Dyspnoea
- Chest pain
- Haemoptysis
- Pulmonary hypertension
- Cyanosis.

Ventricular septal defect (VSD)

A hole connecting the ventricles which may be due to a congenital cause, it can also be acquired following a myocardial infarction. The signs are dependent on both the size and site; small holes tend to produce loud murmurs, while larger holes are linked with pulmonary hypertension.

Coarctation of the aorta

A congenital narrowing of the descending aorta, and more common in males. Signs include: radio-femoral delay, hypertension, weak femoral pulse and systolic murmurs.

Inherited cardiac conditions (ICCs)

ICCs are caused by mutations in the components of the heart's electrical and contractile system. It should be stressed that there are numerous conditions, including: arrhythmia syndromes, cardiomyopathies; inherited arteriopathies; muscular dystrophies and disorders of lipid metabolism caused by an inherited genetic defect known as familial hypercholesterolaemia (FH) (NICE, 2008; Burton et al., 2009). Affected individuals are at risk of serious cardiac events and sudden death. Some examples from these categories include:

- *Long QT syndrome (LQTS)* – is characterized by a lengthening of the QT interval (measured from the beginning of the QRS to the end of the 'T' wave) on the ECG. This places the patient at risk of ventricular tachyarrhythmias, which may develop into syncope, cardiac arrest or sudden death. Standard Time of the QT Interval is 0.35–0.42 (secs) (see *Mental Health Assessment, Chapter 15*).
- *Brugada syndrome* – is a disorder associated with one of a number of ECG patterns that are characterized by incomplete RBBB and ST

elevations in the anterior precordial leads. Patients are likely to be young males who are otherwise healthy and may have normal CVS physical examination. Like LQTS, they are prone to develop ventricular tachyarrhythmias and the associated problems of these.
- *Hypertrophic cardiomyopathy (HCM)* – is a disease affecting the myocardium and there are three main types. HCM also known as HOCM, dilated cardiomyopathy (DCM), and arrhythmogenic right ventricular cardiomyopathy (ARVC).

In the UK, 4 out of 5 sudden deaths are due to cardiac arrythmias. NICE recommends the use of implantable cardioverter defibrillators in treating people who have familial cardiac conditions, such as long QT syndrome; brugada syndrome; hypertrophic cardiomyopathy and arrhythmogenic right ventricular dysplasia (NICE, 2014d).

Valvular heart disease

Either through disease or age, the valves of the heart can and do become ineffectual and fail to close correctly and consequently leak (*regurgitant*) or they become narrow (*stenotic*) or both. The common consequences of this are acquired left ventricular valve problems: aortic or mitral stenosis, or aortic or mitral regurgitation.

Mitral stenosis: signs and symptoms
- Exertional dyspnoea
- Productive cough of blood-tinged sputum and may be streaked with haemoptysis
- Malar flush on upper cheeks (*dusky pink discoloration*) occurs in severe stenosis
- Irregular pulse (*as a result of atrial fibrillation*)
- A loud first heart sound (S_1) is heard on auscultation at the apex.

Mitral regurgitation: signs and symptoms
- Pulmonary oedema (*acute regurgitation*)
- Exertional dyspnoea, fatigue and lethargy (*chronic regurgitation*)
- The first heart sound (S_1) is soft.

Aortic stenosis: signs and symptoms
- Patients usually have no symptoms until the valve is reduced to one third of its size
- Angina
- Exertional syncope
- Congestive heart failure
- Carotid pulse may be slow rising (*plateau pulse*)

- ECG shows evidence of LVH (*if severe and demonstrating a LV strain pattern*)
- ECG may show depressed ST segment and inversion of the 'T' wave in leads I, AVL, V5 and V6.

Aortic regurgitation: signs and symptoms
- Patients with chronic regurgitation remain asymptomatic, and then develop:
  - Dyspnoea and orthopnoea
  - Fatigue (*due to LVF*)
  - Collapsing pulse (*with wide pulse pressure*)
  - ECG displays evidence of LVH.

OTHER CONSIDERATIONS

Cardiovascular involvement and sepsis

Sepsis is responsible every year for approximately 37,000 deaths and 100,000 hospital admissions in the UK (Daniels, 2011), and for patients with severe sepsis the overall mortality rate is 35%. This is nearly five times higher than for ST elevation myocardial infarction and stroke (NICE, 2015b).

However, evidence produced seven decades ago described the relationship between cardiac dysfunction and sepsis, recognizing **red flag** sepsis, with its characteristics of a full bounding pulse, flushing, pyrexia, oliguria and hypotension (Waisbren, 1951).

Three decades later, the Society of Critical Care Medicine (SCCM) and the American College of Chest Physicians (ACCP) introduced a definition for systemic inflammatory response syndrome (SIRS). The ideology behind defining SIRS was to express a clinical response to a non-specific insult of either infectious or non-infectious origin (Kaplan, 2015). They defined SIRS as two or more of the following variables:

- Fever >38°C, or, <36°C
- Heart rate >90 beats per minute
- Respiratory rate >20 breaths per min, or, arterial carbon dioxide tension ($PaCO_2$) <32 mmHg
- White blood cell (WBC) count (>12,000/iL or >10% immature [band] forms).

They also explained that SIRS is non-specific and can be caused by inflammation, ischaemia, infection, trauma or several insults combined; consequently SIRS is not always related to infection.

Evidence published in the same decade identified that it was apparent that some patients did not significantly increase their cardiac output in response to expansion of their circulating volume, suggesting they had some element of myocardial dysfunction (Calvin et al., 1981).

During the previous decade the heart and cardiovascular system dysfunction have been studied with regards to **red flag** sepsis and septic shock, although the reason for the effects remain relatively unclear. A common theme throughout the available literature studies postulates that there is little or no evidence to suggest that global ischemia may not be an underlying cause of this dysfunction, but that some septic patients may have undiagnosed cardiac characteristics which may serve to confuse the patient assessment. Merx and Weber (2007) stated that circulating myocardial depressant factors in sepsis could potentially include cytokines, prostanoids and nitric oxide.

Current evidence clearly identifies that early recognition and treatment of sepsis, severe sepsis, septic shock and red flag sepsis will significantly reduce the mortality of these patients (Parliamentary and Health Service Ombudsman, 2013; UK Sepsis Trust, 2014; 2015). NICE have already produced guidance on neutropenic sepsis (NICE, 2012), and are currently formulating guidance on sepsis, recognizing and treating severe sepsis, which is due for publication in July 2016 (NICE, forthcomming).

Sepsis is a time critical condition and occurs when the body's reaction to infection causes systemic effects that are evident as two or more criteria of the systemic inflammatory response syndrome (SIRS), which have been activated by a new infection (see Table 3.1). Some patients will develop end-organ

Table 3.1 Systemic Inflammatory Response Syndrome (SIRS) is present if the patient has two or more criteria

Criteria
Temperature <36.0°C or >38.3°C
Pulse rate >90/beats per minute
Respiratory rate >20/breaths per minute
New confusion/drowsiness
Blood glucose >7.7 mmol/l (not if diabetic)
White blood cell (WBC) >12 or <4.0 × 10^9/l

Adapted from The UK Sepsis Trust (2014).

Cardiovascular assessment

Table 3.2 Defining the severity of sepsis – sepsis risk stratification

Severity	Definition	Criteria
Uncomplicated sepsis	SIRS + presumed or confirmed infection	
Severe sepsis	Sepsis + one or more organ dysfunction criteria (other than shock)	Organ dysfunction • Need for O_2 to maintain SpO_2 >90% • Lactate >2.0 mmol/l
Septic shock	Sepsis + shock	Shock criteria • Lactate >4 mmol/l at any time point • Hypotension (SBP <90 mmHg) persisting after 30 mL/kg intravenous fluid • Mean blood pressure <65 mmHg, or a reduction of >40 mmHg from the patient's usual systolic blood pressure

Adapted from The UK Sepsis Trust (2014).

dysfunction, indicating severe sepsis. Septic shock is a subset of severe sepsis, recognized as sepsis through sepsis with hypoperfusion which is resistant to fluid therapy (see Table 3.2).

Paramedics should undertake sepsis screening as a two-stage process:

- Stage 1: Initial screening for SIRS prompted by clinical signs and suspicion of infection.
- Stage 2: Screening the level of severity of sepsis, or a Sepsis Risk Stratification.

Once the paramedic has confirmed sepsis, then they should perform a Sepsis Risk Stratification.

Red Flag Sepsis

While assessing Stage 2 screening, there is an added obligation to ascertain if **red flag sepsis** (RFS) is present. This condition is identified from the inclusion of the following criteria:

> **Table 3.3** Red flag sepsis: sepsis risk stratification
>
> **Stage 1:** SIRS is present if the patient has two or more criteria
>
> **Stage 2:** Red flag sepsis is identified if **ANY ONE** of the following is present.
>
> - Systolic B.P <90 mmHg
> - Heart rate >130 per minute
> - Respiratory rate >25 per minute
> - Oxygen saturations <91%
> - Responds only to voice or pain/unresponsive
> - Purpuric rash
> - Lactate >2 mmol/l (where available)

- Heart rate of >131
- Respiratory rate of >25
- Oxygen saturations <91%
- AVPU score <Alert (e.g. Verbal, Pain, Unresponsiveness).

After undertaking the Stage 1 screening of SIRS, the following provides a sepsis risk stratification for sepsis patients who the paramedic may deem to be at significant risk of this condition (see Table 3.3).

If you suspect you are dealing with a patient with severe sepsis, septic shock or potential **red flag** sepsis, then early recognition, fluid therapy and rapid transfer to hospital are indicated to enable the Sepsis Six care bundle to be achieved within the first hour.

Caution should always be given to the administration of fluids in patients with coronary heart disease (CHD), but if you are unsure, advice should be sought on the amounts while carefully monitoring your patients.

> ### Possible actions to be taken:
>
> - Commence the administration of Sepsis Six (*as appropriate to skill/local guidelines*). Sepsis Six actions are:
>   1. Administer high-flow oxygen.
>   2. Take blood cultures and consider infective source.
>   3. Administer intravenous antibiotics.
>   4. Give intravenous fluid resuscitation.
>   5. Check haemoglobin and serial lactates.
>   6. Commence hourly urine output measurement.
> - Pre-alert the receiving emergency department or specialist unit.

The UK Sepsis Trust Pre-hospital Sepsis Screening and Action Tool is reproduced below with kind permission from the UK Sepsis Trust (Figure 3.6).

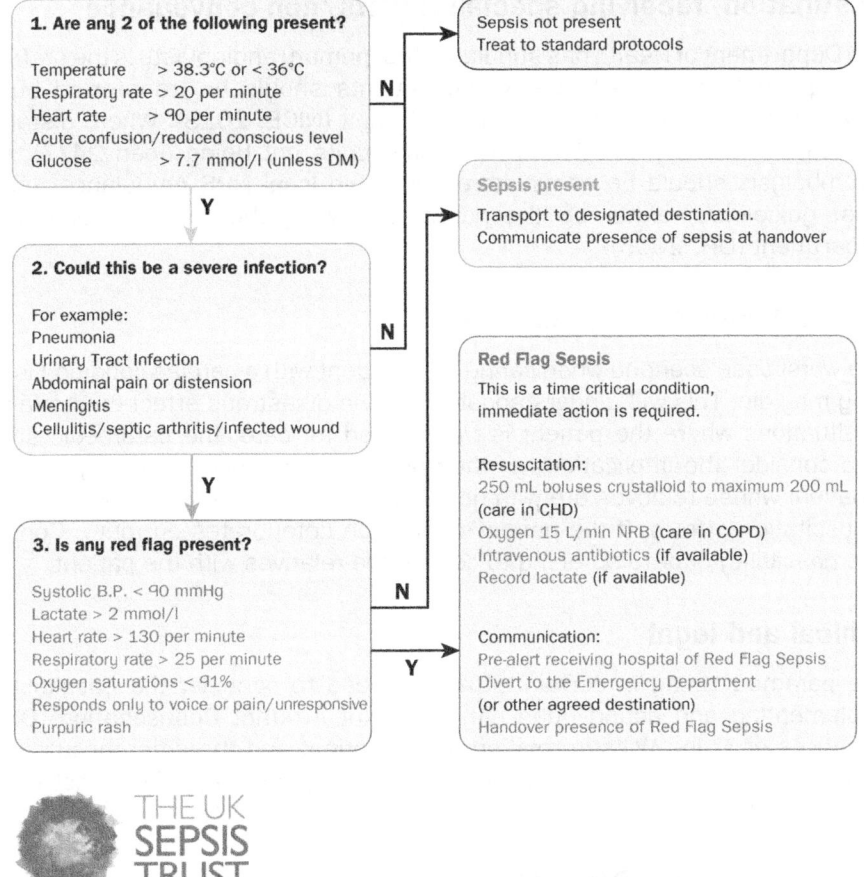

Figure 3.6   The UK Sepsis Trust Pre-hospital Sepsis Screening and Action Tool

Ethnicity

Ethnicity is recognized as a risk factor for developing coronary heart disease (Astin and Atkin, 2010). A gene mutation that almost guarantees the development of heart disease is carried by 60 million people of Asian origin.

Communication

Patients whose first language is not English, when confronted with pain or stress, can and do revert to their native language. By assessing a CVS emergency effectively, the paramedic should consider this factor and manage accordingly.

Destination/receiving specialist units/non-conveyance

The Department of Health has stipulated that primary angioplasty is the preferred management of a heart attack and patients should be transferred by the paramedic to a 24/7 primary angioplasty unit (NICE, 2013). Where distances or local variations prevent this (i.e. some units not being open 24/7), then thrombolysis should be administered (if within local NHS Ambulance Service Trust guidelines) either by the paramedic or by the receiving emergency department (DH, 2005).

Social/family/carer/guardian

The worst case scenario when caring for a patient with a cardiac condition is that they may die. This will, understandably, have a disastrous effect on the family. In situations where the patient is transported for care, the paramedic should also consider the implications of their actions. Remember you may transport a patient whose relatives are with you, but they may also have to witness your resuscitation efforts, if the patient's condition deteriorates en route. Consider this possibility prior to agreeing to convey the relatives with the patient.

Ethical and legal

The paramedic may in certain situations need to consider the possibility of implementing and acting upon either Do Not Attempt Resuscitation (DNAR) directives or Living Wills in relation to the patient and the emergency cardiac situation, and or having to implement the Recognition of Life Extinct (ROLE) procedure (AACE, 2013c).

CHAPTER KEY POINTS

- Identify time critical problems within the primary survey and manage appropriately.
- Undertake and interpret the 12-lead ECG.
- Undertake a complete secondary survey and history, including the cardiovascular physical examination.
- Decide on the appropriate and opportune time to move the patient to hospital.

REFERENCES

Association of Ambulance Chief Executives (2013a) *UK Ambulance Services Clinical Practice Guidelines 2013 Pocket Book: Implantable Cardioverter Defibrillator.* Bridgwater: Class Professional Publishing.

Association of Ambulance Chief Executives (2013b) *UK Ambulance Services Clinical Practice Guidelines 2013 Pocket Book: Pain Assessment Model.* Bridgwater: Class Professional Publishing.

Association of Ambulance Chief Executives (2013c) *UK Ambulance Services Clinical Practice Guidelines 2013 Pocket Book: Recognition of Life Extinct (ROLE).* Bridgwater: Class Professional Publishing.

Astin, F. and Atkin, K. (2010) *Ethnicity and Coronary Heart Disease: Making Sense of Risk and Improving Care.* Better Health Briefing 16. Available at: http://better-health.org.uk/briefings/ethnicity-and-coronary-heart-disease-making-sense-risk-and-improving-care (accessed. 25 May 2015).

Bickley, L.S. and Szilagyi, P.G. (2012) *Bates' Guide to Physical Examination and History Taking* (11th edn). Philadelphia, PA: Lippincott Williams & Wilkins.

British Thoracic Society (2015) *Emergency Oxygen Use in Adult Patients Guideline.* Available at: https://www.brit-thoracic.org.uk/searchresults/?txtSearch=2015+Oxygen+Guidelines&search= (accessed 25 May 2015).

Burnett, L.B. (2015) *Cocaine Toxicity in Emergency Medicine.* Available at: http://emedicine.medscape.com/article/813959-overview (accessed 23 May 2015).

Burton, H., Alberg, C. and Stewart, A. (2009) *Heart to Heart. Inherited Cardiovascular Conditions Services: A Needs Assessment and Service Review.* Available at: www.phgfoundation.org/file/4668/ (accessed 22 May 2015).

Calvin, J.E., Driedger, A.A. and Sibbald, W.J. (1981) An assessment of myocardial function in human sepsis utilizing ECG gated cardiac scintigraphy. *Chest* 80: 579–86.

Camm, A.J. and Bunce, N.H. (2012) Cardiovascular disease. In: Kumar, P. and Clark, M. (eds) *Clinical Medicine* (8th edn). Edinburgh: Saunders Elsevier.

College of Paramedics (2015) *Paramedic Curriculum Guidance* (3rd edn) (Revised). Bridgwater: College of Paramedics.

Daniels, R. (2011) Surviving the first hours in sepsis: getting the basics right (an intensivist's perspective). *Journal of Antimicrobial Chemotherapy* 66 (Suppl. ii): 11–23.

DH (Department of Health) (2005) *The National Service Framework for Long-term Conditions.* London: Department of Health Publications.

DH (Department of Health) (2009) *Reference Guide to Consent for Examination or Treatment* (2nd edn). London: Department of Health.

Fisher, J., Brown, S.N. and Cooke, M. (eds) (2013) *UK Ambulance Services Clinical Practice Guidelines 2013: Altered Level of Consciousness.* Bridgwater: Class Professional Publishing.

Kaplan, L.J. (2015) *Systemic Inflammatory Response Syndrome.* Available at: http://emedicine.medscape.com/article/168943-overview (accessed 25 May 2015).

Longmore, M., Wilkinson, I.B., Baldwin, A. and Wallin, E. (2014) *Oxford Handbook of Clinical Medicine* (9th edn). Oxford: Oxford University Press.

Merx, M.W. and Weber, C. (2007) Cardiovascular involvement in general medical conditions: sepsis and the heart. *Circulation* 116: 793–802.

NICE (National Institute for Health and Clinical Excellence) (2008) *Identification and Management of Familial Hypercholesterolaemia.* Available at: http://www.nice.org.uk/guidance/cg71 (accessed 25 May 2015).

NICE (National Institute for Health and Clinical Excellence) (2010a) *Transient Loss of Consciousness ('Blackouts') Management in Adults and Young People.* NICE clinical guideline 109. Available at: www.nice.org.uk/guidance/CG109 (accessed 23 May 2015).

NICE (National Institute for Health and Clinical Excellence) (2010b) *Chronic Heart Failure: National Clinical Guideline for Diagnosis and Management in Primary and Secondary Care.* NICE clinical guideline 108. Available at: http://www.nice.org.uk/guidance/cg108/evidence (accessed 24 May 2015).

NICE (National Institute for Health and Clinical Excellence) (2012) *Neutropenic Sepsis: Prevention and Management of Neutropenic Sepsis in Cancer Patients.* NICE clinical guideline 151. Available at: http://www.nice.org.uk/guidance/cg151/evidence (accessed 23 May 2015).

NICE (National Institute for Health and Clinical Excellence) (2013) *Myocardial Infarction with ST-Segment Elevation.* NICE clinical guideline 167. Available at: http://www.nice.org.uk/guidance/cg167/evidence (accessed 23 May 2015).

NICE (National Institute for Health and Clinical Excellence) (2014a) *CVD Risk Assessment and Management.* Available at: http://cks.nice.org.uk/cvd-risk-assessment-and-management#!topicsummary (accessed 23 May 2015).

NICE (National Institute for Health and Clinical Excellence) (2014b) *Atrial Fibrillation: The Management of Atrial Fibrillation.* NICE clinical guideline 180. Available at: http://www.nice.org.uk/guidance/cg180/evidence (accessed 24 May 2015).

NICE (National Institute for Health and Clinical Excellence) (2014c) *Acute Heart Failure: Diagnosing and Managing Acute Heart Failure in Adults.* NICE clinical guideline 187. Available at: http://www.nice.org.uk/guidance/cg187/evidence (accessed 24 May 2015).

NICE (National Institute for Health and Clinical Excellence) (2014d) *Implantable Cardioverter Defibrillators and Cardiac Resynchronisation Therapy for Arrhythmias and Heart Failure (Review of TA95 and TA120).* NICE TA134. Available at: http://www.nice.org.uk/guidance/ta314/chapter/1-Guidance (accessed 25 May 2015).

NICE (National Institute for Health and Clinical Excellence) (2015a) *Cardiovascular Conditions.* Available at: https://www.nice.org.uk/guidancemenu/conditions-and-diseases/cardiovascular-conditions (accessed 23 May 2015).

NICE (National Institute for Health and Clinical Excellence) (2015b) *Sepsis: The Recognition, Diagnosis and Management of Severe Sepsis.* Available at: https://www.nice.org.uk/guidance/indevelopment/gid-cgwave0686 (accessed 23 May 2015).

NICE (National Institute for Health and Clinical Excellence) (forthcoming) *Sepsis: The Recognition, Diagnosis and Management of Severe Sepsis.* http: www.nice.org.uk/guidance/indevelopment/gid-cgwave0686 (accessed 30 December 2015).

Olshansky, B. (2015) *Atrioventricular Nodal Re-entry Tachycardia (AVNRT): Treatment and Medication.* Available at: http://emedicine.medscape.com/article/160215-treatment (accessed 23 May 2015).

Parliamentary and Health Service Ombudsman (2013) *Time to Act: Severe Sepsis: Rapid Diagnosis and Treatment Save Lives.* London: Parliamentary and Health Service Ombudsman.

Porth, C.M. (2014) *Essentials of Pathophysiology: Concepts of Altered Health States* (4th edn). London: Lippincott Williams & Wilkins.

Resuscitation Council (UK) (2011) *Advanced Life Support* (6th edn). London: Resuscitation Council. Reprinted in 2012 (with corrections).

Salomone, J.P. and Pons, P.T. (2014) *Pre-Hospital Trauma Life Support (PHTLS)* (8th edn). Maryland Heights, MO: Mosby Elsevier.

Swanton, R.H. and Banarjee, S. (2008) *Swanton's Cardiology: A Concise Guide to Clinical Practice (Pocket Consultant)* (6th edn). Oxford: Blackwell Publishing Ltd.

The UK Sepsis Trust (2014) *Pre-Hospital Screening and Action Tool*. Available at: http://sepsistrust.org/wp-content/files_mf/1409315077PHScreening2014.pdf (accessed 25 May 2015).

The UK Sepsis Trust (2015) *Toolkit: Prehospital Management of Sepsis*. Available at: sepsistrust.org/wp-content/files_mf/1409315090PHToolkit2014FINAL.pdf (accessed 25 May 2015).

Tidy, C. (2011) Bradycardia. Available at: http://www.patient.co.uk/doctor/bradycardia (accessed 23 May 2015).

Waisbren, R.A. (1951) Bacteremia due to gram-negative bacilli other than the Salmonella: a clinical and therapeutic study. *AMA Archive of Internal Medicine*. 88: 467–88.

World Health Organization (2014) *The 10 Leading Causes of Death*. Available at: http://www.who.int/mediacentre/factsheets/fs310/en/ (accessed 24 May 2015).

4 Abdominal and gastro-intestinal assessment
Chris Baker

The gastro-intestinal (GI) and urinary system organs are incorporated within the abdominal pelvic region, however, the *alimentary canal* commences at the mouth and progresses down through the 'thoracic' cavity before it reaches the abdominal cavity. The National Institute for Health and Clinical Excellence (NICE) has published several guidelines on digestive tract conditions (NICE, 2015a). Due to the complex anatomy which varies between genders, assessment is often approached with concern by the paramedic. However, by following the format described, problems that may be of serious concern can be identified. This chapter aims to provide a structured systematic approach to the abdominal and GI assessment and will assist the paramedic in identifying abnormalities.

SCENE ASSESSMENT

As with any scene, paramedics can gain a great deal of information from the initial assessment, such as at an accident, where the mechanism of injury (MOI) can highlight an index of suspicion of damage to the abdominal organs and systems. When approaching a patient who has been involved in a road traffic collision (RTC), consideration must be given to the MOI and the phases of the collision itself, specifically the deceleration forces on the vehicles, the patient, their organs and any subsequent collision and the manner in which these affect the body (Pilbery, 2014).

Alternatively, it could involve attending a patient with an illness, where positioning or movement of the patient may provide clues to the condition before the first question is asked. The patient may be either very still and deliberately ensuring minimal movement while experiencing pain, as in the case of peritonitis, or be unable to remain in one position, and writhing in agony as seen in uteric or biliary colic. Alternatively the paramedic may see or identify:

- Medications pertinent to conditions affecting the gastro-intestinal and urinary system.

- Receptacles containing vomit, it is important to note consistency and colour, for example, vomit may appear as dark ground coffee dregs (*indicative of bleeding*).
- There may be specific smells which could suggest gastro-intestinal or urinary upsets, such as a urinary tract infection (UTI), or diarrhoea.
- Signs of long-term alcohol abuse (*alcohol abuse occurring within the home environment or outside*), which can have serious effects on the liver, kidneys and lining of the digestive tract.
- Evidence of smoking and its long-term use should prompt the paramedic to consider potential problems such as peptic ulcers, or cancers affecting the GI system, including stomach, colon, pancreas or liver. Smoking can also affect the liver's ability to process toxins and remove them from the body which can also mean that higher doses of medication will be required in order to return a therapeutic effect (National Institute of Diabetes and Digestive and Kidney Disease, 2014).

Smokers are at a higher risk of developing:

- Crohn's disease
- Gallstones
- Gastritis (*smokers >50 years of age*)
- Increased pain in patients with irritable bowel syndrome (IBS).

The paramedic should also be aware of:

- Obvious signs of pregnancy, vaginal bleeding, or miscarriage in females of child-bearing years. Ectopic pregnancy must also be considered. If the patient is within the relevant age range, consider pregnancy, and pregnancy testing if indicated.
- Does the patient look as if they are able to care for themselves? Are they well groomed, with a good level of personal hygiene? Are they well nourished?

PRIMARY SURVEY

The initial scene assessment may allow the paramedic the opportunity to begin making a decision on whether the patient is **time critical** or non-time critical. The clinical signs gained during the primary survey will assist in this diagnosis; however, the experienced paramedic will often know that a patient's condition is either serious or time critical from the moment they set eyes on them.

Even if the patient initially appears well, remember, as with any time critical conditions, deterioration can be rapid. The paramedic should remember that patient assessment is a fluid process and ensure that they undertake the abdominal/GI primary survey properly to make certain that subtle signs will not be overlooked, and obtain the evidence to identify if the patient has a time critical condition or not.

Consider the use of the current abdominal trauma guidelines, ensuring consideration for time critical features (Fisher et al., 2013), such as:

- Major ABC problems
- Haemodynamic compromise
- Decreased level of consciousness
- Neck and back injuries.

DANGER

The matter of safety must be considered, as with any scene or emergency. The appropriate personal protective equipment (PPE) must always be worn and the paramedic must consider any risks involved and other resources required.

Abdominal injuries and illnesses of the gastro-intestinal and urinary systems have an increased risk of body fluids, whether they are of either a vomit or blood-borne origin. Consider the possible dangers during your initial assessment of the scene and consider the relevant steps to take in order to minimize these dangers. Take necessary precautions, including universal precautions, and decide if any further professional assistance may be required.

RESPONSE

As the paramedic introduces themselves to the patient, they note the patient's ability to respond using verbal communication. Questions such as 'What happened?' and, 'Why have you called us today?' offer the conscious patient the opportunity to introduce their presenting complaint. Remember that patients in severe pain may have difficulty communicating fluently. Consideration can once again be given to the position of the patient, and the movement (*or lack of movement*) of the patient, and the unresponsive or unconscious patient who will require rapid intervention to protect their airway. At this stage an assessment using the AVPU scale will suffice.

AIRWAY

When attending a patient presenting with a problem of gastro-intestinal origin, the patency of the airway can be affected by the risk of aspiration of gastric contents. Remember that intermittent projectile vomiting in adults refers to periodic episodes of vomiting that are unusually violent or forceful. However, conditions such as bleeding oesophageal varices and ruptured peptic (*gastric and duodenal*) ulcers may also lead to the risk of blood, causing obstruction to the airway. With blood in the airway, consider how this can be atomized as the patient exhales, or coughs, and the need to wear protective eyewear when treating such a patient.

> **Possible actions to be taken:**
> - Consider causes of airway obstruction (*vomit and/or blood*)
> - Suction as appropriate
> - Position patient appropriately
> - Consider 'C' spine techniques if appropriate
> - Wear appropriate personal protective equipment (PPE), including eye protection.

BREATHING

Pain pathologically increases the respiratory rate. Consider GI conditions that could increase or slow the respiratory rate such as hyperventilation or Kussmaul respirations (*deep sighing respirations*) classically seen in diabetic ketoacidosis (DKA) (Longmore et al., 2014). Alternatively, is the patient presenting with hypoventilation due to vomiting and excessive loss of gastric hydrochloric acid (HCl) (Thomas, 2015)?

- Remember that GI problems can and do present as chest pain. 'Heart attack' pain sometimes feels like indigestion or heartburn, or patients present with nausea and vomiting.
- Can you smell hepatic foetor on their breath (*indicates liver disease and smells like pear drops*)?
- Consider the respiratory effort and ascertain if they are using accessory muscles or if they have diaphragmatic breathing.
- If the patient presents with a SpO_2 of 94% or below, then oxygen should be administered appropriately (British Thoracic Society, 2015).
- When listening to breathing sounds, consider the anatomical relationship between the thoracic and abdominal cavities (*during respiration the external markings for the abdomen change and the organs move up and down within the cavities*).
- Damage to the diaphragm may result in the contents of the abdominal cavity entering the thoracic cavity, such as a hiatus hernia (*occurs when part of the stomach pushes up into the chest*). Alternatively, the patient may have an injury to the thoracic cavity which leaks through the damaged diaphragm and causes irritation/damage to the abdominal cavity contents.

> **Possible actions to be taken:**
> - Identify cause of dyspnoea (manage appropriately)
> - If respiratory rate <10 or >29 breaths per minute, assist ventilations (<12 in traumatically injured adult patients)
> - Ensure the patient is not hypoxic and administer oxygen appropriately to patient's illness or injury.

CIRCULATION

Having assessed the pulse and blood pressure, including rate, regularity and efficiency, consider the conditions which could cause visible changes to the integumentary and/or circulatory system and are relative to the gastro-intestinal and genito-urinary systems. On approach, the paramedic will have already made an initial assessment of the patient's colour; it must be remembered that some patients are naturally pale while others are naturally flushed. This can be verified by asking relatives and friends of the patient if this colour is normal for them. Alternatively, are they presenting with other visible signs of abdominal GI problems or complaining of specific related signs and symptoms?

- Does the patient present with hot, flushed skin suggestive of pyrexia and possible infection (Raftery et al., 2014)?
- Do they appear jaundiced (*icterus: yellowish discoloration of the skin associated with increased levels of bilirubin circulating, due to liver conditions and haemolytic anaemia*) (Bickley and Szilagyi, 2013)?
- Are they presenting with haematemesis?
- Are they complaining of haematuria?
- Or complaining of melaena?
- Is the patient in a dehydrated state?
- Consider underlying structures in trauma. Damage to spleen, liver, and underlying major blood vessels could lead to exsanguination of patient. Always consider the mechanism of injury, and potential damage.

Haematemesis

This is often described as particles resembling coffee grounds in appearance. It must be remembered that this will be blood which has been partially digested by gastric juices after being in the stomach for some time. Fresh haematemesis (*bright red blood*) will be due to recent bleeding high in the gastro-intestinal system, such as bleeding in the oesophagus or mouth, and care should be taken to consider the patient history and possibility of the blood originating within the respiratory system. Consider the causes of the bleeding which include:

- Peptic ulcers
- Cancers of the digestive tract
- Blood-thinning medications
- Oesophageal varices.

If the patient has had recent facial trauma, or suffered a nose bleed, is there the possibility that the particles resembling coffee grounds are due to blood swallowed after either of these events, rather than blood originating in the digestive system?

Haematuria

May be visible and occur in genito-urinary trauma, but this is not always the case. The source of the bleeding may be suggested by a careful history; haematuria that occurs at the start of micturition is normally associated with urethral disease, while in haematuria that occurs at the end of micturition, the prostrate or bladder base may be the source. However, if the bleeding is seen as an even discoloration throughout the urine, then the origin could be either in the bladder or above (Ballinger, 2012).

Genito-urinary damage is likely to occur in patients with blunt or penetrating trauma to the back or flanks. Special attention should be paid to patients with bruises, contusions or tenderness around these areas, as damage may have occurred to the kidneys or ureters (Greaves et al., 2012).

Damage to the bladder or urethra may lead to haematuria while other causes include glomerulonephritis (*inflammation of the glomeruli within the nephron of the kidneys*), which may be due to infection or long-term use of non-steroidal anti-inflammatory drugs (NSAID). Cancer anywhere along the urinary tract, kidney and bladder stones, and use of medications that can thin the blood (*aspirin*, *clopidogrel*) are also causative factors.

Melaena

Bleeding from the lower part of the gastro-intestinal tract, which is seen as dark tarry stools, while the term haematochezia may be used to describe red or maroon-coloured stools due to fresh blood, as would be associated with a bleeding rectal pile. Melaena signifies the loss of at least 60 ml of blood into the gastro-intestinal tract, usually from the oesophagus, stomach, or duodenum. This may be due to peptic ulcers, gastritis, esophageal or gastric varices, reflux oesophagitis, or tears due to retching and vomiting (Bickley and Szilagyi, 2013).

Dehydration

The physical signs of dehydration are usually only apparent with moderate to severe dehydration. The first physical symptom is thirst, and the patient has a dry and parched mouth. The tongue can be inspected to see if it is wet, and the eyes should be glistening. Skin turgor is lost with marked dehydration (Epstein et al., 2009). Skin turgor can be assessed by pinching the skin on the neck or the anterior chest wall, although many practitioners check the skin on the back of the hand as this is less intrusive for the patient. When pinched and released, hydrated skin should immediately spring back to its original location, while dehydrated skin returns slowly. This test is unreliable in those whose skin may be losing its elasticity as part of the natural process of ageing.

Movement and positioning

Consider how the patient is positioned. Conditions such as pancreatitis often prevent the patient from being able to lie supine, but instead they present leaning forward, with the abdomen flexed, and incapable of finding a comfortable position (Bickley and Szilagyi, 2013).

> **Possible actions to be taken:**
> - If haematemesis is present, ascertain if dark or fresh (*manage airway as appropriate*)
> - If no external haemorrhage visible but signs and symptoms of shock are present, consider internal haemorrhage and manage as appropriate (see *Trauma Assessment, Chapter 7*)
> - Ascertain the colour and frequency of the haematuria (*record findings*)
> - Ascertain the colour and frequency of the melaena (*record findings*)
> - Assess skin turgor (*lost in marked dehydration*) (*manage shock accordingly, see Trauma Assessment, Chapter 7*).

DISABILITY

Assess the patient's level of consciousness and record the appropriate element of the AVPU framework. Assess the pupils and ascertain if they are PERRLA: Pupils Equal and Round; React to Light and Accommodation. Specifically assess the patient's blood glucose levels. Consider if the abdominal GI condition has affected their ability to undertake normal and well activities of daily living (ADLs) (*a normally fit person can become incapacitated due to severe diarrhoea or haematemesis*), consider the effects on an elderly person living alone or a single parent with small children.

EXPOSE/EXAMINE/EVALUATE

Expose and examine the patient, look for scars, visible pulsations (*aneurysm*), masses, distension, striae (*stretch marks*), hernia, bruising, and if trauma has occurred, check for evidence of penetrating injury or eviscerated organs. Remember to consider consent, especially in emergency situations (DH, 2009). With abdominal trauma, examine for signs of injury, including pattern bruising, such as that caused by a seat belt in a road traffic accident. When assessing traumatic injury to the abdomen, consider the three anatomical areas of the abdomen;

- Abdominal cavity
- Pelvis
- Retro-peritoneal area (Fisher et al., 2013).

Careful attention must be given to the sections of the abdomen and pelvis which could have been susceptible to damage, and the structures within these areas. The paramedic is reminded that the thorax and the abdomen contain the majority of the body's vital organs. Contemplating injuries to the abdomen will lead the paramedic to being armed with an index of suspicion as to potential findings upon examination. By dividing the abdomen into quadrants (see Figure 4.1), and then considering the organs of the GI and urinary systems located within

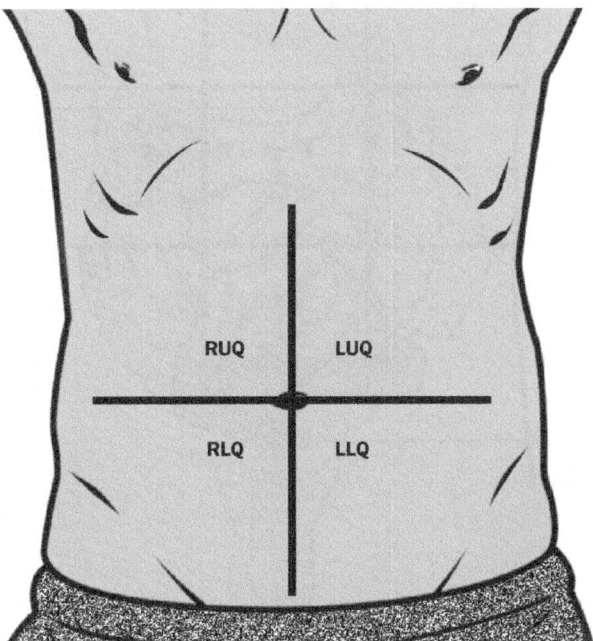

Figure 4.1 Abdominal quadrants

them, the paramedic will be assisted in looking for specific signs and symptoms related to problems of the organs contained therein.

Or if the paramedic prefers to be more specific, the following nine abdominal regions can be identified and specified in any subsequent documentation (see Figure 4.2).

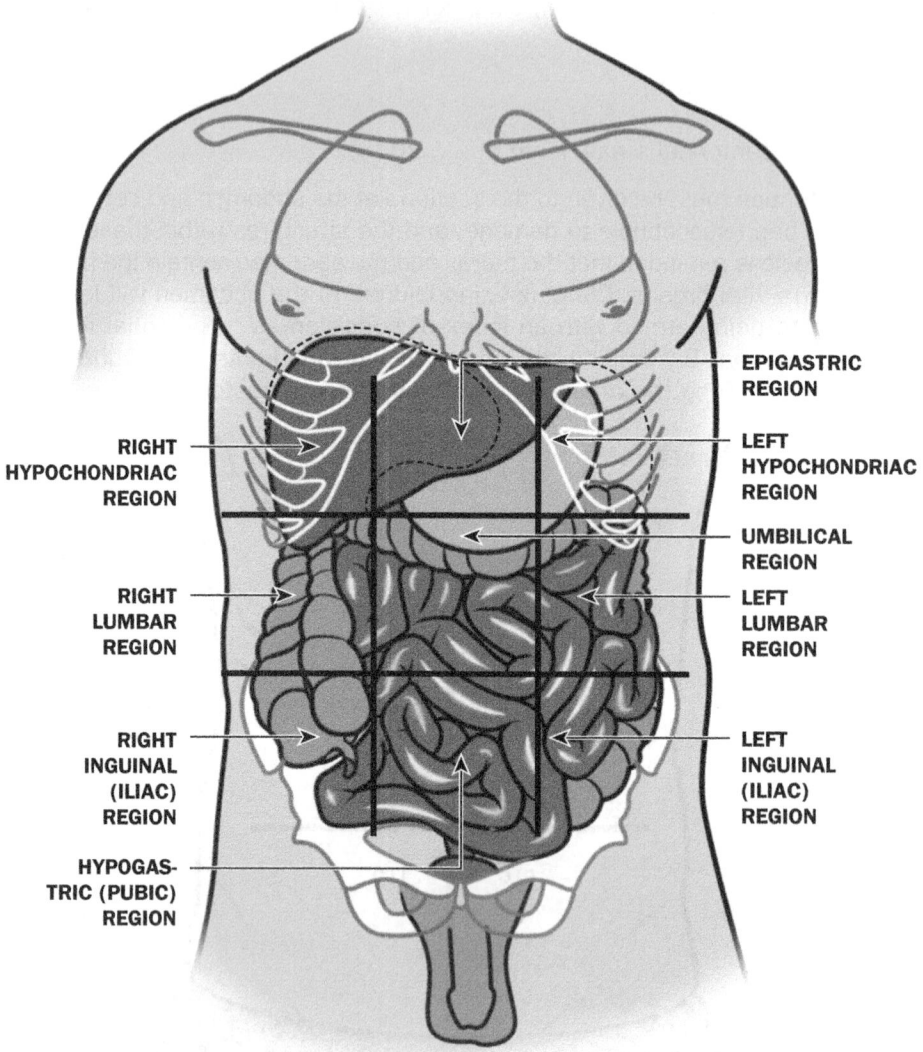

Figure 4.2 The nine abdominal regions

> **Possible actions to be taken:**
> - Remember the patient's dignity and obtain consent from the patient prior to exposing them for the examination
> - Expose the abdomen and look for evidence (*scars, masses, distension, visible pulsations, etc.*)
> - Evidence of trauma: ascertain if there are any penetrating injuries or eviscerated organs (*manage appropriately, see Trauma Assessment, Chapter 7*)
> - Assess each quadrant and be aware of the potential damage which may have occurred to underlying organs
> - Evaluate – transfer to the appropriate treatment centre (*if time critical*), or move on to the secondary survey.

SECONDARY SURVEY

An abdominal examination should be undertaken in a structured format. It can be undertaken in a rapid and systematic manner when the patient presents with a life-threatening condition, however, there is little in the way of interventions which can be undertaken in the out-of-hospital arena. Undertaking a focused history and assessment of the abdomen, gastro-intestinal (GI) and genito-urinary (GU) systems will enable the paramedic to establish illnesses and problems that have not been identified within the primary survey. Due to the nature and complexity of both illnesses and injuries involving these systems, the paramedic may find assessing and diagnosing them a daunting task. However, by using the following structured format and examination process, the paramedic will be provided with the opportunity of detecting signs and symptoms of underlying medical conditions to the systems and associated organs.

HISTORY

As discussed, the history of the presenting complaint is a short story about how the patient has come to be unwell, and how their problem is progressing. The key elements of obtaining a patient history are discussed and an example of how the elements could be recorded is described:

- PC: 42 ♀ C/O pain in the upper right abdomen
- HPC: After eating breakfast about 3 hours ago, the patient developed an acute pain which gradually worsened, pain worsens on inspiration, and the patient states that it radiates towards her right shoulder.

Presenting complaint

Ascertain the reason why the patient has requested the attendance of a paramedic, it may be trauma or illness-related, but may be as vague as *a pain in my stomach*. It may be the patient presents with symptoms that the paramedic identifies, and from these, the paramedic may gain some insight into the questions they consider relevant asking to enable them to make a differential diagnosis and form an initial impression.

The presenting symptoms are and can be related to either the GI or GU problem. Patients with a GI history may present with the following symptoms:

- Abdominal pain
- Mouth ulcers, dysphagia, indigestion, dyspepsia
- Appetite or weight changes
- Nausea, emesis, haematemesis
- Changes to bowel habits: diarrhoea, constipation
- Bleeding per rectum (PR), melaena
- Pruritus, dark urine, pale stools.

However, with a GU history, the patient may present with the following symptoms:

- Fever
- Loin pain, dysuria, haematuria
- Urethral or vaginal discharge
- Painful intercourse, dyspareunia
- Menses (*discharge from the uterus during menstruation*)
- Menarche (*the first appearance of menstruation*)
- Menopause (*period when ovaries cease functioning and menstruation stops*) (Longmore et al., 2014).

History of presenting complaint

What is the history of the presenting complaint? The patient who complains of acute abdominal pain, which has increased since eating a meal a few hours ago, may have an entirely different diagnosis to the patient who complains of abdominal pain but has a two-day history of vomiting and diarrhoea. If the patient presents with abdominal pain, the paramedic should use the SOCRATES framework, to assist them in gaining a more thorough impression of the presenting complaint:

    S – Site. Where exactly is the pain?
    O – Onset. Ask if the pain developed slowly or rapidly, was it over the course of minutes, hours or days?
    C – Character. Ask them to describe the pain, do they explain it as a: vague, stabbing, sharp, dull, crushing, cramping, burning or colicky pain?

Abdominal and gastro-intestinal assessment

R – Radiate. Does the pain move anywhere?
A – Associated symptoms. Has the pain been associated with bowel movements, urination, flatulence or vomiting? Did it build up in a crescendo and then drop off?
T – Time/duration. How long has the pain lasted? What was the patient doing when the pain began? Did the pain wake the patient, or follow a particular event? Is there any history of trauma that the pain may be related back to?
E – Exacerbating/relieving factors. Ask about what eases or makes it worse? Look at the positioning of the patient, and the amount they are moving to confirm this.
S – Severity. Obtain an initial pain score (*0 = no pain, 10 = worst pain ever*).
(AACE, 2013; Longmore et al., 2014).

The paramedic, when clarifying the history of the presenting complaint, should ask relevant questions to ascertain the appropriate information. The following questions may be appropriate for a patient who presents with abdominal pain and vomiting:

- Did the vomiting precede the pain?
- Did they feel nauseous before they vomited?
- Frequency – how many times have they vomited?
- What is the consistency and character of the vomit: watery, bile, faecal, blood, coffee dreg particles?

The following questions may be appropriate for an elderly patient who is complaining of abdominal pain and constipation:

- When did you last open your bowels?
- Did you have any pain on passing stools?
- Has the patient or their relatives/carers noticed a change in the smell of their faeces, changes in colour? If so, how long have these changes been taking place over?
- Was there any blood present? If so, was it fresh blood, or black and tarry?
- Does the patient have an absolute constipation associated with 'colicky' pain?
- Is there an associated swelling of the abdomen?
- Has the patient recently changed their lifestyle? For patients who have given up smoking, this may be the cause of the constipation.

Colic is defined as severe pain resulting from periodic spasm in an abdominal organ and is often associated with the peristaltic wave moving through the digestive system (*the involuntary movements of the muscles of the digestive tract as they move food through the digestive system*).

Past medical history

Does the patient have a history of GI or GU problems? Do they still have their appendix? Has the patient had recent surgery, or previous operations?

Ask if the patient has any recurring or previous GI or GU illnesses, including ulcers (*peptic or duodenal*), gallbladder disease, inflammatory bowel disease, jaundice, hepatitis, urinary tract infections, renal colic, gout, analgesic use, hypertension or GI bleeding. Ask female patients about their last menstrual period (LMP) (Rushforth, 2009). When considering GI bleeds, the following guidance may be of benefit:

- Is there unexplained syncope? (*should raise suspicion of concealed GI bleed*)
- Does the visible bleed originate from the upper or lower GI tract?
- When did the bleeding begin?
- Is there a history of GI disease?
- Is there a history of aspirin or non-steroidal anti-inflammatory drug (NSAID) use?
- Does the patient take beta-blockers or calcium-channel blockers? (*which can mask tachycardia in the shocked patient*)
- Does the patient take iron tablets or have they consumed beetroot/drinks containing red dye? (*may alter the colour of stools*)
- Is there a history of anti-coagulatory or anti-platelet therapy?
- Is there a history of liver disease/abdominal surgery or alcohol abuse?
- Did the haematemesis present after an increase in intra-abdominal pressure (*from retching or coughing*), or several episodes of non-bloody emesis?
- What are the character and quantity of the blood loss?

If blood loss is not visible, ask the patient or relatives to estimate colour/volume (*bleeding PR is difficult to estimate*). The blood acts as a laxative, but repeated blood/liquid stool, or just blood, is associated with more severe blood loss than maroon/black solid stool.

Drug/medication history

Some medications will cause issues with the GI system, such as antibiotics leading to diarrhoea, pain killers leading to constipation. Does the patient need to take medication for a problem with another body system which has a direct effect upon the gastro-intestinal or urinary system, such as furosemide, which would result in excessive urination, or antibiotics which could lead to thrush, due to lowering of the defensive fauna contained within the urinary tracts? Ask if they have used or currently use: steroids, non-steroidal anti-inflammatory

Abdominal and gastro-intestinal assessment

drugs (NSAIDs), or the contraceptive pill, if female. Also ask if they have recently had any dietary changes, especially as those who have changed to a high fibre diet may present with a swollen abdomen and excessive flatulence.

Social/family medical history

Does the patient require care at home? Are they receiving this care, or are they a potentially *vulnerable adult*? Is there a family history which may be of relevance to the presenting complaint, such as a parent who suffers from Crohn's disease (Rushforth, 2009)? The paramedic should consider that certain GI conditions may be hereditary and therefore the patient should be questioned regarding their family history of the following conditions:

- Colon cancer
- Polyps
- Irritable bowel syndrome
- Stomach ulcers
- Jaundice
- Diabetes
- Alcoholism
- Crohn's disease
- Ulcerative colitis – an inflammatory condition affecting the colon. It always involves the rectum and spreads continuously for a variable distance. The history will reveal blood in diarrhoea, mucus and pus being passed rectally, loss of weight, anaemia and abdominal pain (Brooker, 2008).

Regarding the patient's social history, the paramedic should ascertain information about the following:

- Smoking
- Alcohol
- Overseas travel
- Tropical illnesses
- Occupational exposures
- Sexual orientation (Longmore et al., 2014).

EXAMINATION

When considering the examination of the patient, it is important to consider the modesty of the patient, and the fact that certain patients may find some of the questions somewhat embarrassing. It is also important to note that in order to gain an accurate impression, the paramedic will need to ask some of the embarrassing questions in a skilful and tactful manner. The history will have led the paramedic to the site of any abdominal pain. Tell the patient to let you know if you cause them pain during the physical examination. Exposure of the abdomen in order to inspect, auscultate, palpate and percuss remains an important aspect, but consider gaining the trust of the patient, their consent to the examination, and to the location in which you choose to undertake the examination. When operating as a solo responder, the paramedic may find it necessary to use the relative or carer as a chaperone for the benefit of the patient (*depending on gender of the patient*) and also as children and young adults may find it harder to answer questions related to digestive and urinary habit, sexual activity or menstrual cycle.

The examination of the abdomen should be undertaken with the patient lying flat, arms at their side, using inspection, auscultation, palpation and then percussion, as palpation of the abdomen prior to auscultation may have an effect upon the frequency and location of bowel sounds (Rushforth, 2009).

Inspection

Does the abdomen appear symmetrical?; is it a normal shape with no protrusions? Bulges may be due to distension of the bladder above the level of the symphysis pubis, if low in the abdomen, or be due to a hernia. The bulge or *mass* may be seen to be pulsatile, suggesting that the patient may have an abdominal aortic aneurysm, for this reason, a bulge should not be overlooked. If the patient is conscious, they may well be aware of a hernia, and of the normal appearance of this protrusion. Ask the patient in these instances whether the hernia has changed shape or size. Patients may also be aware of aortic aneurysms, and of their normal size, possibly even prognosis. An aneurysm is usually painless, so be aware that pain may be an indicator of the imminent or actual rupture of the aorta. Also examine the abdomen for rashes, dilated veins showing near the surface due to venous obstruction, and the presence of jaundice due to liver conditions.

Striae, or stretch marks on the patient's abdomen, may be different colours for different reasons. If the patient has previously lost weight or had skin stretched due to pregnancy, then these lines will be silver in colour. New striae can be pink or blue, and may be seen with weight gain, and in patients with darker skin, these may be dark brown in colour. Cushing's syndrome is caused by an excess of cortisol production by the adrenal glands or by excessive use of cortisol or other similar steroid hormones (Pilbery, 2014). This condition causes thinning of the skin and easy bruising, and can lead to pink or purple striae on the abdomen. These may also be seen on the thighs, breasts and shoulders. These patients are likely to have previously presented with life-threatening illnesses, including asthma, rheumatoid arthritis and some allergies, which will have been ascertained during the gaining of the patient history.

Abdominal and gastro-intestinal assessment

The abdomen may be protruding, and the size and shape of the rest of the patient require consideration when this is the case. In a person of average weight, the abdomen is normally non-protruding, becoming rounded as more weight is carried. When the abdomen is protruding or distended, it may be due to patient obesity, or pregnancy. When considering swelling of the abdomen, the five 'F's' should be considered as causes. These are:

- *Flatus* – or gas in the intestinal tract.
- *Faeces* – contained within the digestive system. This may be palpated when undertaking deep palpation in the lower left quadrant of the abdomen. This is quite normal prior to a bowel movement, and should be soft if palpated.
- *Foetus* – will involve questions about the patient's sexual activity, contraception and menstrual cycle.
- *Fat* – may bring considerations as to patient's diet, but can make a thorough palpation of the abdomen difficult.
- *Fluid* – ascites, ovarian cyst.

Ascites is simply free fluid in the abdominal cavity due to an underlying oedema, and when palpating the abdomen a palpable fluid wave may be observed (Brooker, 2008). Ascites is most typically seen in patients who suffer from liver disease, but it can also be appreciated with underlying malignancy and, to a certain extent, with renal and cardiac insufficiency (Pilbery, 2014).

Other waves which may be witnessed when inspecting the abdomen include that of peristalsis, although these are normally slight and more prominent in individuals with low body fat. When easily visible, stronger rippling waves can be seen that may be an indicator of a bowel obstruction, and would be associated with absent bowel sounds beyond the point of the movement. These will often be associated with colicky pain.

Undertake 'The cough test': **Assessment** – look at the patient's face and ask them to 'cough'. If this causes pain, flinching or they move their hands to protect the abdomen, all of which are positive signs, then suspect peritonitis (Longmore et al., 2014).

When inspecting the abdomen of trauma patients, the paramedic should consider certain bruising patterns which are worthy of note. These include both Cullen's sign and Grey Turner's sign. Cullen's sign is bruising around the umbilicus, whilst Grey Turner's sign is bruising along the flank, due to retroperitoneal bleeding. The latter is indicative of blunt force haemorrhage, aortic leaking, pancreatic or renal bleeding. Both these signs should alert the paramedic to retro-peritoneal haemorrhage. Seat belt marking and pattern bruising may be present in road traffic incidents and related trauma. Once again, it is important for the paramedic to consider the organs which may be damaged.

In addition to this, the assessment may be made more difficult when the patient is unconscious, has spinal cord injury (*due to loss of sensation*), major distracting injuries, and for patients who have ingested drugs or alcohol (Greaves et al., 2012).

> **Possible actions to be taken:**
> - Inspect the abdomen and ascertain evidence of either visible pulsations, scars, masses, hernia, peristalsis, striae or distension
> - If distension is present identify the cause (*five 'F's*)
> - Undertake the cough test
> - In trauma patients, look for Cullen's and Grey Turner's signs
> - Manage conditions accordingly (see *Trauma Assessment, Chapter 7*).

Auscultation

Unlike other assessments, the abdominal assessment takes place in a different order. After inspection comes auscultation. Auscultation provides important information about bowel sounds and movement. It is important to listen to the abdomen before performing percussion or palpation, as these manoeuvres may alter the frequency of bowel sounds. This provides important information about the movement of fluid and gases within the abdominal cavity. Listening for bowel sounds can be a confusing subject for the paramedic, with various texts suggesting differing optimal times spent listening to the abdomen between 10 seconds and 7 minutes. The latter is unlikely to be of benefit in the emergency situation, and would certainly not be pertinent to consider in a patient with a potentially time critical condition. For each patient, a time versus benefit analysis will need to be made in order to decide how long each quadrant will be listened to, and what the paramedic can gain from such an examination. In addition to this issue, and as with any auscultation of a patient, the environment needs to be quiet enough to allow the sounds to be heard. Finally, regular practice is required in order to ensure that the paramedic/clinician has gained a baseline of normal abdominal sounds.

When a patient complains of pain in a specific quadrant of the abdomen, best practice is to commence the auscultation in the quadrant immediately adjacent to the pain quadrant in a clockwise direction. For example, if the pain is experienced in the left upper quadrant, then commence the assessment in the left lower quadrant (see Figure 4.3). This will ensure that this routine will be

Abdominal and gastro-intestinal assessment

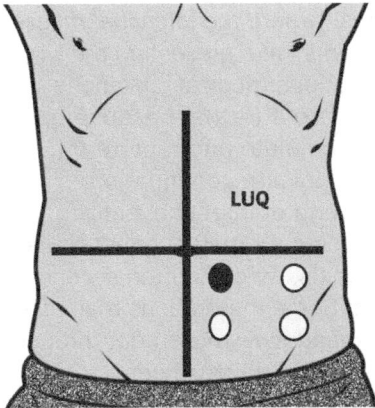

Figure 4.3 Auscultation of abdominal quadrants if the patient reports pain in their left upper quadrant (LUQ)

followed when undertaking percussion and palpation of the abdomen and the purpose of this will be discussed shortly.

- Use the diaphragm of the stethoscope and begin by placing it in the chosen quadrant nearest to the umbilicus.
- Good practice dictates that both the stethoscope head and the hands of the paramedic are warm enough to ensure patient comfort.
- When time is of the essence, divide the quadrant into a further four quadrants, and then place the stethoscope in the centre of each of these smaller quadrants and auscultate for 15 seconds, beginning in the quadrant closest to the umbilicus and moving in a clockwise fashion. In the time critical patient, this assessment is of limited benefit (Rushforth, 2009).
- When time is not of the essence, the stethoscope is placed in each of the four quadrants spending at least 2 minutes in each quadrant in order to allow enough time to hear sounds (*although a period of up to 7 minutes may be required*).

If the pain presents in left upper quadrant (LUQ):

- Commence auscultation in left lower quadrant (LLQ)
- Continue in a clockwise direction auscultating the 'pain' quadrant last
- If time is of the essence, divide each quadrant into four, commencing nearest to the umbilicus and continue in a clockwise direction, and then place the stethoscope in the centre of each of these smaller quadrants and auscultate for 15 seconds.

The majority of bowel sounds are normal. Normal bowel sounds are gurgling sounds (*usually occurring 5–35 per minute*) that can be heard with the diaphragm of a stethoscope. The paramedic needs to be able to identify abnormal sounds that will assist with the assessment of the patient's health. Abnormal sounds are described as absent, hypoactive or hyperactive.

- *Absent bowel sounds* – is when the paramedic is unable to hear any bowel sounds after listening to the abdomen, and indicates a lack of intestinal activity. It is also known as 'ileus' (*where the intestinal muscle ceases movement and bowel contents remain in situ, presenting the same problems found with a bowel obstruction*). Various medical conditions can lead to this but it is important to evaluate it further because gas, secretions and intestinal contents can accumulate and rupture the bowel wall, although absent sounds often indicate constipation.

- *Hypoactive bowel sounds* – indicates a slowing of intestinal activity. This may be normal as it occurs while sleeping, or may suggest bowel obstruction, peritonitis, or generalized peritonitis, which is often secondary to a disease in the abdominal-pelvic organs. Some medications may affect bowel movements, for instance, narcotics may slow movement through the digestive system, as will drugs designed to halt diarrhoea.
- *Hyperactive bowel sounds* – are described as an increase in intestinal activity (*loud and high-pitched*). These are associated with progressive bowel obstruction, large amounts of fluid and gas accumulating in the bowel, and are an ominous sound which could suggest impending bowel paralysis. They are also associated with diarrhoea, hunger or after meals, so consider asking the patient about the timing of their last meal.

Auscultate for hepatic bruits in patients with liver disease. Listen for bruits over the renal, iliac and femoral arteries as well as the aorta (see Figure 4.4). Renal

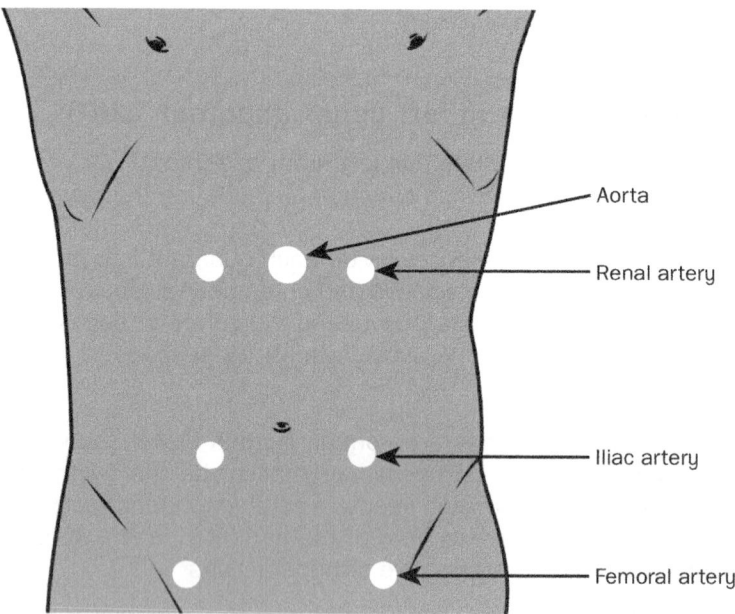

Figure 4.4 Auscultation of bruits

artery stenosis may be the cause of hypertension. Auscultate for flow bruits over the femoral arteries, as patients with intermittent claudication (*cramp in the leg caused by artery obstruction*) may have arteries that have become narrowed due to atheroma.

Abdominal sounds should always be evaluated in conjunction with symptoms such as nausea, vomiting, the presence or absence of bowel movements or gas. When hypo- or hyper-active bowel sounds are present with abnormal symptoms, the paramedic must remember that continued evaluation is important.

Possible actions to be taken:

- Identify the area of pain; commence auscultation in the next clockwise quadrant
- Listen between 2 and 7 minutes, continue in a clockwise direction
- If time is of the essence, sub-divide the quadrant into four and auscultate each area for 15 seconds
- Identify and record any absent, hypo- or hyper-bowel sound activity
- Auscultate for bruits over the renal, iliac and femoral arteries
- Record findings.

Palpation

Palpation of the abdomen is undertaken using a light and deep palpation technique in each of the four quadrants. Initially palpate each quadrant lightly (*1-2 cm depth*). Light palpation involves placing your hand onto the patient's abdomen, and then flexing your fingers so that your fingertips push into their abdomen. The abdomen should be soft to the touch, and there should be no tenderness upon palpation. Then, if appropriate, increase the palpation depth (*4-6 cm depth*). When considering this action in an obese patient, the paramedic could apply one hand on top of the other to assist with this aspect of the examination.

Commence palpation in the appropriate quadrant, away from the site of pain. While palpating, observe the patient's face for signs of pain and establish if the palpation hurts them, due to any of the following:

- *Tenderness* – this can be superficial, deep or rebound
- *Rebound tenderness* – occurs from movement of inflamed viscera of peritonitis against parietal peritoneum. **Assessment** – To check for rebound tenderness (*pain increased on release rather than on deep*

*palpatio*n), palpate (*press*) slowly on the tender area and then quickly release
- *Guarding* – reflex contraction of the abdominal muscles as you palpate
- *Rigidity* – sustained tension of abdominal muscles which become hard and inflexible (*indicative of peritonitis*).

Palpation should identify which organs are enlarged or tender, whether additional fluid is accumulating within the cavity, or if there are any masses, and whether these are solid or pulsatile. Locating pulsatile masses while palpating requires careful consideration as to the need for deep palpation. This could lead to damage to the weak artery walls and a contained mass becoming an exsanguinating haemorrhage.

As has previously been stated, considerable care should be taken if a pulsatile mass is felt, and deliberation should also be given to palpating a rigid abdomen. Palpating a rigid abdomen due to peritoneal inflammation could cause increased pain or, more importantly, rupture an inflamed abdominal organ.

Percussion

The purpose of percussion in the abdominal assessment is to discover the borders of the abdominal organs, their size, density and location, and if they contain air or fluid. Hollow organs produce tympany, like the sound of a drum, while solid organs produce dull sounds. Dullness may be due to faeces, fluid or a solid mass, it may also be due to a tumour. For instance, dullness over the ovaries could be due to a large ovarian cyst. Percussion is used to ascertain the size of the liver and spleen and to ascertain if there is air in the stomach or bowel.

To percuss the liver and estimate its size, start in the right mid-clavicular line and percuss below the umbilicus with tympany and percuss upward towards the liver, when it changes to dullness. Mark to indicate the liver border. Then in the same mid-clavicular line, percuss down from lung resonance to liver dullness. This indicates the lower border of the liver. Mark this and measure between the two lines. This is the height of the liver.

When the spleen enlarges, it does so anteriorly, downwards and medially. As it does so, it replaces the tympany of the stomach and colon with dullness. Percuss in the lowest interspace in the left anterior axillary line for tympany.

Ask the patient to take a deep breath and percuss on inspiration. The percussion note should remain tympanic, if it changes to dullness, this suggests splenomegaly (*enlarged spleen*), and is known as a positive splenic percussion sign.

Abdominal and gastro-intestinal assessment

Possible actions to be taken:

- Palpate and percuss the four quadrants
- Percuss and identify the size and borders of the liver and the spleen
- Ascertain if there is air in the stomach or bowel
- Percuss in several directions away from tympany or resonance to dullness to outline edges
- In the LUQ, a large dull area suggests splenomegaly.

REVIEW OF SYSTEMS AND VITAL SIGNS

When assessing a patient with inflammatory gastro-intestinal conditions, the pulse and temperature are likely to be elevated. When the respiratory rate is also raised, the likelihood is that there is an additional infection of the chest, or that internal blood loss may be causing the signs of shock.

When reviewing genito-urinary conditions the paramedic should consider undertaking a urinalysis assessment, which includes examining the patient's urine for the appearance, concentration and content. An abnormal reading may indicate either illness or disease, such as:

- Cloudy urine may be indicative of an infection (UTI).
- Raised levels of protein may be indicative of kidney disease.

Pregnancy testing is currently not part of paramedic practice, however, paramedics should consider that any woman of childbearing age with abdominal pain should be presumed to be pregnant, until proven otherwise by pregnancy testing. Remember that there is a risk of a recent course of antibiotics preventing the patient's contraceptive medication from being effective (NHS Choices, 2014).

OTHER CONSIDERATIONS

Ethical and legal

The pre-hospital environment may not be the correct place to undertake an assessment of the genitalia, rectum and anus. This can create ethical and legal issues, as well as affecting professional practice. In the majority of instances, there is usually no reason to undertake an examination of the genitalia unless the patient specifically complains of pain or discomfort in this area, or blood is noted in this area through clothing. Although a bleed in the genitalia can be extensive, gaining informed consent is an absolute necessity, with thorough documentation as to why it was undertaken and that consent had been gained from the patient (Pilbery, 2014). If a persistent erection is seen through clothing in a male patient, damage to the spinal cord should be suspected, but questioning as to the use of sildenafil (*Viagra*) is also relevant. The patient may be embarrassed to admit to having used this drug, but it may prove to be an important part of the history taking and treatment plan.

Clothing associated with a sexual assault or rape victim must be handled as per local and national guidelines, in close liaison with (*and taking the advice of*) the local police service. The patient may need to be taken to a specialist treatment centre, and consideration to having a paramedic of the same sex available to examine the patient if necessary is appropriate.

Rectal examinations may be seen in hospital assessments of trauma patients, but are rarely seen out of hospital unless there are doctors, such as GPs, or BASICS team attending the patient. For the majority of paramedics, a rectal exam is seldom indicated, and the same guidance given for examination of the genitalia should be followed.

Destination/receiving specialist units/non-conveyance

The paramedic will be guided by local protocols as to the hospital destination of choice. In cases of trauma, it is often more relevant to convey the patient to a regional trauma centre, even though it may involve a longer travelling time, to ensure the best possible patient outcome. In cases of non-local conveyance, protocols must always be adhered to, with a thorough assessment having been undertaken.

The National Institute for Health and Clinical Excellence (NICE) offers specific guidance in the following conditions that affect the digestive tract:

- Cholelithiasis and cholecystitis
- Coeliac disease
- Colorectal cancer
- Diarrhoea and vomiting
- Digestive tract conditions: general and other
- Faecal incontinence
- Gastro-oesophageal reflux disease (GORD, including Barrett's oesophagus
- Haemorrhoids and other anal conditions
- Hernia
- Inflammatory bowel disease
- Irritable bowel syndrome
- Lower gastro-intestinal lesions

Abdominal and gastro-intestinal assessment

- Oesophogeal cancer
- Pancreatic cancer
- Pancreatitis
- Stomach cancer
- Upper gastro-intestinal bleeding (NICE, 2015a).

NICE has also published clinical guidelines that cover the following conditions and diseases:

- Acute kidney disease (NICE, 2013)
- Acute upper gastro-intestinal bleeding management (NICE, 2012)
- Diarrhoea and vomiting in children younger than 5 (NICE, 2009)
- Dyspepsia and GORD (NICE, 2014)
- Dyspepsia and GORD in children and young people (NICE, 2015b)
- Irritable bowel syndrome in adults (NICE, 2015c).

Professional

Although the Health and Care Professions Council (HCPC) has no specific guidance concerning abdominal pain and GI and GU assessment, the paramedic must ensure that consent is gained prior to any assessment. As has already been stated, consideration must also be given to the relevance of an examination of the genitalia and rectal area to avoid any accusations of professional misconduct.

Figure 4.5 presents the main gastro-intestinal and genito-urinary conditions and the area of presentation.

COMMON ABDOMINAL CONDITIONS (See Figure 4.5)

Appendicitis

Inflammation of the vermiform appendix. The pain of appendicitis classically begins near the umbilicus, then shifts to the right lower quadrant (RLQ), and coughing increases it. Elderly patients report this pattern less frequently than younger ones.

Signs and symptoms
- Slight fever
- Nausea
- Vomiting
- Loss of appetite
- Constipation
- Diarrhoea
- Localized tenderness (*anywhere in the RLQ, or even in the right flank*)

105

Right Upper Quadrant	Epigastrium	Left Upper Quadrant
Acute cholecystitis	Pancreatitis	Ruptured spleen
Duodenal ulcer	Myocardial infarct	Gastric ulcer
Hepatitis	Peptic ulcer	Aortic aneurysm
Congestive heptomegaly	Acute cholecystitis	Perforated colon
Pyelonephritis	Perforated oesophagus	Pyelonephritis
Appendicitis		(L) Pneumonia
(R) Pneumonia		

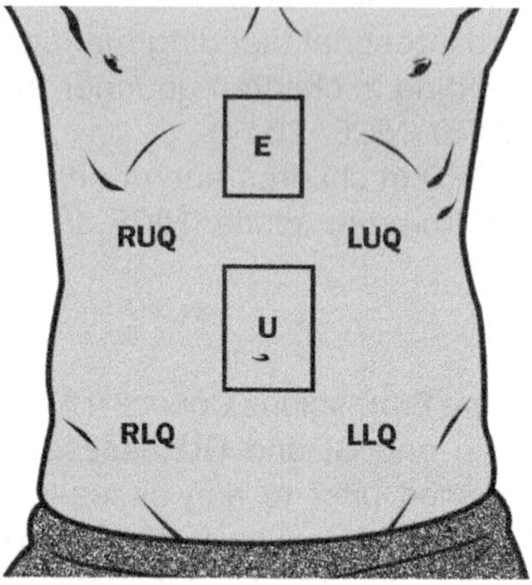

Right Lower Quadrant	Umbilical	Left Lower Quadrant
Appendicitis	Intestinal obstruction	Sigmoid diverticulitis
Salpingitis	Acute pancreatitis	Salpingitis
Tubo-ovarian abscess	Early appendicitis	Tubo-ovarian abscess
Ruptured ectopic pregnancy	Mesentric thrombosis	Ruptured ectopic pregnancy
Renal/ureteric stone	Aortic aneurysm	Strangulated hernia
Strangulated hernia	Diverticulitis	Perforated colon
Mesenteric adenitis		Crohn's disease
Meckel's diverticulitis		Ulcerative colitis
Crohn's disease		Renal/ureteric stone
Perforated caecum		
Psoas abscess		

Figure 4.5 Gastro-intestinal and genito-urinary conditions and area of presentation

- Early voluntary guarding may be replaced by involuntary muscular rigidity
- Right-sided rectal tenderness.

Acute cholecystitis

Cholecystitis is inflammation of the gall bladder. Acute cholecystitis should be suspected whenever there is acute right upper quadrant (RUQ) or epigastric pain.

Signs and symptoms
- Pain in the RUQ
- The pain is usually constant and severe
- The pain may radiate to the right flank or right scapular region
- This pain may occur after eating greasy or fatty foods
- Fever
- Diarrhoea
- Nausea and/or vomiting.

Ectopic pregnancy

In ectopic pregnancy a fertilized egg is implanted somewhere outside the uterus, most commonly the fallopian tubes. The patient will generally exhibit some of the normal signs of pregnancy, including cessation of periods, enlarged and tender breasts, but without the ability to increase in size as the embryo grows, pain is felt by the patient as pressure is placed on the fallopian wall. Rupture of the fallopian tube will lead to shock and death if not recognized and treated urgently.

Signs and symptoms
- Pain in the pelvic region (*typically severe, sharp and possibly stabbing*)
- Pain may present in the shoulder tip, caused by internal bleeding irritating the diaphragm when breathing in and out
- Spotting, or abnormal bleeding, which may be lighter or heavier than a normal period, and more prolonged. This bleeding is often dark in colour and watery (*similar to prune juice*)
- Light-headedness, transient loss of consciousness, syncope
- Pain in the lower back
- Hypotension
- Experience of some early symptoms of pregnancy (*missed or late period, enlarged and tender breasts*).

Intestinal and bowel obstruction

Intestinal and bowel obstruction are common abdominal emergencies, often requiring surgery. Causes may be mechanical or due to compromised blood supply, and, as has previously been mentioned, the patient history is important when ascertaining the location and likelihood of intestinal obstruction.

Small bowel obstruction: signs and symptoms
- Central colicky pain
- Vomiting (*which may be food, bile or even possibly faecal*)

- Abdominal distension (*unlikely to be tender on palpation*)
- History of abdominal surgery with associated scars.

Large bowel obstruction: signs and symptoms
- Central or lower abdominal colicky pain
- Constipation
- Abdominal distension (*tense and tympanic on percussion*)
- Absent bowel sounds
- Vomiting is more likely to be a late sign
- Changes in bowel habit and bleeding per rectum (PR) may suggest carcinoma.

Pancreatitis

This is an acute inflammatory condition of the pancreas, with variable involvement of other regional tissues or remote organ systems. Common causes include:

- Gallstones
- Alcohol
- Idiopathic (*of unknown origin*)
- Trauma-related, generally blunt trauma.

This condition usually presents with abdominal pain (*epigastric radiating through to the back*) and vomiting. In the case of gallstones, there may also be jaundice, though this is rare. These patients are often agitated, and will present with abdominal epigastric tenderness. Consider:

- Severe abdominal pain, usually rapid onset
- Poorly localized in the epigastrium and left upper quadrant
- Radiating to the back
- Aggravated by lying down, relieved by sitting forward
- Vomiting (*may be severe*)
- Patient looks unwell
- Jaundiced
- Shock more commonly in the elderly
- Abdominal tenderness, usually diffuse, guarding and rebound
- Bruising may rarely be noticed in the flanks or around the umbilicus.

Trauma

The abdomen may be affected by blunt or penetrating trauma, and there may be evisceration of the abdominal organs. When patients present with abdominal evisceration, there may be little pain. Care should be taken not to apply dressings which may adhere to the abdominal contents, but covering the wound with a non-adherent dressing will assist in preventing the site becoming infected, or paralysed due to a cold external environment.

Abdominal and gastro-intestinal assessment

When objects are impaled in the abdomen, the object should not be removed, as it may be preventing a severe bleed by remaining in situ. Although this may prove challenging, the impaled object should remain in place, and be secured in the most stable manner possible.

When assessing the GI system in such instances, consider the likelihood of damage of organs obstructing the route the object will have taken. Assess for signs of shock, and also consider whether the object may have caused damage to other systems, for instance, penetrating the diaphragm (see *Respiratory Assessment, Chapter 2 and Trauma Assessment, Chapter 7*) or vascular damage (see *Cardiovascular Assessment, Chapter 3*).

As per current clinical guidelines, do not push eviscerated organs back into the abdominal cavity, but cover them with moist and, where possible, warm, dressings (Fisher et al., 2013). As has been mentioned, consideration must be given to the underlying organs, and how this may lead to serious internal bleeding. Signs and symptoms of shock must be considered, as internal haemorrhage can be masked until the signs of decompensation are observed.

Undertake a full secondary survey of the abdomen, as has previously been discussed. Revisit, considering where the injury may lie, and underlying damage. Marry this to signs and symptoms of the stages of shock. Remember that this is only a guide. Patients taking certain medications, such as beta-blockers or anti-depressants, may not demonstrate the signs and symptoms listed here. For this reason, it is imperative that the paramedic considers the mechanism of injury, and risk of a time critical bleed.

CHAPTER KEY POINTS

- Decide whether the patient is time critical or non-time critical.
- Examine using IAPP (inspect, auscultate, palpate and percussion) in order to adhere to a logical, systematic methodology.
- Use the SOCRATES framework when assessing pain.
- A thorough knowledge of the anatomy of the GI and GU structures, their location and function, aids accurate diagnosis and treatment.
- Undertake a thorough secondary survey and gain a complete patient history, as soon as time allows.
- Consider the necessity for an assessment of the rectum and genitalia, and the legal and ethical issues around undertaking such an assessment, especially in children.
- In trauma patients, consider the mechanism of injury.
- Is the patient vulnerable, and are further steps required?

REFERENCES

Association of Ambulance Chief Executives (2013) *UK Ambulance Services Clinical Practice Guidelines 2013 Pocket Book: Pain Assessment Model*. Bridgwater: Class Professional Publishing.

Ballinger, A. (2012) *Essentials of Kumar and Clark's Clinical Medicine (Pocket Essentials)* (5th edn). Edinburgh: Saunders Elsevier.

Bickley, L.S. and Szilagyi, P.G. (2013) *Bates' Pocket Guide to Physical Examination and History Taking* (7th edn). Philadelphia, PA: Lippincott Williams & Wilkins.

British Thoracic Society (2015) *Emergency Oxygen Use in Adult Patients Guideline*. Available at: https://www.brit-thoracic.org.uk/searchresults/?txtSearch=2015+Oxygen+Guidelines&search= (accessed 22 May 2015).

Brooker, C. (2008) *Churchill Livingstone Medical Dictionary* (16th edn). London: Churchill Livingstone.

Department of Health (2009) *Reference Guide to Consent for Examination or Treatment* (2nd edn). London: Department of Health.

Epstein, O., Perkin, D.G., Cookson, J., Watt, I.S., Rakhit, R., Robins, R, and Hornett, G.A.W. (2009) *Pocket Guide to Clinical Examination* (4th edn). London: Mosby Elsevier.

Fisher, J., Brown, S.N. and Cooke, M. (eds) (2013) *UK Ambulance Services Clinical Practice Guidelines 2013: Abdominal Trauma*. Bridgwater: Class Professional Publishing.

Greaves, I., Wright, C., Porter, K., Hodgetts, T. and Woollard, M. (2012) *Pocketbook of Emergency Care: A Quick Reference Guide for Paramedics*. Edinburgh: Saunders Elsevier.

Longmore, M., Wilkinson, I.B., Baldwin, A. and Wallin, E. (2014) *Oxford Handbook of Clinical Medicine* (9th edn). Oxford: Oxford University Press.

National Institute of Diabetes and Digestive and Kidney Disease (2014) *Smoking and the Digestive System*. Available at: http://www.niddk.nih.gov/health-information/health-topics/digestive-diseases/smoking/Pages/facts.aspx (accessed 4 June 2015).

NHS Choices (2014) *Will Antibiotics Stop My Contraception Working?* Available at: http://www.nhs.uk/Conditions/contraception-guide/Pages/antibiotics-contraception.aspx (accessed 5 June 2015).

NICE (National Institute for Health and Clinical Excellence) (2009) *Diarrhoea and Vomiting Caused by Gastroenteritis: Diagnosis, Assessment and Management in Children Younger than 5 Years*. NICE clinical guideline 84. Available at: http://www.nice.org.uk/guidance/cg84/evidence (accessed 5 June 2015).

NICE (National Institute for Health and Clinical Excellence) (2012) *Acute Upper Gastrointestinal Bleeding Management*. NICE clinical guideline 141. Available at: http://www.nice.org.uk/guidance/cg141/evidence (accessed 5 June 2015).

NICE (National Institute for Health and Clinical Excellence) (2013) *Acute Kidney Injury: Prevention, Detection and Management Up to the Point of Renal Replacement Therapy*. NICE clinical guideline 169. Available at: http://www.nice.org.uk/guidance/cg169/evidence (accessed 5 June 2015).

NICE (National Institute for Health and Clinical Excellence) (2014) *Dyspepsia and Gastro-Oesophageal Reflux Disease: Investigation and Management of Dyspepsia, Symptoms Suggestive of Gastro-Oesophageal Reflux Disease, Or Both*. NICE clinical guideline 184.

Available at: http://www.nice.org.uk/guidance/cg184/evidence (accessed 5 June 2015).

NICE (National Institute for Health and Clinical Excellence) (2015a) *Digestive Tract Conditions*. Available at: https://www.nice.org.uk/guidancemenu/conditions-and-diseases/digestive-tract-conditions (accessed 3 June 2015).

NICE (National Institute for Health and Clinical Excellence) (2015b) *Gastro-Oesophageal Reflux Disease in Children and Young People. Gastro-Oesophageal Reflux Disease: Recognition, Diagnosis and Management in Children and Young People*. NG 1. Available at. http://www.nice.org.uk/guidance/NG1/evidence (accessed 5 June 2015).

NICE (National Institute for Health and Clinical Excellence) (2015c) *Irritable Bowel Syndrome in Adults: Diagnosis and Management of Irritable Bowel Syndrome in Primary Care*. NICE clinical guideline 61. Available at: http://www.nice.org.uk/guidance/cg61/evidence (accessed 5 June 2015).

Pilbery, R. (2014) *Nancy Caroline's Emergency Care in the Streets: United Kingdom* (7th edn). Burlington, VA: Jones & Bartlett Learning.

Raftery, A.T., Lim, E. and Östör, A.J.K. (2014) *Churchill's Pocketbook of Differential Diagnosis* (4th edn). London: Churchill Livingstone Elsevier.

Rushforth, H. (2009) *Assessment Made Incredibly Easy* (UK edn). Philadelphia, PA: Lippincott Williams & Wilkins.

Thomas, C.P. (2015) *Metabolic Alkalosis*. Available at: http://emedicine.medscape.com/article/243160-overview#a0101 (accessed 4 June 2015).

5 Neurological assessment
Jaqualine Lindridge

The neurological system is a control and communication system which connects with each of the other body systems. Due to its complex anatomy, assessment is often approached with trepidation by the paramedic, but although the examination itself appears complicated, its component tests are simple to perform and their results are objective.

This chapter aims to provide a systematic approach to assessment of the neurological system and to assist the paramedic in identifying neurological abnormalities.

SCENE ASSESSMENT

As you approach the scene try to gain an overview of events:
- Evidence of trauma?
- Overturned furniture consistent with a fall or collapse?
- Mobility aids?

Observation of the patient's position is vital; after all, it is the neurological system which coordinates the body's movements as well as consciousness.

- Where is the patient located?
- Are they sitting or standing?
- Observe the general muscle tone of the patient.
- Are they able to sit upright?
- Are they leaning to one side?
- Is there any obvious muscle flaccidity to the face or limbs?
- Is this bilateral or unilateral?
- Are they moving, or still?
- Are their movements purposeful?
- Is the patient suffering a seizure?

PRIMARY SURVEY

Even if at first sight the patient appears well, deterioration can be rapid. If not properly assessed and reviewed, subtle signs will be overlooked; this is particularly true of the neurological system.

DANGER

Initially assess for actual danger that may have caused the patient's injury or illness. If unconscious – are there contaminated needles/syringes, or potentially faulty gas appliances? Will these affect the paramedic, their colleagues, the patient or bystanders? It is essential that the paramedic remains alert for potential dangers, for example, the patient's symptoms may be the result of a deliberate release of a neurological agent, such as Sarin. The paramedic must consider their own safety, especially where multiple casualties present with clusters of neurological signs and symptoms, and should withdraw to prevent or limit their own exposure to any dangers present. Initiate Step 1, 2, and 3 patients for an unspecified CBRNE incident (AACE, 2013a) (*see Respiratory Assessment, Chapter 2*).

Patients who are fitting may need protection. Nearby furniture should be moved away from the patient's body to prevent injury during the seizure, and if possible place padding around the head to prevent injury from a hard floor.

RESPONSE

Assess the patient's level of response using the AVPU scale; if their level of consciousness is reduced, further evaluation may take place during the secondary survey.

AIRWAY

Assess the airway for patency and consider the patient's ability to maintain and protect their own airway. In the unresponsive patient, always consider the possibility of injury to the cervical spine. Any insult to the cervical vertebrae has the potential to cause spinal cord injury (SCI), which at this anatomical level may paralyse some of the respiratory muscles.

In the unconscious patient, the tongue will become **flaccid** and fall posteriorly into the oropharynx, thus occluding the airway. This can be corrected by manual airway manoeuvres ('C' spine appropriate) used in conjunction with patient positioning and airway adjuncts. It is important to remember that the unconscious patient is also at risk of aspiration, even if manual airway manoeuvres are used effectively (AACE, 2013b).

It cannot be assumed that the conscious patient will be able to protect their own airway; the paramedic must be alert to the possibility that the patient may need assistance in clearing secretions, blood or vomit, particularly in patients whose neurological complaint may inhibit the gag **reflex**, such as a stroke.

If present, seizures can also inhibit airway management. Many patients who suffer seizures will exhibit trismus (*inability to open mouth fully*). In such cases, consideration should be given to the use of nasopharyngeal adjuncts.

Possible actions to be taken:

- Open and maintain airway (*considering 'C' spine*)
- Consider appropriate stepwise airway management (see *Respiratory Assessment: Chapter 2*).

BREATHING

Disruption to the respiratory centre of the brainstem can disturb the rate and regularity of breathing and damage to the peripheral nervous system may cause dysfunction of the respiratory muscles. The phrenic nerve originates from the spinal cord at the level of C3–C5 and stimulates the diaphragm; if the cord is damaged above this level, the impulses needed to initiate diaphragmatic contraction are blocked and respiratory arrest will result (Jenkins and Tortora, 2013), hence the popular saying 'C3, 4 and 5 keep the diaphragm alive.' Conditions such as stroke or intra-cerebral haemorrhage can affect the respiratory centre, causing respiratory depression or arrest, whereas conditions such as Guillain-Barré syndrome may cause temporary paralysis of the respiratory muscles (NHS UK, 2015a). Assess for the presence of breathing and evaluate the rate, depth and pattern of breathing and evaluate the need to assist ventilations.

Possible actions to be taken:

- If patient is not responding: look, listen and feel for breathing for 10 seconds
- Consider the need to ventilate
- Ensure that the patient is not hypoxic
- Manage breathing/**hypoxia** effectively before moving to the next element.

CIRCULATION

The neurological system is essential for autonomic control of blood pressure and disruption can be caused by septic shock secondary to neurological infections, such as meningococcal **meningitis** as well as injuries causing neurogenic shock. High cord injuries can produce bradycardia and hypotension as sympathetic tone is lost and vagal activity is unopposed. Although these responses are of delayed onset and therefore infrequently seen in the pre-hospital arena (Guly et al., 2007), they are important causes of cardiovascular compromise in the trauma patient and should be considered in patients who present with signs of shock without evidence of hypovolaemia. Where neurogenic shock is suspected, avoid endotracheal intubation and suctioning unless essential to preserve the airway as these manoeuvres may produce unopposed vagal stimulation.

DISABILITY

Examine the patient to confirm the absence of seizure activity. Observe for jerky movements of the limbs and test the joints for tone. Briefly observe the patient's muscle tone and movement. Look for any flaccid limbs, these will need protection to prevent injury, also note if the muscles are moving the limbs; this is particularly important in the trauma patient. Note any abnormal posturing, such as decerebrate (see Figure 5.1). In decerebrate rigidity, there is an abnormal extensor response; note the extension at the elbows with pronation and flexion at the wrists, or decorticate positions (see Figure 5.2).

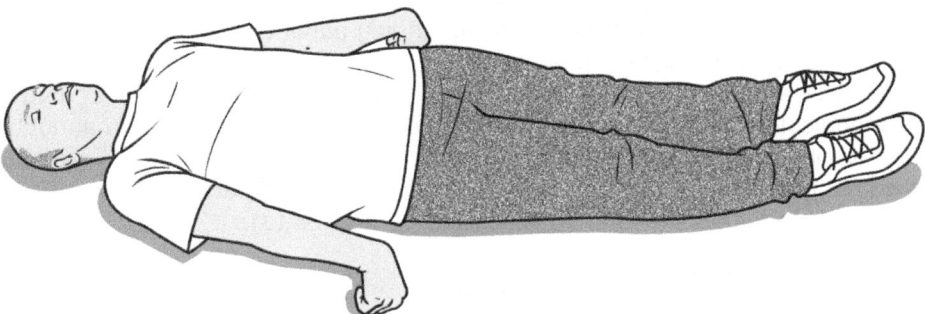

Figure 5.1 Decerebrate positioning – abnormal extensor response

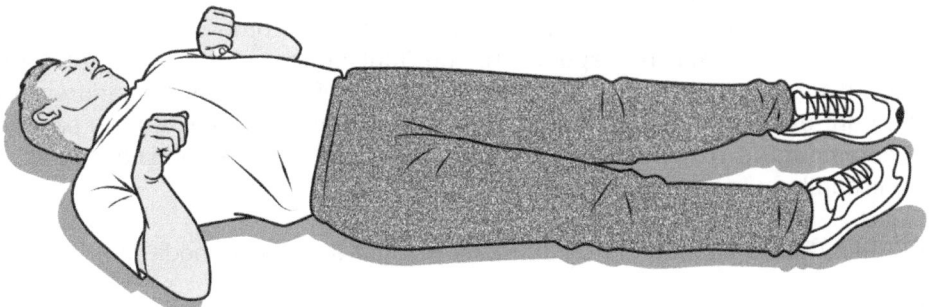

Figure 5.2 Decorticate positioning – abnormal flexor response

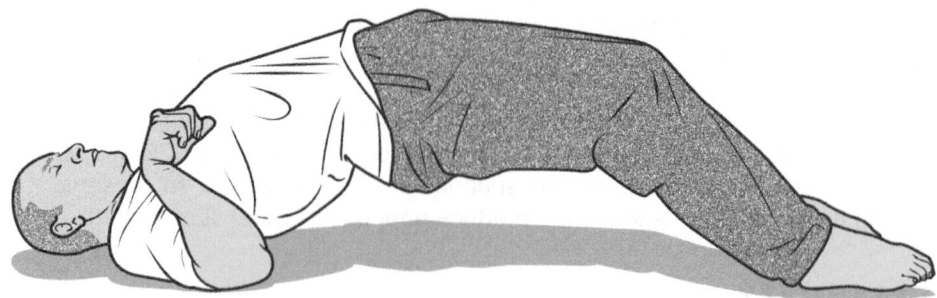

Figure 5.3 Opisthotonus positioning

In decorticate rigidity, there is an abnormal flexor response; note the **flexion** at the elbows.

Alternatively the patient may demonstrate opisthotonus. In opisthotonus the back can be seen to characteristically arch in extreme hyper-extension and may result from brain injury, meningism or tetanus (see Figure 5.3).

Exclude the possibility of **hypoglycaemia** in any patient with a reduced level of consciousness. Hypoglycaemia can present with neurological signs, including hemiparesis, coma and seizures. Prolonged neuroglycopenia can cause neurological deficit and the importance of identifying hypoglycaemia cannot be over-emphasized. Keep in mind the common framework: **ABC 'DEFG'** – 'airway, breathing, circulation, *don't ever forget glucose*'. This is particularly important in paediatric patients (*see Child Assessment: Chapter 11*).

Test the pupils for light reaction

Using a suitable pen-torch, shine the light briefly into the patient's left pupil and observe the pupil's reaction to the light; it should briskly constrict when confronted with the light, and briskly dilate when the light is removed. Shine the light into the left eye a second time, this time observe the right eye; it should react in response to the light shone into the contralateral eye; this is known as the *consensual light reflex*. Repeat this procedure with the right eye. The assessment of 'accommodation' occurs when the patient accommodates to a near object, they converge their eyes and constrict their pupils.

PERRLA (Pupils Equal and Round; React to Light and Accommodation)

While bilaterally dilated pupils are suggestive of hypoxia or poisoning (benzodiazepines and tricyclic anti-depressants), unilaterally dilated and

Neurological assessment

unresponsive pupils are suggestive of a significant cerebral event. If a lesion places pressure on the cranial nerves responsible for movement of the pupils, then dilation may be seen; this is a significant sign and the paramedic should prepare for the possibility of deterioration.

Highly constricted ('pin-point') pupils are associated with certain types of poisoning. Classically, constricted pupils in poisoning are caused by opiates, such as codeine and heroin. Vision problems, sudden trouble seeing in one or both eyes are also associated with pontine stroke (Palande, 2011).

Also observe for any evidence of photophobia, suggestive of meningism and test for the presence of neck stiffness.

Consider the need to assess the patient's temperature. Serious neurological disorders can present with derangements of temperature. Derangements of temperature can cause neurological symptoms. In the paediatric patient, seizures may be the result of fever; if the paramedic can confirm the presence of pyrexia at an early stage, then the correct treatment modality can be initiated. Profoundly raised (hyperthermic) (**hyperthermia**; *core temperature >40°C*) or lowered (hypothermic) (**hypothermia**; *core temperature <35°C*) body temperatures can be life-threatening and both will affect the neurological system *in extremis*. The combination of abnormal body temperature with abnormal neurology indicates a serious problem.

> **Possible actions to be taken:**
> - Assess and document (LOC)
> - Assess and document blood glucose levels
> - Assess and document size and equality of pupils (*consensual/ accommodating*)
> - Undertake a Face, Arms, Speech Test (FAST) (NCCfCC, 2008; NHS UK, 2015b)
> - Assess and record the temperature
> - Pre-alert and transfer to a hyper-acute stroke unit.

EXPOSE/EXAMINE/ENVIRONMENT

Taking environmental and chaperone issues into account, expose the patient. Specifically expose the patient and examine for a rash. In meningococcal septicaemia, look for a non-blanching petechial rash, the rash will develop rapidly from one or two small spots and is a late sign, but if the rash is obvious, then the meningococcal septicaemia is at an advanced stage. Thoroughly examine the patient ensuring that the axillae are included, and in infants the nappy requires removal to examine the gluteal folds.

- Check for evidence of intravenous drug use and medical patches. In the case of the intravenous drug user, 'track-marks' may not be obvious, although often found in the antecubital fossa, the web spaces of fingers and toes are also used, among other sites.
- Look for medical alert tags; these will often reveal information about the patient's past medical history or supply a telephone number where this information can be obtained.

Possible actions to be taken:

- Check for evidence of intravenous drug use and medical patches
- Look for medical alert tags
- Examine and expose and assess as appropriate
- If the patient does not have a **time critical** condition, then undertake an appropriate secondary survey.

SECONDARY SURVEY

Having completed the primary survey, the paramedic should be aware of any immediately life-threatening conditions. If the primary survey is 'positive' for such conditions, the paramedic must evaluate and treat simultaneously, but in the less time critical patient, it is necessary to gain an understanding of their condition in greater detail. This begins by taking a history.

Presenting complaint

The presenting complaint need only be two or three words, examples from a neurological perspective include 'headache' or 'dizziness', with a brief descriptor of the patient.

History of presenting complaint

The history of the presenting complaint is a short story of how the patient has come to be unwell or injured, and how their problem is progressing. For example, for a patient presenting with dysarthria their documentation might read:

- PC: 80 ♀ C/O slurred speech.
- HPC: Sudden onset of slurred speech, at approximately 14.45 hrs, accompanied by weakness of the right arm and leg. Patient's husband states the left side of the patient's face appears 'droopy'. No change since onset.

Here we have a brief story of what has happened to the patient. There are some key elements which are particularly important in the neurological history; the speed of onset should be noted, always observe if the onset is abrupt or insidious. Also note any improvements or deterioration; this information will assist in formulating differential diagnoses later.

Past medical history

The neurological system interacts with all of the other systems of the body so it is essential to note a complete history, not just the elements which are obviously neurological in origin. For example, the patient may report they suffer with the cardiovascular disorder called Hughes syndrome. Hughes syndrome, otherwise known as *antiphospholipid syndrome or antiphospholipid antibody syndrome*, is a disorder of coagulation that causes blood clots (thrombosis) in both arteries and veins as well as pregnancy-related complications such as miscarriage, stillbirth, preterm delivery, or severe pre-eclampsia. The syndrome occurs due to the auto-immune production of antibodies against phospholipid (aPL) (a cell substance), and has an increased tendency to form emboli, so they are at an increased risk of ischaemic stroke; such information can be taken into consideration when evaluating any presenting neurological symptoms.

Drug/medication history

Enquire about the medications the patient is taking. Be sure to include *all* types of drugs, and not just those prescribed to the patient by other health care practitioners, including the use of illicit drugs. While it is recognized that this is a potentially awkward question, it must be addressed. Many neurological signs and symptoms can be caused by illicit drug use.

Always ask about allergies at an early stage; remember if the paramedic/clinician omits to gain this information and the patient loses consciousness, then the opportunity to gain this vital piece of history is lost and the patient may be at risk from avoidable harm.

Social/family medical history

Enquire as to whether there is a familial history of neurological complaints; conditions such as stroke and migraine may have a familial link.

REVIEW OF SYSTEMS AND VITAL SIGNS

It is important to differentiate between signs and symptoms. Keep in mind that symptoms provide subjective data; symptoms are things which the patient *feels*, whereas signs present objective data; signs are something which the clinician can feel, see or hear. The purpose of the review of systems (ROS) is to 'interrogate' the patient's *symptoms*; it is an information-gathering exercise designed to identify which symptoms the patient has or has not experienced.

If the patient is in pain, they usually will wish to discuss this first.

Pain

When assessing a patient's pain, use the SOCRATES framework (AACE, 2013c):

- **S** – Site. Where exactly is the pain? (*e.g. frontal, occipital lobe*)
- **O** – Onset. Ask if it came on suddenly or gradually. (*The speed of onset in neurological evaluation is vital in assessing the likely causes; a sudden onset of severe headache should raise the paramedic's suspicion of a serious pathology, such as a sub-arachnoid haemorrhage.*)
- **C** – Character. What does the pain feel like? (*Asking the patient what the pain is like will usually reward the paramedic with a comment on its severity only. Ask the patient to describe what it feels like, only providing examples (i.e. sharp or dull) if necessary. The quality of pain in migraine will normally be consistent with previous episodes; a change in quality should raise suspicions.*)
- **R** – Radiate. Where does the pain start and finish? (*Find out where the source of the pain is located, is it unilateral or bilateral? Does it radiate into any other portion of the head or neck (or vice versa!)? Pain arising from an irritated nerve (radicular pain) will often radiate the length of that nerve, such as in sciatica, where the pain usually radiates along the tract of the sciatic nerve from the gluteal region to the foot.*)
- **A** – Associated symptoms. Has the pain been associated with any other symptoms? (*If so, ask the patient to explain what these are.*)
- **T** – Time/duration. How long have they had the pain? (*Try to gain an understanding of the relationship of the pain with other findings. What was happening when the pain started? What time of day do the headaches tend to occur? Is there a pattern forming which will aid diagnosis? Is this an apparent 'first and worst' headache, or is there a slower, more insidious crescendo?*)
- **E** – Exacerbating/relieving factors. Does anything make the pain better or worse? (*Provocation by sudden movements of the head, coughing or sneezing, may indicate raised intracranial pressure (Fuller, 2013). Palliation by rest or dimmed lights may be more suggestive of migraine.*)

Neurological assessment

S – Severity. Obtain an initial pain score (*0 = no pain, 10 = worst pain ever*). *(Only the patient can decide how severe the pain is! If possible, the paramedic should use a validated pain scoring system to help understand how severe the pain is to the patient. A good paramedic never disregards a high pain score based on their own opinion of how much pain a patient is really suffering, and always investigates and manages severe pain.)*

Also enquire about other common symptoms:

- Dizziness. Distinguish from vertigo; if the patient is experiencing light-headedness, or feels as though they may faint, this is suggestive of dizziness. If, however, the patient reports a sensation of the room 'spinning' around them, this is more likely to be vertigo.
- Seizures, syncope, or any type of 'black-out'. If syncope is present, ask about any patterns, e.g. during exercise, or if any prodromal symptoms were present.
- Sensory symptoms, such as pins and needles or loss of sensation.
- Motor symptoms, such as weakness or paralysis, and if there have been any involuntary movements, such as tremors or tics (Bickley, 2013).

After obtaining a through history, the paramedic should approach the physical examination of the neurological system systematically and examine the following four areas: mental status, cranial nerves, sensory system and motor system.

Mental status

The evaluation of mental status comprises an assessment of level of consciousness, behaviour and appearance, speech and cognitive function.

Assess the patient's level of consciousness:
- Are they alert and responding readily?
- Do they need frequent stimulation to elicit a response (*stuporous*)?
- Are they *lethargic* and slow to respond with a tendency to drift off to sleep?
- Take the time to perform the test called the Glasgow Coma Scale (GCS) properly, and never attempt to guess the results! Best Eye (4), Best Motor (5), and Best Verbal (6), with a respective maximum score of 15, and minimum score of 3 (AACE, 2013d).
- In the UK the majority of fatal head injury outcomes are in the moderate (GCS 9–12) or severe (GCS 8 or less) groups (NICE, 2014).

Observe the patient's general appearance and behaviour:
- Are they well kempt?

- Behaviour consistent with social or cultural norms?
- Flights of speech or ideas suggesting a psychiatric aetiology?

Listen to their speech:

- Word-finding difficulties (dysphasia)?
- Is their speech slurred (dysarthria)?

Assess recall; use an appropriate tool in respect to the patient, e.g. the abbreviated mental test (AMT) for elderly patients is a useful tool, see Table 5.1.

Table 5.1 Mini mental status examination (<8/10 suggests confusion)

1	Age?
2	Time? (to nearest hour)
3	Address to recall at end of test, e.g. 42 West Street
4	Year?
5	Name of this place?
6	Identification of two persons? (e.g. paramedic, carer)
7	Date of birth?
8	Start of WWI? (Age of patient – start of WWII)
9	Name of present monarch
10	Count backwards 20 to 1?
	Address recall correct (3 above)

Source: (Hodkinson, 1972)

Cranial nerves

Assessing the cranial nerves is not as difficult as it sounds, and some of the cranial nerves have already been examined as part of the primary survey. A series of simple tests will confirm if the cranial nerves are intact.

Smell
The olfactory nerve (CN I) is not routinely tested in pre-hospital care.

Eyes and vision
The optic nerve (CN II):

- Visual acuity (VA) can be informally tested by reading newspaper text, starting with the headline and moving on to smaller fonts (formal examination requires a VA chart not usually appropriate to pre-hospital care).
- Visual fields are examined using a technique known as confrontation. The paramedic sits face-to-face with the patient, approximately 60 cm (2 ft) away. Both the paramedic and patient should cover corresponding

Neurological assessment

eyes (e.g. if the patient covers the left eye, the paramedic should cover their right), the paramedic then 'confronts' the patient's vision by bringing their moving fingers into the peripheral vision of the patient in each quadrant bilaterally, comparing findings with their own vision.
- If trained, fundoscopy should be performed to assess for papilloedema.
- Observe the eyelids for ptosis (*the inability to elevate the eyelid*) and examine the pupils for consensual light reflex, and accommodation.
- Assess the extra-ocular movements. The oculomotor nerve (CN III), trochlear nerve (CN IV) and the abducens nerve (CN VI) are all involved in controlling the movements of the eyes and are examined together. Ensuring the patient's head remains still, ask the patient to follow your finger through the cardinal positions of gaze; left and right superior, left and right lateral and left and right inferior. This is done by drawing a wide, imaginary 'H' in front of the patient with your finger. Allow your finger to trace this shape, slowly hold each position of view briefly, watching for nystagmus (*an involuntary rapid movement of the eyeball*).

The face
The trigeminal nerve (CN V):

- Sensory assessment: apply light touch to the forehead, maxillae and mandible bilaterally.
- Motor assessment: with the patient's teeth clenched, palpate the temporal and masseter muscle mass. The facial nerve (CN VII). Assess the motor function of CN VII by assessing the symmetry of the following facial movements:
  - Frown
  - Smile (*showing teeth*)
  - Tightly close the eyes and open them against (*gentle*) resistance
  - Puff out the cheeks against resistance (see Figure 5.4).

The ears
The vestibocochlear nerve (CN VIII) is responsible for hearing (cochlear division); it is also involved in balance and equilibrium (vestibular division).

- Stand behind the patient and rub your fingers together, or whisper quietly, asking the patient to repeat what you say (*cochlear division*).
- On the review of systems, complaint of balance disturbance, dizziness or vertigo may implicate the vestibular division of CN VIII.

The mouth
The glossopharyngeal (CN IX) and **vagus** (CN X) nerves are tested together.

- Ask the patient to open their mouth and say 'aahh': the uvula should remain midline.

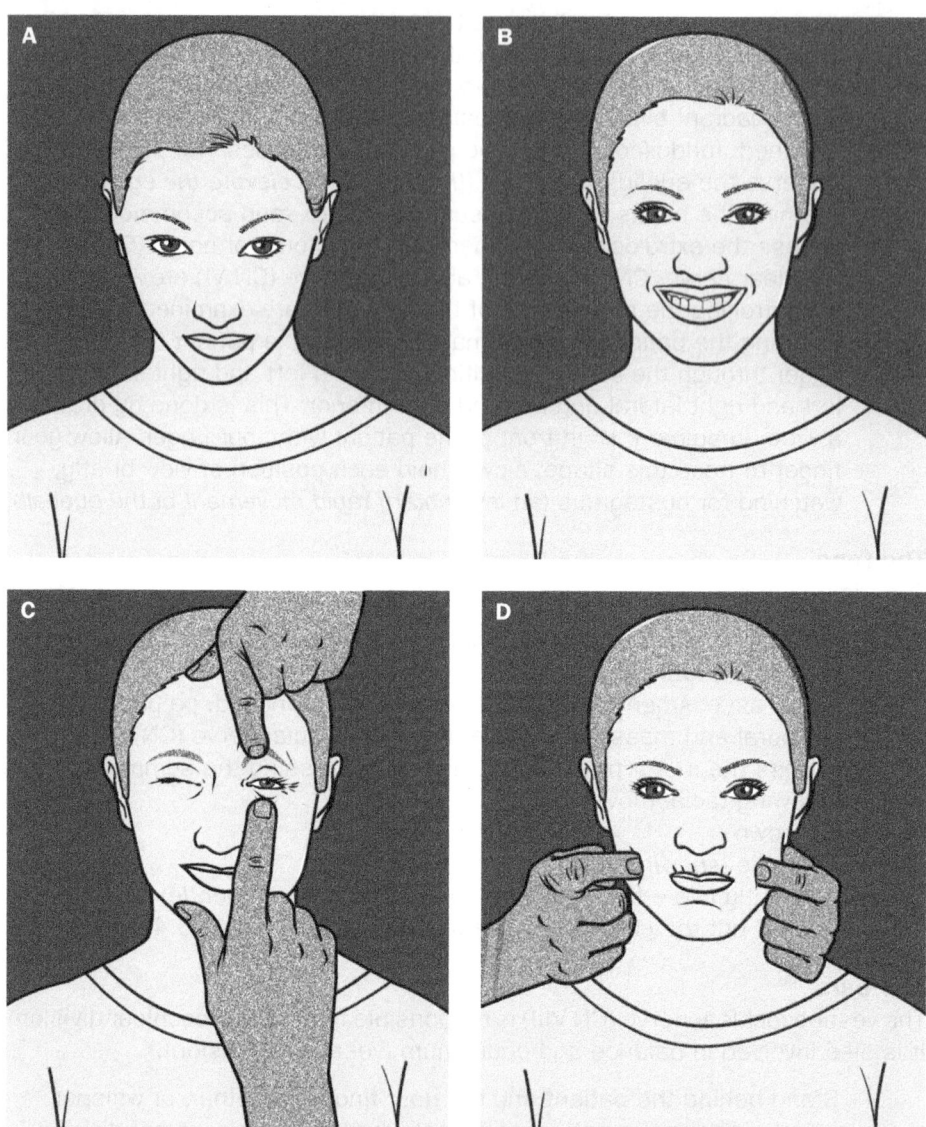

Figure 5.4 Demonstration of the motor function of facial nerves

The hypoglossal nerve (CN XII) controls the tongue.

- When *stuck out*, the tongue remains midline.
- Observe the patient's speech. If it appears abnormal, ask the patient to attempt a tongue twister, such as this commonly used phrase: 'round the rugged rock that ragged rascal ran'.

Neurological assessment

The shoulders

The accessory nerve (CN XI):

- Turn their head against resistance.
- Shrug their shoulders (see Figure 5.5).

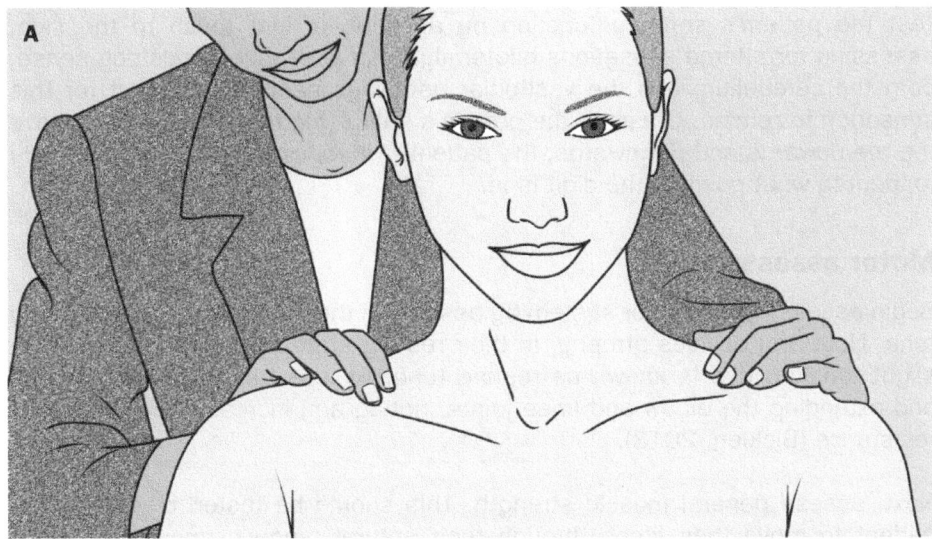

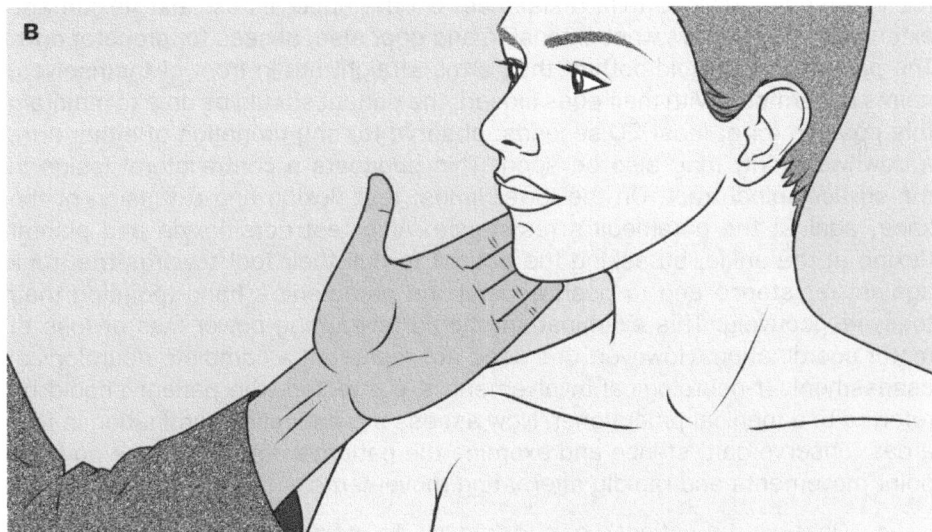

Figure 5.5 Testing of trapezius and left sternocleidmastoid muscles with 5.5a showing trapezius and 5.5b showing left sternocleidomastoid

Examination of the cranial nerves is now complete; although it may seem that there is much to do here, when practised, the entire assessment will take only a minute.

Sensory assessment

Test the patient's sensory function by applying a light touch to the skin, assessing for altered sensations bilaterally. Also assess joint position sense; both the cerebellum and the vestibular pathways need to be intact for this sensation to remain. Grasping the patient's hallux (*big toe*) at the sides, move the toe upwards and downwards; the patient (*with eyes closed*) should be able to identify what position the digit is in.

Motor assessment

Begin assessing the motor system by assessing the patient's muscle bulk and tone. Note any obvious atrophy. In their resting state, muscles should retain slight tension; this is known as resting tone. Assess tone by gently flexing and extending the elbow and knee joints, noting any increased or decreased resistance (Bickley, 2013).

Next, assess general muscle strength. This should be tested by asking the patient to move their limbs through their natural range of movement while the paramedic provides mild resistance. On the upper limbs: test flexion and extension at the elbow, wrist extension and grip. Also, assess for pronator drift. The patient should hold both of their arms straight out in front of themselves, palms uppermost. With their eyes closed, the patient should be able to maintain this position for at least 20 seconds; observe for any pronation of either arm, a downward drift may also be seen. This suggests a contra-lateral lesion in the cortico-spinal tract. On the lower limbs: test flexion and extension of the knee, against the paramedic's resistance. Also test dorsiflexion and plantar flexion at the ankle, by asking the patient to pull their foot towards the trunk against resistance and to push against the paramedic's hand (pointing their toes) respectively. This examination should reveal any power loss or loss of motor coordination. However, this does not represent a complete neurological assessment. If neurological involvement is suspected, the patient should be referred to a medical practitioner. Now assess the patient's coordination in four areas: observe gait, stance and examine the patient's ability to make point-to-point movements and rapidly alternating movements.

- Observe the patient's gait for ataxia. An ataxic gait refers to a gait which lacks coordination; this is often due to cerebellar disease. It is also seen in acute intoxication; however, this should never be the

Neurological assessment

paramedic/clinician's initial assumption. Asking the patient to walk 'heel to toe' may reveal more discrete ataxias (Bickley, 2013).
- Perform the Romberg test. Ask the patient to stand with their feet together (ensuring their safety) and close their eyes for 20–30 seconds (Bickley, 2013). In cerebellar disease, the patient will be unable to maintain their stance with eyes open and closed. In a positive Romberg test, the patient stands fine with their eyes open, but is unable to maintain their stance with eyes closed; this is due to a loss of joint position sense.
- Assess point-to-point coordination. The paramedic should hold their finger steady within easy reach of the patient and ask the patient to touch the end of this finger, followed by the patient's own nose. After a few repeats of this, ask the patient to close their eyes and continue. In the absence of cerebellar disease, these movements should be smooth and accurate. If cerebellar damage has occurred, the patient's movements may appear clumsy and inaccurate; this will worsen when the patient closes their eyes and loses the compensation of vision. Also ask the patient to run their heel from the contra-lateral knee down to the ankle; failure to complete this test accurately suggests cerebellar disease, however, inability to *find* the knee without looking is more suggestive of a loss of joint position sense.
- Examine the patient's ability to perform rapidly alternating movements; the paramedic should demonstrate slapping the back of their own hand against their own thigh, followed by swiftly turning their hand over and slapping the palm of their hand against their thigh. The patient should copy this movement and increase the speed of movement until they are performing the movements as rapidly as possible. If cerebellar disease is present, the patient will be unable to perform these movements in a swift coordinated fashion and they will appear slow and clumsy (dysdiadochokinesis); it is important to note that the dominant hand may perform better in this task and this is quite normal (Bickley, 2013).

Once the paramedic has completed the physical examination, the information can be added to that gleaned from the history and differential diagnoses considered. There are a number of common neurological complaints which the paramedic will see in practice, these are outlined below.

COMMON NEUROLOGICAL CONDITIONS

Stroke

Stroke can have an ischaemic or haemorrhagic aetiology; differentiation requires imaging and accurate diagnosis will take place in the hospital setting.

Usually there is a sudden onset to the presentation and the patient's previous medical history may reveal risk factors for emboli, such as atrial fibrillation, valvular heart disease, hypertension or diabetes mellitus.

Headache is rare in stroke; if present, it is usually severe and consistent with a haemorrhagic cause. The stroke patient will more commonly present with one or more of the following symptoms:

- Unilateral facial palsy (forehead sparing)
- Hemiparesis or hemiplegia of the limbs (*usually* contralateral to the facial palsy)
- Dysphasia/dysarthria.

If the patient remains ambulant, gait abnormalities may be observed due to hemiparesis of the lower limbs; an ataxic gait may suggest cerebellar involvement.

Vital signs

The respiration rate is usually normal; if the respiratory centre of the brainstem is affected, irregular **bradypnoea** may be seen. Hypertension is a common risk factor for stroke and can result in a full pulse. Haemorrhagic strokes can produce profoundly raised intracranial pressure; Cushing's Triad may also be seen, whereby bradycardia and hypertension are added to irregular respirations.

Assessment of the ECG results may reveal atrial fibrillation; this arrhythmia is often the cause of the embolus in ischaemic stroke. Although blood glucose is largely unaltered by stroke, hypoglycaemia must be excluded as a cause of sudden onset of neurological symptoms.

Usually the patient will present with an unaltered level of consciousness. Unconsciousness is unusual in stroke and should raise suspicions of a haemorrhagic cause.

Pupillary reaction is usually normal; ipsilateral dilatation of the pupils may be seen in severe cases. Bilaterally pinpoint pupils raise suspicions of pontine damage.

Transient ischaemic attack

The presentation of the transient ischaemic attack (TIA) patient is identical to that of an ischaemic stroke. TIA differs from stroke in that the neurological symptoms consistent with stroke syndrome completely resolve within 24 hours of onset. Many TIAs resolve within a few minutes, and dependent on their risk stratification, may not need to be seen immediately in secondary care. However, the paramedic must be diligent in assessing these patients to ensure that no continuing symptoms are missed, and that the patient is safe to be referred to a less acute pathway; TIAs are often a precursor to a completed stroke and it is essential these patients are properly assessed and referred.

> **Possible actions to be taken:**
> - Exclude hypoglycaemia as a cause of sudden onset neurological symptoms
> - Undertake a Face, Arms, Speech Test (FAST) (NCCfCC, 2008; NHS, UK, 2015b)
> - Pre-alert and transfer to a hyper-acute stroke unit.

Sub-arachnoid haemorrhage

Sub-arachnoid haemorrhage (SAH) occurs when an aneurysm ruptures, leaking blood into the arachnoid space below the arachnoid mater. SAH presents classically with sudden onset of first and worst occipital headache, often described as a thunderclap.

Additional signs and symptoms
- Nausea and vomiting
- Meningism
- Drowsiness
- Seizures
- Reduced level of consciousness or coma.

Vital signs
- If the brainstem is affected, irregular bradypnoea may be seen.
- Patients with SAH are prone to arrhythmias and may present with bradycardia, tachycardia or a normal pulse.
- ECG changes frequently occur after a SAH, including ST segment, T waves, U waves and QT prolongation (Van den Bergh et al., 2004).
- Hypertension is common, either as an existing risk factor, or as a result of raised intracranial pressure.
- The level of consciousness varies according to the severity of the haemorrhage; the patient may present with a GCS of 15/15 or may be moribund.
- Pupils may be normal; unilateral dilatation may progress to bilaterally fixed and dilated pupils as coma deepens.
- Temperature is usually normal in early presentation, though may rise over a period of days following the initial event.

Head injury

In practice, the paramedic will see both major and minor head injuries, resulting in both primary and secondary brain injuries. Primary brain injury results from the mechanism at the time of the injury. The paramedic can do little to reverse primary injuries; their focus is reducing the potential for secondary brain injury. Secondary brain injury is caused by a range of factors, many of which are preventable (Wyatt et al., 2012). The paramedic should seek to ensure that any primary survey problems are identified and corrected, this will assist in preventing secondary brain injury as a result of hypoxia, hypovolaemia (*leading to inadequate cerebral perfusion*) and seizures. The brain-injured patient is particularly sensitive to changes in pCO_2, and it is essential to ensure that when ventilating the patient, hypercapnia is avoided as this will raise intracranial pressure further (Wyatt et al., 2012).

The patient may complain of headache, of varying severity, be alert for the possibility of contra-coup patterns of injury developing. When taking a history, the paramedic should specifically ask about symptoms suggestive of intracranial pathology:

- Nausea and vomiting
- Limb weakness or abnormal sensations
- Visual disturbances.

Record a set of vital signs at an early stage, paying particular attention to the patient's mental status.

- The Glasgow Coma Score should be re-assessed frequently, decline in a GCS score of two or more points may indicate an increased inter-cranial pressure (Salomone and Pons, 2014), whereas some types of brain injury (*in particular subdural and epidural haemorrhage*) are associated with lucid intervals (Kumar and Clark, 2008).
- Bradycardia and hypertension are associated with raised intracranial pressure. As the intracranial pressure rises as a result of haemorrhage or oedema, the blood pressure must rise also to 'overcome' this and achieve cerebral perfusion. Irregular bradypnoea and Cheyne-Stokes ventilation are associated with damage to the brainstem, possibly as a result of herniation.
- Blood glucose measurement is indicated in any patient with a reduced level of consciousness and should be corrected; in the head-injured patient, prolonged hypoglycaemia can contribute to secondary brain injury.
- Pupil examination may reveal unilateral dilation and loss of reaction to light; in the head-injured patient this is a significant sign which may progress to bilaterally dilated pupils in herniation (Kumar and Clark, 2008).

Neurological assessment

Assess for evidence of facial or skull fractures and look for signs of base of skull fracture:

- Periorbital ecchymosis (*purple discoloration*)
- Bruising to the mastoid process (*Battle's sign, late sign*)
- Otorrhoea
- Rhinorrhoea.

Where appropriate, assess the remaining cranial nerves, cerebellar function and the limbs for tone, power and sensation. Cranial nerve abnormalities may reflect primary or secondary injury as a result of compression of the affected nerves. Abnormalities in the limbs may reflect primary injury, or development of raised intracranial pressure; developing widespread paralysis may reflect herniation (Kumar and Clark, 2008).

Meningitis

Meningitis is a condition which produces inflammation of the **meninges**. The patient will usually be pyrexic, with a history of malaise. Meningitis presents classically with meningism as a result of irritation to the meninges.

Signs and symptoms
- Headache
- Photophobia
- Neck stiffness
- Kernig's sign (*with the patient supine, begin with the hip and knee in 90° of flexion, when the knee is extended pain is elicited in the neck*)
- Brudzinski's sign (*passive neck flexion produces an involuntary flexion of the hip*)
- Raised fontenelle in infants (see *Figure 11.1, Child assessment, Chapter 11*)
- Severe cases, opisthotonus (*tetanic spasm causing hyperextension of the back, see Figure 5.3*)

Signs of raised intracranial pressure may also be seen:

- Headache, often severe
- Reduced level of consciousness
- Irregular respirations/bradypnoea
- Bradycardia
- Hypertension.

If septicaemia complicates meningitis, classic findings can be a very late, potentially pre-terminal sign:

- Rash, classically a non-blanching, petechial rash
- Macular rash may be seen in the early stages.

As the patient deteriorates, profound shock may occur and tachycardia, hypotension, seizures and coma may be seen.

- Pulse oximetry may be reduced, reflecting poor perfusion of the extremities in developing shock.

Patients with neurological signs on presentation have a 50%–90% mortality rate (Tidy and Knott, 2014). It is essential to remember that the classic signs of neck stiffness and non-blanching rash are usually absent in the early stages. Where meningitis is suspected, particularly in a paediatric patient, look for the following signs (Thompson et al., 2006):

- Cold hands and feet (despite fever)
- Abnormal skin colour
- Leg pain.

Possible actions to be taken:

- Be alert!
- Meningitis is a time critical emergency
- Presentation may be deceptively mild
- In children or young people with suspected or confirmed bacterial meningitis or meningococcal septicaemia, their temperature, respiratory rate, pulse, blood pressure, urine output, oxygen saturation and neurological condition should be monitored at least hourly until stable (NICE, 2010).

Seizures

Seizures are a common presentation in pre-hospital care, and are often associated with epilepsy. However, there are many causes of seizure activity beyond epilepsy and seizures can herald serious neurological pathology. The paramedic should also consider, and if possible reverse, the following causes:

- Hypoxia
- Hypoglycaemia
- Electrolyte imbalance
- Eclampsia
- Intracranial pathology such as brain injury
- Poisoning
- Pyrexia
- Psychogenic causes.

Although there are several classifications of seizure, the tonic clonic seizure is the most common presentation to the paramedic and requires prompt identification and management. Prolonged tonic clonic seizures are associated with hypoxia and neuronal damage; seizures lasting longer than 30 minutes or multiple seizures with incomplete recovery over 30 minutes are classified as status epilepticus and represent a serious emergency (Reiser, 2011).

A tonic clonic seizure is associated with loss of consciousness, followed by a brief tonic phase. During this tonic phase the body's muscles contract firmly for a few seconds before the clonic phase begins. During the clonic phase, rhythmical and often violent muscular contractions occur throughout the musculoskeletal system, although due to the underdeveloped musculature of the paediatric patient, clonic activity can be more discrete in children. The length of the clonic phase is variable, and dependent on the pathology of the seizure. Often the patient will bite their tongue and become incontinent during the seizure, although a lack of these finding does not in itself preclude a seizure.

Vital signs
- Effectiveness of ventilation is reduced although accurate assessment is extremely difficult in a patient exhibiting clonic activity.
- Cyanosis is common.
- SpO_2 will be reduced.
- Hypoxia may lead to tachycardia.
- Blood glucose levels may be lowered; glycogen reserves may be depleted during prolonged seizure activity or represent the cause of the fit.
- Pupils are unresponsive during tonic clonic activity.

During a tonic clonic seizure, the patient will be unresponsive to stimuli; after cessation of the fit, it is common for the patient to exhibit confusion and a reduced level of consciousness for some time; this is known as the post-ictal period. In all cases of seizure, once the patient has been stabilized, the paramedic should endeavour to discover the cause of the ictus, as well as examine the patient for injuries which may have been caused by a fall or accident during the tonic phase, or injuries caused by violent muscular contractions themselves.

Possible actions to be taken:
- Protect patient from injury
- Assess and manage hypoxia and hypoglycaemia accordingly
- Pre-alert and transfer to hospital as appropriate.

Impressions

It will not always be possible, or appropriate, to come to a diagnosis in pre-hospital care. However, the paramedic should use their history and examination skills to produce an impression of the patient's conditions. Try to include the patient's circumstances in this impression; it should reflect more than a list of differential diagnoses. There are many conditions which can be managed at home, however, the paramedic may feel that this is inappropriate and this should be recorded in the impression; for example, the patient who presents with a minor head injury may have the added complication of living alone, and may be a reason to admit to emergency department for observation.

OTHER CONSIDERATIONS

Communication

Many neurological disorders present with communication difficulties. Some patients will have difficulty making themselves understood and may also have cognitive difficulties affecting their ability to understand the paramedic. The paramedic should recognize this and tailor their communication accordingly, avoiding complex terms and seeking to communicate with the patient in the language they are most comfortable with at the time; for example, some neurological patients may have been speaking fluent English as a second language for decades, but after a stroke may communicate better in their first language. The paramedic should also recognize the emotional impact that communication problems may have on the patient and approach communication in a patient and conscientious manner.

Social/family/carer/guardian

Consider the patient's social support needs; many neurological patients will need support when discharged and the paramedic should evaluate any obvious need for formal assessment and referral to social support agencies. In particular, conditions such as minor head injury and epilepsy, where early discharge from hospital, or even out-of-hospital care, are common, the availability of support at home can be a defining factor in the safety of such discharges, as can the structure of the home environment when considering discharge of the neurologically impaired patient.

Ethical and legal

Where consciousness is impaired, capacity issues immediately come to the fore. The paramedic should be careful to assess the patient who is thought to lack capacity in line with the Mental Capacity Act 2005 (Department of Health,

2005) (see Mental Health Assessmet: Chapter 15) and ensure that they act in the best interests of the patient. In the case of the unconscious patient, the doctrine of necessity usually provides that paramedics will act in the best interests of the patient, and effect any treatments deemed necessary by the paramedic to sustain life. This doctrine would only normally be overridden where a valid advance decision exists pertaining to life-sustaining care or where the patient has nominated a lasting power of attorney (personal welfare) under the Act, and their capabilities extend to making such decisions. Many patients with degenerative neurological conditions will make such advance plans; the paramedic has a responsibility to familiarize themselves with such points of law and adhere to them where appropriate.

Destination/receiving specialist units/non-conveyance

Conveyance to the emergency department is usually the default for the neurological patient. In some cases, patients presenting with minor neurological complaints, such as minor head injury or symptoms consistent with an ongoing problem (such as epilepsy) may not benefit from attendance at the emergency department. In such cases the paramedic must make a full assessment of the patient before making this decision. Paramedics should feel the weight of responsibility in discharging patients from their care and ensure any decisions not to convey are safe and robustly made. If any doubt exists, seek assistance from, or consider referring the patient to a specialist and/or advanced paramedic. Any decision not to convey a patient must reflect any national standards set, such as the National Institute for Health and Care Excellence (NICE) *Head Injury-Triage, Assessment, Investigation and Early Management of Head Injury in Children, Young People and Adults* (NICE, 2014). Many hospitals are now providing specialist services for some neurological conditions, such as head injury and stroke. Refer to local and national guidance for more information.

Professional

The neurological patient is often a vulnerable patient. The paramedic should in particular ensure that they meet their professional obligation to act in the best interests of service users. As previously discussed, the extent of the neurological evaluation included in this chapter does not reflect the complete assessment required by many neurological patients; the paramedic must therefore honour their professional obligation to ensure they do not exceed their scope of practice and make referrals where appropriate.

Facts and figures

In the UK, every year there are approximately 152,000 strokes, which equates to one stroke every three and a half minutes. Most people affected are over

65, but anyone can have a stroke, including children and even babies (Stroke Association, 2015). Thus, stroke is a common presentation to the paramedic and prompt recognition of stroke syndrome in the out-of-hospital environment contributes to reducing mortality and morbidity from this condition; remember time is brain. As a leading cause of mortality and morbidity, the paramedic should be alert to this potential diagnosis and act quickly to admit the patient.

CHAPTER KEY POINTS

- When assessing the neurological patient; be systematic and thorough.
- Ensure primary survey problems are identified, managed and reviewed.
- **DO NOT** expect everything to be obvious – serious pathology can be subtle.
- Ensure patients are referred appropriately.

REFERENCES

Association of Ambulance Chief Executives (2013a) *UK Ambulance Services Clinical Practice Guidelines 2013 Pocket Book: Chemical, Biological, Radiological, Nuclear and Explosive Incidents*. Bridgwater: Class Professional Publishing.

Association of Ambulance Chief Executives (2013b) *UK Ambulance Services Clinical Practice Guidelines 2013 Pocket Book: Airway and Breathing Management*. Bridgwater: Class Professional Publishing.

Association of Ambulance Chief Executives (2013c) *UK Ambulance Services Clinical Practice Guidelines 2013 Pocket Book: Pain Assessment Model*. Bridgwater: Class Professional Publishing.

Association of Ambulance Chief Executives (2013d) *UK Ambulance Services Clinical Practice Guidelines 2013 Pocket Book: Glasgow Coma Scale*. Bridgwater: Class Professional Publishing.

Bickley, L.S. (2013) *Bates' Pocket Guide to Physical Examination and History Taking* (7th edn). Philadelphia, PA: Lippincott Williams & Wilkins.

Department of Health (2005) *Mental Capacity Act*. London: The Stationery Office.

Fuller, G. (2013) *Neurological Examination Made Easy* (5th edn). London: Churchill Livingstone Elsevier.

Guly, H.R., Bouamra, O. and Lecky, F.E. (2007) The incidence of neurogenic shock in patients with isolated spinal cord injury in the emergency department. *Resuscitation* 76: 57–62.

Hodkinson, H.M. (1972) Evaluation of a mental test score for assessment of mental impairment in the elderly. *Age and Ageing* 1(4): 233–8. Available at: http://www.patient.co.uk/doctor/abbreviated-mental-test-amt (accessed 21 February 2015).

Jenkins G.W. and Tortora, G.J. (2013) *Anatomy and Physiology from Science to Life* (3rd edn). International Student Version. Hoboken, NJ: John Wiley & Sons, Inc.

Kumar, P. and Clark, M. (eds) (2008) Neurology. In Ballinger, A. and Patchett, S. (eds) *Pocket Essentials of Clinical Medicine* (4th edn). Edinburgh: Saunders Elsevier.

NCCfCC (National Collaborating Centre for Chronic Conditions) (2008) *Stroke: National Clinical Guideline for Diagnosis and Initial Management of Acute Stroke and Transient Ischaemic Attack (TIA)*. London: Royal College of Physicians.

NHS UK (2015a) *Symptoms of Guillian-Barré Syndrome*. Available at: http://www.nhs.uk/Conditions/Guillain-Barre-syndrome/Pages/Symptoms.aspx (accessed 18 February 2015).

NHS UK (2015b) *Stroke – Act F.A.S.T.* Available at: http://www.nhs.uk/actfast/Pages/stroke.aspx (accessed 19 February 2015).

NICE (National Institute for Health and Care Excellence) (2010) *Bacterial Meningitis and Meningococcal Septicaemia: Management of Bacterial Meningitis and Meningococcal Septicaemia in Children and Young People Younger Than 16 Years in Primary and Secondary Care*. NICE clinical guideline 102. Available at: http://www.nice.org.uk/guidance/CG102 (accessed 21 February 2015).

NICE (National Institute for Health and Care Excellence) (2014) *Head Injury: Triage, Assessment, Investigation and Early Management of Head Injury in Children, Young People and Adults.* NICE clinical guideline 176. Available at: http://www.nice.org.uk/guidance/cg176 (accessed 21 February 2015).

Palande, L. (2011) *Pontine Stroke*. Available at: http://www.buzzle.com/articles/pontine-stroke.html (accessed 19 February 2015).

Reiser, R.C. (2011) Seizures. In Aghababian R.B. (ed.) *Essentials of Emergency Medicine* (2nd edn). Sudbury: Jones & Bartlett Learning.

Salomone, J.P. and Pons, P.T. (2014) *Pre-Hospital Trauma Life Support (PHTLS)* (8th edn). Maryland Heights, MO: Mosby Elsevier.

Stroke Association (2015) *About Stroke*. Available at: http://www.stroke.org.uk/about-stroke (accessed 21 February 2015).

Thompson, M.J., Ninis, N., Perera, R., Mayon-White, R., Phillips, C., Bailey, L., Harnden, A., Mant, D., and Levin, M. (2006) Clinical recognition of meningococcal disease in children and adolescents. *The Lancet* 367(9508): 397–403.

Tidy, C. and Knott, L. (2014) Meningitis. Available at: http://www.patient.co.uk/doctor/Meningitis.htm (accessed 30 November 2014).

Van den Bergh, W.M., Algra, A. and Rinkel, G.J.E. (2004) Electrocardiographic abnormalities and serum magnesium in patients with subarachnoid hemorrhage. *Stroke* 35: 644–8. Available at: http://stroke.ahajournals.org/content (accessed 21 February 2015).

Wyatt, J.P., Illingworth, R.N., Clancy, M. J., Munro, P.T. and Robertson, C.E. (2012) *Oxford Handbook of Accident & Emergency Medicine* (4th edn). Oxford: Oxford University Press.

Useful websites

http://www.elu.sgul.ac.uk/cso/
SGUL Physical Examination Videos
http://www.epilepsy.org.uk
The British Epilepsy Association
http://www.evidence.nhs.uk/topic/stroke
NHS Evidence: Stroke
http://www.gbs.org.uk

Guillain-Barré Syndrome Group (past patients offer visiting and counselling services)
http://www.mssociety.org.uk
The Multiple Sclerosis Society
http://www.parkinsons.org.uk
Parkinson's Disease Society
http://www.patient.co.uk/patientplus
Provides well-referenced articles on many conditions and injuries. It is free of charge with no registration necessary.
http://www.stroke.org.uk
The Stroke Association (UK) (information resource for patients and health care professionals)
http://www.theabn.org/public/patientcarer.php
Lists all the individual websites for patients and carers with various neurological conditions.
https://www.youtube.com/playlist?list=PLGESeMFkgqnxC3Yvkgq7_sdfUszaRvlpr
McLeod's Clinical Assessment Videos

6 Spinal injuries assessment
Nigel Ward

This chapter will discuss the considerations given by the paramedic when presented with a patient with possible spinal injuries. It is estimated that the incidence of spinal cord injury in the UK is between 12 and 16 per million, the majority of which are caused by trauma (NHS England, 2015).

SCENE ASSESSMENT

The existence of possible spinal injuries may be suspected by the paramedic even before a primary survey is possible. Initial information regarding mechanism of injury and the history of events is often available before arrival at the scene of an incident. In addition, the scene presented on arrival, including both position and location of the patient, can provide evidence of actual or potential spinal injuries.

Remember, spinal injuries are not only caused by road traffic collisions (RTCs). Damage to vertebrae and the spinal cord can result from other trauma and major causes of spinal injury and include sports injuries, shallow water incidents, motorcycle crashes and falls from height. It is worth noting that around 20% of falls from height greater than 15 feet (4.57 metres) will result in an associated lumbar spine fracture (Salomone and Pons, 2014).

PRIMARY SURVEY

Particular attention should be paid to the methods of assessing and maintaining a patent airway in patients with suspected cervical spine injuries ('C' spine). The paramedic should understand that if they assess and subsequently manage the patient's C spine incorrectly, it has the potential to cause spinal cord injury (SCI).

At the time of publication, the National Institute for Health and Clinical Excellence (NICE) has commissioned the National Clinical Guideline Centre (NCGC) to develop trauma guidance on spinal injury assessment and this is due for publication in February 2016 (NICE, 2016).

DANGER

Danger considerations will vary greatly depending on the mechanism of injury and the location of any traumatic injury. On arrival at the scene, the paramedic should liaise with other emergency services present; if not already on scene and required, then they should request their attendance, via emergency operations control. Full personal protective equipment (PPE) should be worn.

When attending incidents on building and other industrial sites and railways, the paramedic will be subject to, and must comply with, health and safety legislation specific to those sites (Health and Safety at Work Act 1974, part 1, section 7) (Legislation.gov.uk, 2015). It is worth noting that under CIMAH (Control of Industrial Major Accident Hazards) regulations, emergency planning on industrial sites is the responsibility of local Fire and Civil Defence Associations and that rendezvous points (RVPs) will be pre-designated (Health and Safety Executive, 1999).

When attending potential spinal injury incidents, the paramedic should consider the cause(s) of the injury when assessing the risk of danger to self, colleagues and others at the scene. Possible sources of danger to the paramedic include (but are not limited to):

- Traffic and moving motor vehicles
- Fire and chemical hazards
- Falling objects from above
- Unstable or unsecured machinery or vehicles
- Unsafe walls and ceilings
- Assailants on scene
- Incidents that have occurred in water (diving).

Possible actions to be taken:
- Wear personal protective equipment (PPE)
- Request fire/police service assistance
- Request Hazardous Area Response Team (HART) or Special Operations Response Team (SORT)
- Ensure the safety of others at the scene.

RESPONSE

Ordinarily, the approach to a patient would include an assessment of their response to verbal commands and questions. A conscious patient would, naturally, turn their head and face a paramedic initiating contact verbally. For this reason a patient with suspected spinal injury should, whenever possible, be approached

Spinal injuries assessment

from the front. Ideally this assessment will be undertaken by two personnel, the paramedic and colleague, the former will make direct eye contact with the patient and tell the patient to 'look at me', while the second will then undertake the appropriate stabilization/neutral alignment of the 'C' spine. Bring the patient's neck into the neutral inline position. If there is any increased pain or neurological deficit or if there is resistance to movement, this procedure should be ceased and the patient maintained in the position they are in (Trauma.org, 2002). A brief explanation can now be given describing what assessment will follow.

Possible actions to be taken:

- Approach the patient from the front
- Explain your actions clearly and concisely
- Obtain and maintain neutral alignment
- Assess and record the patient's level of consciousness (AVPU).

AIRWAY

The airway should be assessed and, if not already patent, should be opened and assessed for patency. The paramedic has the responsibility of recognizing the potential for spinal injury from the initial scene assessment and the need to employ the appropriate 'C' spine method of airway management (see Figure 6.1).

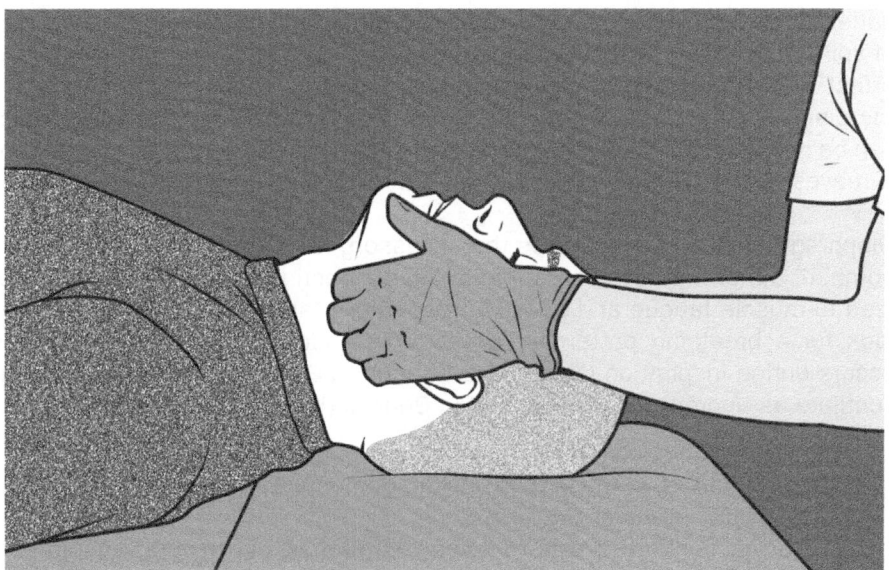

Figure 6.1 Jaw thrust manoeuvre

Studies have shown that between 3% and 25% of spinal injuries are exacerbated by excessive and unnecessary movement of the patient within the emergency department (Banit et al., 2000). This may be reduced if the paramedic instigates the correct handling of the patient at the onset of treatment before arrival at the trauma unit.

Movement should be minimal as any pressure on the spinal cord from misaligned or fractured vertebrae may cause neurological damage. In order to avoid this, the initial airway management is manual but may be assisted later, by oropharyngeal airway, supra-glottic airways or **endotracheal tube (ETT)** if required (Salomone and Pons, 2014).

> **Possible actions to be taken:**
> - Recognize the possibility of 'C' spinal injury, use the jaw thrust manoeuvre
> - Stepwise airway management as appropriate (see *Respiratory Assessment, Chapter 2*)
> - Ensure airway is patent before proceeding to next element.

BREATHING

When assessing the patient's breathing, the first concern should be 'is the patient breathing?' Poor or inadequate breathing may, in itself, be as a result of spinal cord injury (SCI). Damage to the spinal cord above C5 will have a direct effect on the mechanism of respiration caused by weakness or paralysis of the diaphragm, and usually require mechanical ventilation. Their vital capacity can be reduced to 10%–20% of normal, with either weak or ineffective coughing (Greaves et al., 2008).

Diaphragmatic paralysis causes the accessory respiratory muscles to take up some, or all, of the work of respiration by contracting more intensely. This can lead to muscle fatigue and possibly respiratory failure. The paramedic should look for a breathing pattern of paradoxical abdominal wall retraction which occurs during inspiration (Nader and Shahriar, 2009). If the patient is **apneic**, ventilate as appropriate (Resuscitation Council (UK), 2010).

- Inadequate ventilations (rate <12 per minute) should be assisted using bag valve mask (BVM) with additional oxygen therapy to maintain SpO_2 levels at 94%–98%.
- Normal ventilation rate (between 12 and 20 per minute) should be monitored and oxygen therapy considered in the case of the trauma patient.

- Fast ventilations (20–30 per minute) should also be monitored. The cause of increased respiration is increasing levels of carbon dioxide or reducing levels of oxygen in the blood. This should be addressed with oxygen therapy at high levels.
- Abnormally fast ventilations (above 30 per minute) may be a result of hypoxia and oxygen therapy at high levels should be commenced. It may be necessary for the paramedic to assist ventilation using BVM and to find and reverse the cause of increased respiration (Salomone and Pons, 2014).

NB: *The above breathing rates are based on an adult patient. Adjustments should be made when dealing with infants and children.*

Possible actions to be taken:
- Assess breathing rate and function
- Ventilate apnoeic patients or those who have weak or diaphragmatic breathing as appropriate
- Administer oxygen accordingly (British Thoracic Society, 2015)
- Assist inadequate ventilations, too fast as well as too slow
- Manage and reverse the causes of hypoxia
- Transfer to appropriate trauma unit.

CIRCULATION

- Control any obvious external haemorrhaging. Nearly 80% of patients with spinal injury have multiple injuries. Symptoms of shock should not be attributed to the spinal injury until all haemorrhaging has been excluded (Greaves et al., 2008) (see *Trauma Assessment: Chapter 7*).
- Assess the colour and general appearance of the skin. Vasoconstriction and poor peripheral circulation can provide an idea of the perfusion of vital organs. A conscious patient who is clearly cerebrally perfused with warm normal skin implies that the patient is not in shock. However, the opposite can also be the case.
- Assess blood pressure and if the patient is hypotensive (*systolic <90 mmHg*), implement correction management.
- Injury at or above thoracic (T6) can lead to considerable loss of sympathetic autonomic control. This results in hypotension and bradycardia due to heightened vagal responses. (*In effect, the 'accelerator' is not functioning and only the 'brakes' work.*) Peripheral vasodilation, hypotension and bradycardia caused

by the disruption of sympathetic nervous control are termed 'neurogenic shock'. However, hypovolaemia must be excluded before you attribute the cause of the hypotension to 'neurogenic shock' (Greaves et al., 2008).

Possible actions to be taken:
- Control external haemorrhage
- Monitor and record capillary bed refill and pulses
- Assess appearance and temperature/colour of skin
- If hypotensive, assess and exclude hypovolaemia as the cause
- Treat shock due to hypovolaemia in order to prevent secondary injury from hypoperfusion (see *Trauma Assessment: Chapter 7*).

DISABILITY

Symptoms of spinal cord injury can vary, depending on the location and severity of the injury. Full dissection will result in complete loss of function but in the case of a partial dissection some motor or sensory function may be retained. Injury to the neck will affect the arms, legs and torso, and thoracic (*chest level*) injuries will affect the legs. The spinal cord does not go beyond the first lumbar vertebra, so injuries below this point are not spinal cord injury, but may cause 'cauda equina syndrome' which is damage to the nerve roots in this region.

- Assess neurological symptoms by asking the patient if they are experiencing any loss of feeling or movement. The paramedic should assess and observe the patient's breathing, numbness or sensory changes, increased muscle tone, pain and limb weakness, and in the unconscious patient assess for any loss of bowel control (Zieve and Hoch, 2010).
- Assess the patient's level of consciousness (AVPU).
- Assess the blood glucose levels.
- Assess the patient's pupils (PERRLA).
- Abnormal posturing may be observed and is a sign of serious damage to the central nervous system. The following may be seen:
  - **decerebrate posture** – rigid **extension** of the arms and legs, downward pointing of the toes, and backward arching of the head (see *Neurological Assessment, Chapter 5*), or
  - **decorticate posture** – rigidity, **flexion** of the arms, clenched fists, and extended legs (see *Neurological Assessment, Chapter 5*).

Possible actions to be taken:

- Assess and document LOC (AVPU)
- Assess and document blood glucose levels, and neurological symptoms
- Assess and document size and equality of pupils (PERRLA)
- Note abnormal postures (decerebrate/decorticate).

EXPOSE/ENVIRONMENT/EVALUATE

- Continued patient assessment requires the paramedic to expose and examine the injured patient by removing clothing or other materials covering the body. This should be performed with reference to previous findings to establish an evaluation of the patient's condition and ongoing prognosis.
- How much, or how little, to remove is a decision based on the environment and the ongoing findings. Remove as much as is necessary to ascertain either the presence or absence of injuries. While patient modesty is a consideration, it should not interfere with an examination. Consent must, however, be obtained (Department of Health, 2009).
- Look for pre-existing injuries or injuries which might have caused subsequent trauma. For example, an assault may have led to a fall from height in the patient's attempts to flee their assailant. A thorough examination after a relatively minor fall may lead to the discovery of a penetrating injury.
- Be aware of the patient's modesty and also the risk of hypothermia. Cover the patient with blankets during and after the examination and evaluation process (Salomone and Pons, 2014).
- Examine the patient with an open mind and be prepared to find the unexpected injury. If you don't look, you won't find. (*Complete a head-to-toe examination as part of the secondary survey.*)

Possible actions to be taken:

- Expose, Examine, Evaluate
- DO NOT be blinkered, keep an open mind
- Consider dignity and hypothermia, blankets are an important part of patient assessment
- Transfer the patient to the appropriate trauma unit.

SECONDARY SURVEY

Having completed a primary survey and documented the observations a secondary survey is initiated to ascertain if the patient requires spinal immobilization. This involves a head-to-toe examination (see Trauma Assessment: Chapter 7) which includes every side of the patient, top, bottom, back, front and the left and right (Greaves et al., 2008). This will enable the paramedic to gather more detailed information about the patient's condition and ascertain what happened to cause the injury. Ascertain and confirm if the patient has any of the following:

- Decreased level of consciousness or is unable to cooperate fully with the examination.
- Is under the influence of alcohol or drugs (*including illicit or prescribed*).
- Complains of spinal pain (*tenderness isolated to muscles of the side of the neck is not spinal pain*).
- Vertebral tenderness or deformity on palpation.
- Neurologic deficit.
- Painful or distracting injuries (AACE, 2013a).

After undertaking this and evaluating the appropriate information, the paramedic will be able to decide whether or not to proceed to immobilization of the patient.

Presenting complaint

- What is the mechanism of injury? Is the patient in pain? Where is the pain? The presence of pain to the spinal region is a clear indicator of the possibility of spinal injury. However, the lack of pain to the spine should not rule out injury until it has been established that pain is not being masked by pain from another injury. Assess the pain using the SOCRATES framework (AACE, 2013b).
- Is the patient able to move their limbs individually?
- Does this cause further pain?
- Are there any abnormal sensations in the limbs or trunk?
- The nervous system is so complex and the range of symptoms associated with spinal cord injury or damage so varied that any unusual sensory or motor sensation should be taken seriously (Greaves et al., 2008).

History of presenting complaint

The exact history of the injury is important when assessing the patient with a spinal injury and deciding whether or not to fully immobilize them. The paramedic should assess each patient with an open mind: there are some

Spinal injuries assessment

dangerous mechanisms of injury which require an X-ray or a CT scan to exclude spinal injury in patients with head or neck pain. These are:

- a fall from height greater than 5 metres (or two to three times the patient's height)
- a fall down five stairs or more
- impact to the head causing axial load to the spine, e.g. rugby scrum or diving into shallow water
- motor vehicle collision with high speed impact, roll-over or ejection of the passenger; a motor cycle and bicycle collision; collision involving recreational vehicles (quad bikes, etc.)
- impact from behind by bus, lorry or high speed vehicle or shunt into oncoming, moving traffic (Wardrope et al., 2004).

Past medical history

The past medical history (PMH) of the patient may have a bearing on their treatment and could provide valuable clues to the history of the presenting complaint in the confused or concussed patient. It can also lead the paramedic to suspect alternative events to those being described and expand the range of observations in their secondary survey.

- What predisposing medical conditions does the patient have?
- Diabetic patients may need a glucose challenge to correct hypoglycaemia. Indeed, a hypoglycaemic episode may have been the cause of the initial trauma.
- Cardiac patients who may initially have had some chest pain may be distracted from this fact by overriding pain from impact injuries. It is worth considering if an arrhythmia may have led to a loss of consciousness and, subsequently, to the resultant mechanism of injury.

Possible actions to be taken:

- Undertake a full assessment and history
- Immobilize the patient appropriately
- Obtain information regarding the PMH and predisposing illnesses
- Ascertain if the patient has diabetes
- Be thorough in patient observations and only make exclusions with evidence
- Transfer to an appropriate trauma unit.

Drug/medication history

The patient may have taken/ingested alcohol or drugs that may reduce or mask the patient's perception of pain. Ascertain if the patient has other conditions for which they take medications, or if they have any allergies to any drugs.

OTHER CONSIDERATIONS

Patient-specific factors may indicate a higher level of risk of spinal injury. Older adults over the age of 65 and those suffering from bone disorders such as osteoporosis, ankylosing spondylitis and rheumatoid arthritis are among these (Wardrope et al., 2004).

An older patient who has fallen may be unable to distinguish between old and new neck pain. Older patients may also find it difficult to recall or describe a mechanism of injury, especially those with dementia. If there is any doubt, the patient should be immobilized and transported to hospital. Some older people develop kyphosis, a spinal curvature, and it may be impossible to immobilize them and apply a cervical collar. In such cases, the patient's head should not be forced into a neutral alignment. The patient should be made comfortable using blankets and other padding. Confusion may make spinal immobilization distressing for patients and it may be appropriate to loosen belts and head blocks in order to minimize movement in the patient, remember to reassure them. Spinal injury or SCI should not be excluded in an intoxicated patient with a significant mechanism of injury (Clubb, 2007).

Communication

If communication barriers prevent reliable response to direct questioning and there is a significant mechanism of injury, the patient should be treated for spinal injury until this can be excluded. Consider assistance from translator services if necessary and if locally available.

Ethical and legal

In some cases of spinal trauma, the police will be attempting to obtain statements from patients. The paramedic's first responsibility is to the patient and their priority is to assess and immobilize the patient. Police may travel with the patient as this provides a continuity of evidence should there be any criminal proceedings as the result of the injuries sustained.

Destination/receiving specialist units

A patient not in cardiac arrest should be conveyed to an appropriate trauma centre, depending on local guidelines. The first regional trauma centre was introduced in London in 2010, followed by the regional network of trauma centres, which have now established research in trauma systems (Trauma Audit and Research Network, 2015).

Facts and figures

Over 40,000 people in the UK and around 270.000 people in the United States are affected by spinal cord injury. Road traffic collisions (account for 37% of these cases with other causes including falls (29%), sports injuries (9%) and violence (14%). Nearly half of all patients are between 16 and 30 years old and 81% are male (*British Medical Journal*, 2015).

CHAPTER KEY POINTS

- When undertaking the assessment of a patient with suspected spinal injury, be systematic and thorough.
- Ensure primary survey problems are identified, managed and reviewed.
- Examine the patient with an open mind and be prepared to find the unexpected injury, remember that the range of symptoms associated with spinal cord damage is so varied that any unusual sensory or motor sensation should be taken seriously.
- Ensure patients are referred to the appropriate trauma unit.

REFERENCES

Association of Ambulance Chief Executives (2013a) *UK Ambulance Services Clinical Practice Guidelines 2013 Pocket Book: Neck and Back Trauma – Immobilisation Algorithm*. Bridgwater: Class Professional Publishing.

Association of Ambulance Chief Executives (2013b) *UK Ambulance Services Clinical Practice Guidelines 2013 Pocket Book: Pain Assessment Model*. Bridgwater: Class Professional Publishing.

Banit, D.M., Grau, G. and Fisher, J.R. (2000) Evaluation of the acute cervical spine: a management algorithm. *Journal of Trauma-Injury Infection & Critical Care*, 49(3): 450–6.

British Medical Journal (2015) *Best Practice: Chronic Spinal Cord Injury*. Available at: http://bestpractice.bmj.com/bestpractice/monograph/1176/basics/epidemiology.html (accessed 27 February 2015.)

British Thoracic Society (2015) *Emergency Oxygen Use in Adult Patients Guideline*. Available at: https://www.brit-thoracic.org.uk/searchresults/?txtSearch=2015+Oxygen+Guidelines&search= (accessed 27 February 2015).

Clubb, R. (2007) Delayed diagnosis of a patient with cervical spine injury resulting in complete cervical spine dislocation without serious or lingering neurological signs: a case report. *The Internet Journal of Emergency Medicine*, 4(1). Available at: https://ispub.com/IJEM/4/1/6391 (accessed 27 February 2015).

Department of Health (2009) *Reference Guide to Consent for Examination or Treatment* (2nd edn). London: Department of Health.

Greaves, I., Porter, K. and Garner, J. (eds) (2008) *Trauma Care Manual* (2nd edn). Boca Raton, FL: Hodder Arnold.

Health and Safety Executive (1999) *Control of Major Accident Hazards Regulations*. Available at: http://www.hse.gov.uk/comah/background/consultcomments.htm (accessed 27 February 2015).

Legislation.gov.uk (2015) *Health and Safety at Work Act etc 1974*. Available at: http://www.legislation.gov.uk/ukpga/1974/37 (accessed 10 May 2015).

Nader, K. and Shahriar, P. (2009) *Diaphragmatic Paralysis*. Available at: http://emedicine.medscape.com/article/298200-overview (accessed 27 February 2015).

National Health Service (NHS) England (2015) *Spinal Cord Injury*. Available at: http://www.england.nhs.uk/commissioning/spec-services/npc-crg/group-d/d13/ (accessed 25 February 2015).

NICE (National Institute for Health and Clinical Excellence) (2016) *Spinal Injury Assessment: Assessment and Imaging, and Early Management for Spinal Injury (Spinal Column or Spinal Cord Injury)*. Available at: https://www.nice.org.uk/guidance/indevelopment/gid-cgwave0645 (accessed 10 May 2015).

Resuscitation Council (UK) (2010) *Resuscitation Guidelines*. Available at: http://www.resus.org.uk/pages/GL2010.pdf (accessed 27 February 2015).

Salomone, J.P. and Pons, P.T. (2014) *Pre-Hospital Trauma Life Support* (PHTLS) (8th edn). Maryland Heights, MO: Mosby Elsevier.

The Trauma Audit and Research Network (TARN) (2015) *Newsletter: Research in Trauma Systems*. Available at: https://www.tarn.ac.uk (accessed 11 May 2015).

Trauma.org. (2002) *Initial Assessment of Spinal Injury*. Available at: http://www.trauma.org/index.php/main/article/380/ (accessed 27 February 2015).

Wardrope, J., Ravichandran, G. and Locker, T. (BMJ.com) (2004) *Risk Assessment for Spinal Injury After Trauma*. Available at: http://www.bmj.com/cgi/content/full/328/7442/721 (accessed 27 February 2015).

Zieve, D. and Hoch, D.B. (2010) *Spinal Cord Trauma*. Available at: http://www.nlm.nih.gov/medlineplus/ency/article/001066.htm (accessed 27 February 2015).

7 Trauma assessment
Stuart Elms and Graham Harris

Trauma is the acute physiological and structural change that occurs in a patient's body when an external source of energy dissipates faster than the body's ability to sustain and dissipate it (Pilbery, 2014). *Major trauma* is seen as the most common cause of loss of life under 40 years of age, and by 2020 on a global perspective through life years lost will be the second place with regards to premature death and disability (Trauma Audit & Research Network (TARN), 2015a).

In 2010, the National Audit Office (NAO) identified that in England alone there were approximately 20,000 incidents of major trauma, of which 5,400 resulted in death or permanent disabilities (NAO, 2010). The commonest cause of death is due to road traffic collision (RTC). The NAO advised that there are around a further 28,000 cases which do not meet the precise definition of major trauma, but still require to be cared for in the same way. Later that year NHS England introduced the first regional trauma centre in London, followed by regional trauma centres and systems throughout England (NHS England, 2010). In 2014, the Chief Executive for NHS England applauded 'a major NHS success story', after TARN published data which demonstrated a 20%–40% in case mix adjusted odds of survival for major trauma in 2013/14 with statistically significant improvement trends (TARN, 2015b).

The aim of this chapter is to provide the paramedic with a structured systematic approach to the assessment of the patient who has sustained trauma, resulting in multiple injuries which potentially could affect one or more bodily systems.

SCENE ASSESSMENT

As you approach the scene take a 'global overview' in order to ascertain the mechanism of injury (MOI) and the potential cause of the trauma. Using the acronym **SCENE** will provide the paramedic with a structured assessment (AACE, 2013a):

- **S – Safety** (perform a dynamic risk assessment)
- **C – Cause including MOI** (establish events leading up to the incident)
- **E – Environment** (any environmental factors that should be considered)
- **N – Number of patients** (how many patients are at the scene)
- **E – Extra resources needed** (request additional resources immediately)

Trauma may have occurred due to one or more of the following reasons:

mechanical	moving vehicle, fall from height
chemical	acid burns or ingested agents
thermal	burns – wet or dry, frostbite
electrical	high voltage electrocution
barometric	sudden pressure changes – explosions

When determining the cause of trauma and the MOI, first consider what form of energy was involved and its magnitude, as each variable produces differing patterns of injury and therefore dictates different management considerations. The energy transfer that the patient is subjected to will result in either or both of these types of trauma – blunt or penetrating:

- *blunt trauma*: where the tissues are not penetrated by an external object (bruising caused by a seat belt during sudden deceleration)
- *penetrating trauma*: where the tissues are penetrated by an external object (gunshot wound (GSW), stabbing or an impaled object).

PRIMARY SURVEY

At the time of publication the National Institute for Health and Clinical Excellence (NICE) has commissioned the National Clinical Guideline Centre (NCGC) to develop five separate pieces of guidance on trauma, and these are due for publication in February 2016, and include the following:

- Complex fractures: assessment and management of complex fractures (including pelvic fractures and open fractures of limbs)
- Fractures: diagnosis, management and follow-up of fractures (excluding head and hip, pelvis, open and spinal)
- Major trauma: assessment and management of airway, breathing and ventilation, circulation, haemorrhage and temperature control
- Spinal injury assessment: assessment and imaging, and early management for spinal injury (spinal column or spinal cord injury)
- Major trauma services: service delivery of major trauma services (NICE, 2016).

Trauma assessment

The primary survey is modified for trauma to include **DR 'C' ABCDE**. This extra element covers major catastrophic haemorrhage which should be controlled during the primary survey phase and follows the evidence-based **C-ABC** algorithm (Hodgetts et al., 2006).

The severity of the trauma and the resulting injuries will determine the possibility of the patient having sustained one or more life-threatening injuries. As these have the potential to cause death or severe disability, the paramedic should undertake the primary survey and implement as appropriate the following:

- Identify major trauma patients at the scene of the incident who are at risk of death or disability.
- Immediate interventions to allow safe transport.
- Rapid dispatch to a major trauma centre for surgical management and critical care (AACE, 2013b).

DANGER

- Ensure the safety of yourself, your colleagues and the patient. Use your vehicle as protection at road traffic incidents.
- If not already on scene, request assistance of other appropriate emergency services: Helicopter Emergency Medical Services (HEMS), Hazardous Area Response Team (HART) or Special Operations Response Team (SORT), fire and rescue (*entrapments, fires*) and police (*traffic or crime scenes*).
- Ensure that personal protective equipment is worn as appropriate to the incident (*high-visibility clothing, gloves, hats*).

Possible actions to be taken:

- Ensure safety of self, colleagues and patients
- Wear PPE as appropriate
- Request other emergency services (*fire service/police*) as appropriate
- Request specialist assistance (HEMS)/(HART or SORT) if available
- Request the assistance of an appropriate specialist, advanced or consultant '*Critical Care*' paramedic (College of Paramedics, 2015).

RESPONSE

- Assess the patient's response using the AVPU scale and record appropriately.

- Remember that alterations in the patient's level of consciousness (LOC) may be due to an injury affecting their airway, breathing or circulation and resulting hypoxia.
- The patient may be unable to respond due to obstruction of the airway.

Possible actions to be taken:

- Assess the patient's level of consciousness (AVPU)
- Record any period of unconsciousness – it may be part of the patient's lucid interval.

CATASTROPHIC HAEMORRHAGE

There will be incidents that paramedics attend where trauma has resulted in catastrophic haemorrhage. If this is not assessed and managed appropriately, then the patient may die.

- Ensure the immediate control of obvious catastrophic bleeding.
- Use the appropriate algorithm in relation to head, neck, torso or limb(s).
- Use and apply appropriate tourniquet(s) or haemostatic dressing(s) (AACE, 2013c).

Possible actions to be taken:

- Control obvious catastrophic haemorrhage
- Apply tourniquets or haemostatic dressings as appropriate
- Ensure haemorrhage is controlled before proceeding to the next element.

AIRWAY

The paramedic should remember that patients with trauma have a higher risk of cervical 'C' spine injuries, and should therefore use the appropriate airway opening techniques. Remember that patients who do require resuscitation often have an obstructed airway (Resuscitation Council (UK), 2011).

- If the patient is unresponsive, open the airway (*with the appropriate 'C' spine manoeuvre*).
- Airway obstruction may be due to oedema of the airway caused by burns, maxillo-facial injuries, or foreign bodies.

- Use stepwise airway management to secure a patent airway (*airway manoeuvre – jaw thrust, suction, oral/nasal airway adjuncts, supraglottic airway devices, endotracheal intubation, needle cricothyroidotomy*) (*see Respiratory Assessment, Chapter 2*).

Possible actions to be taken:
- Use 'C' spine airway manoeuvre if appropriate
- Use airway adjuncts (stepwise airway management), as appropriate (*see Respiratory Assessment, Chapter 2*)
- Ensure airway is patent and secure before proceeding to next element.

BREATHING

There are various life-threatening injuries caused by trauma that affect the patient's breathing; the paramedic should ensure that they identify these as part of their assessment.

- Assess if the patient is breathing: what is the rate?
- Is it adequate?
- Do they have any dyspnoea?
- Assess the SpO_2 levels and administer 15 l/min O_2, if appropriate (British Thoracic Society, 2015).
- Use the Look, Feel, Listen technique (Greaves et al., 2012).
- Auscultate and identify **time critical** respiratory conditions.

The following life-threatening injuries may occur to the thoracic cavity of the trauma patient:

- Aortic dissection
- Tension pneumothorax
- Open pneumothorax
- Massive haemothorax/haemhorrage
- Flail segment
- Cardiac tamponade.

Aortic dissection

Aortic dissection is a condition that presents as a sudden severe tearing retrosternal pain which radiates to the back; the degree of the radiation will depend on the blood vessels involved. If branch arteries are affected, the patient may present with either the absence of pulses or unequal blood pressure recording in each arm.

Signs and symptoms
- Sudden severe tearing retrosternal pain (*may radiate to back*).
- Absence of radial pulses and unequal blood pressure.

Tension pneumothorax

A tension pneumothorax occurs when an opening is created within the pleural lining of the lung. If a one-way valve is created, air will enter the pleural space on inhalation but will not leave on exhalation. This creates an increased intra-pleural pressure, leading to the collapse of the lung. As the tension pneumothorax increases in size, the pressure pushes the contents of the mediastinum to the opposite side of the body obstructing the blood flow of the heart, and reducing the cardiac output. In addition, the tension may compress the diaphragm and the opposing lung.

Without immediate intervention the tension pneumothorax will initially result in respiratory arrest, and if interventions are still not undertaken, this condition will result in the patient suffering a cardiac arrest.

Signs and symptoms
- Blunt or penetrating trauma to the chest
- Dyspnoea/rapid respiratory rate/rapid weak pulse
- Decreasing level of consciousness
- Deviated trachea (*away from the injured side*)
- Absent air sounds on injured side
- Reduced SpO_2
- Surgical **emphysema**.

Open pneumothorax

An open pneumothorax is caused by a penetrating injury to the chest wall causing air to enter the pleural space. The negative pressure created in the thoracic cavity can draw air through the hole in the chest wall. This may present as a sucking chest wound.

Signs and symptoms
- Penetrating trauma to the chest
- Dyspnoea
- Sucking chest wound
- Reduced air entry on affected side
- Surgical emphysema.

Massive haemothorax/haemorrhage

A haemothorax occurs when blood enters the pleural space within the lungs. The pleural space of the lungs can hold up to 3 litres of blood and therefore can represent a significant source of blood loss (Salomone and Pons, 2014). Massive haemorrhage classically presents with the various signs and symptoms of the four stages of shock (see Table 7.1). These signs and symptoms are often subtle and may not always be present.

Table 7.1 Classification of hypovolaemic shock; Classes I–IV (Adults)

Class	Blood loss mLs and % volume	Symptoms
I	<750 ml <(15%)	HR: <100 beats per minute RR: 14–20 breaths per minute BP: Normal Symptoms: Minimal; BP unchanged; tachycardia occurs occasionally.
II	750–1500 ml (15–30%)	HR: >100 beats per minute (*tachycardia*) RR: 20–30 breaths per minute (*tachypnoea*) BP: Normal Symptoms: Pulse pressure decreases (as diastolic ↑); Pallor; Patient may present with anxiety, aggression or be frightened
III	1500–2000 ml (30–40%)	HR: >120 beats per minute (*tachycardia*) RR: 30–40 breaths per minute (*tachypnoea*) BP: Decreased (minimum loss that results in hypotension) Symptoms: Inadequate perfusion: pallor, sweating. Altered mental state; confusion, aggression and anxiety.
IV	>2000 Ml >(40%)	HR: >140 beats per minute (*weak and thready pulse*) (tachycardia may deteriorate to bradycardia) RR: >40 breaths per minute (*tachypnoea – air hunger*) BP: Decreased (Marked ↓Systolic BP, with narrow pulse pressure) Symptoms: lethargy, drowsiness and or unconsciousness

Adapted from: Greaves et al. (2012).

Signs and symptoms
- Mechanism of injury – blunt or penetrating trauma to the chest
- Dyspnoea
- Reduced chest expansion on side of injury
- Reduced air entry on side of injury
- Signs of hypovolaemic shock.

Flail segment

A flail segment occurs when two or more adjacent ribs are broken in two or more places. A paradoxical movement of the lungs occurs due to the free floating flail segment that moves independently of the remainder of the ribs. The flail segment moves in with inhalation and out with exhalation, opposing the normal movement of ribs in respiration, causing inadequate ventilation.

Signs and symptoms
- Significant blunt trauma to the chest
- Paradoxical breathing
- Reduced chest expansion on affected side
- Pain
- Dyspnoea.

Cardiac tamponade

Cardiac tamponade occurs when there is bleeding into the pericardial cavity which can prevent effective contraction of the heart. A high index of suspicion should be held with any penetrating trauma within the *danger zone*. This zone is located between the nipple line and a horizontal line drawn perpendicular with the epigastrum.

Signs and symptoms
- Mechanism of injury (*penetrating injury to the danger zone*)
- Signs of cardiogenic/obstructive shock
- Beck's Triad – hypotension, distended neck veins, muffled heart sounds.

Possible actions to be taken:
- Ensure that breathing is adequate (*respirations <10 or >29 breaths per minute require ventilatory support*)
- Seal sucking chest wounds, stabilize flail segments, decompress tension pneumothoraces accordingly
- Administer oxygen appropriately to patient's injury
- Manage hypoxia appropriately
- Pre-alert and transfer to the nearest regional trauma unit.

CIRCULATION

While the assessment of catastrophic haemorrhage is immediate, the patient who has sustained trauma may also have internal haemorrhage that is not so easily identifiable. It is imperative that paramedics identify at the earliest opportunity patients who have hypovolaemic shock and deal appropriately. Remember these signs and symptoms are often subtle and may not always be present (see Table 7.1).

- Look to see if the patient has any form of haemorrhage, internal or external, and manage accordingly.
- Assessment of the trauma patient's circulatory system includes palpating the radial pulse, or, for penetrating torso injuries, a central pulse.
- Assess peripheral if available, or alternatively assess central capillary refill taken over the sternum or forehead (>2 *seconds indicates poor perfusion*).
- Administer IV fluids appropriately (NICE, 2004, 2014; AACE, 2013d).

Possible actions to be taken:
- Control external haemorrhage
- Assess and manage shock accordingly
- IV access and intravenous fluids en route
- Pre-alert and transfer to the nearest regional trauma centre.

DISABILITY

Remember that trauma patients may have sustained a head injury, or alternatively their injuries affecting the respiratory and circulatory systems may cause hypoxia, and result in altered levels of consciousness.

- Assess the patient's level of consciousness (AVPU).
- Ascertain if the patient has been unconscious – information from witnesses/bystanders (*brain injuries are associated with lucid intervals*).
- Assess the patient's posture, note any decerebrate or decorticate positioning.
- Assess the patient's pupils for both size and reaction, dilation of pupils may be due to intracranial pressure (ICP) (PERRLA).
- Assess and note obvious deformities of limbs.

Possible actions to be taken:

- Assess the patient's LOC (AVPU)
- Record any periods of unconsciousness, it may be part of a lucid interval
- Assess the patient's pupils
- Assess and note posture and any obvious deformities.

EXPOSE/EXAMINE/EVALUATE

In trauma situations it is imperative that injuries are identified and assessed, therefore it may be necessary to remove clothing to expose the injury.

- Expose fully and examine the patient's injury.
- Evaluate and determine the need to transfer to the nearest regional major trauma centre.

Possible actions to be taken:

- Expose and examine injuries and evaluate the findings
- Identify and manage time critical conditions appropriately
- Pre-alert and transfer to the nearest regional trauma unit.

SECONDARY SURVEY

History

History taking is an important skill for paramedics to master in order to provide timely interventions and treatment. In trauma it is vital to understand the mechanism of injury and the resultant possible major life-threatening complications to the patient. Competent paramedics should observe the scene and the patient to create a picture of events. Remember to use witness observations as well as that of the patient.

Presenting complaint

- What has happened to cause these injuries?
- Do you have any pain? If so, where?
- Have you moved from the scene? If so, how?
- Do you remember the events fully?
- Did you lose consciousness?

In trauma, the use of the following acronym may assist the paramedic: ATMIST (AACE, 2013e):

    A – Age
    T – Time of incident
    M – Mechanism
    I – Injuries
    S – Signs and symptoms
    T – Treatment given/immediate needs

History of presenting complaint

A thorough understanding of the mechanism of injury is essential in identifying possible injuries the patient may have.

Road traffic collisions (RTC)
- Were they wearing a seat belt?
- Is there a 'bull's eye' on the front windscreen? If so, is it inwards or outwards?
- Is there any further damage to the vehicle?
- Are there fatalities within the vehicle?
- Was the patient ejected?
- Has the vehicle overturned? (*All of these suggest a high transfer of energy.*)

Fall from height
- What was the distance of the fall?
- What type of surface did the patient land on?
- Which part of the body took the impact of the fall?

Penetrating injuries
- What was the instrument that caused the injury?
- Where are the injuries on the body? (*This should highlight the possible injuries to underlying structures.*)

Burns
- What caused the burn?
- When did the burn happen?
- Where are the burns to the body?
- Did the event happen in an enclosed space? (*This is indicative of inhalation injuries.*)
- Does the patient have any difficulty in breathing (DIB)?

Paramedics should ensure they use a validated objective tool when assessing a patient's pain severity. They should also ensure they use appropriate pain management to minimize the distress of the patients in trauma situations. The SOCRATES framework will assist the paramedic in assessing pain (AACE, 2013f; Longmore et al., 2014):

- **S** – Site. Where exactly is the pain?
- **O** – Onset. When did the injury occur?
- **C** – Character. Describe the pain in your own words, is it a sharp/dull/burning pain?
- **R** – Radiate. Does the pain go anywhere else?
- **A** – Associated symptoms. Is it associated with any other symptoms? For example, nausea and/or vomiting.
- **T** – Time/duration. Was the onset sudden or gradual? And has it changed?
- **E** – Exacerbating/relieving factors. Does anything make the pain better or worse? Is there pain on inspiration or movement?
- **S** – Severity. Obtain an initial pain score (0 = no pain, 10 = worst pain ever).

The following areas are important, but not essential, in patients with life-threatening injuries. The paramedic must also remember that certain patient groups, which include the elderly, the obese and pregnant women, are all at high risk in the trauma situation, therefore a thorough history is beneficial (NCEPOD, 2007). The numbers of elderly and obese persons have increased dramatically in the UK during the twentieth century.

Past medical history

- Have you had any recent operations?
- Do you suffer from clotting disorders?
- Do you have any chronic medical conditions?

Drug/medication history

- Do you take any anti-coagulant medication?
- Do you take beta-blockers?
- Have you taken recreational drugs or alcohol within the past 24 hours?

REVIEW OF SYSTEMS RELATED TO TRAUMA

In the out-of-hospital environment it is essential to review the following systems which may provide additional information on the condition of the patient. The paramedic should recognize that if they reach this point in history taking, it is unlikely the patient's condition is life threatening.

Respiratory

- Can the patient talk in full sentences? (*An inability could be indicative of an airway obstruction or breathing problem.*)
- Does your airway feel tight? (*This may be indicative of inhalation burns.*)
- Do you have any difficulty breathing?
- Do you have any pain on inspiration?

Circulation

In the trauma situation the paramedic will often rely on visual observation of external haemorrhage, and observation of cardiovascular vital signs rather than using questions to understand the circulatory system. See vital signs section below.

Neurological

- Was there any loss of consciousness (LOC)?
- Do you remember what happened?
- Do you have any neck or back pain?
- Can you move your arms and legs?
- Have you vomited?

Musculoskeletal

- Do you have any pain on movement?
- Prior to the traumatic injury, did you suffer from any long-term musculoskeletal pain?

VITAL SIGNS

Vital signs are essential to every patient assessment. They should be used in conjunction with the information found in the history taking and physical examination process, to differentiate between patients with a time critical and non-time critical condition. The paramedic must remember that continual reassessment of the vital signs is an essential part of patient assessment.

Respiratory rate

The paramedic should note the rate, depth and rhythm of respiration to provide a holistic view of the patient's respiratory function. Remember that patients with a respiratory rate of <10 or >29 breaths per minute will require ventilatory support, as both rates are indicative of inadequate minute volumes and respiratory failure.

Pulse oximetry

Pulse oximetry provides a measurement of the arterial blood saturation of oxygen, and the appropriate levels of oxygen should be administered accordingly (BTS, 2015). In the trauma situation the paramedic must be aware of the limiting factors in pulse oximetry, as inaccurate measurements can occur during exposure to movement, bright light, dirt or cold environments. Patients are more likely to be exposed to these environments in trauma situations.

Pulse rate

The pulse rate is a quick and non-invasive method of gaining an insight into the trauma patient's circulatory volume and function. The paramedic should initially assess the radial pulse, if palpable, ascertain if it is strong, weak or thready. A patient demonstrating tachycardia may be indicative of shock, whereas a patient with bradycardia may be demonstrating a pre-terminal sign (Salomone and Pons, 2014).

Capillary bed refill (CBR)

The capillary refill can be taken both peripherally and centrally on the trauma patient. Paramedics should be aware of limiting factors such as shock, which may contribute to a false reading. Undertaking a central capillary refill taken over the sternum or forehead may provide a more accurate indication of a patient's circulatory function.

- Pressure should be applied for 5 seconds and capillary refill should return in less than 2 seconds.
- >2 seconds suggests poor tissue perfusion.

Blood pressure

In the trauma situation, changes in blood pressure are likely to occur due to a decrease in circulating blood volume caused by the injuries sustained and resulting blood loss. The paramedic should be aware of the stages of shock and recognize that hypotension occurs in the latter stages of shock (see Table 7.1).

Capnometry, End tidal CO_2 (EtCO_2)

The paramedic should recognize the significance of using **capnometry** when assessing the trauma patient. It is most often used in the intubated patient to confirm endotracheal tube or supraglottic airway placement. However, end tidal CO_2 with a normal wave form and constituent value is also indicative of an adequate circulatory volume. A poor wave form and a falling constituent value may be an early indicator of a falling circulatory volume due to continuous bleeding (Kodali, 2013).

Glasgow Coma Score (GCS)

Assess the patient's level of consciousness using the Glasgow Coma Score (GCS). It is important to assess the GCS early in the trauma patient and to continue to reassess this as it may highlight underlying injuries, especially to the brain. When providing information about the GCS of individual patients, it should be on the three separate responses on the GCS, e.g. if a patient scores 13 based on scores of 4 on eye-opening, 4 on verbal response and 5 on motor response, this should be communicated as E4, V4, M5 (NICE, 2014).

- Record T if an endotracheal (ET) tube is inserted when scoring Best Verbal (Smith et al., 2011).
- A GCS score of 3–8 indicates a severe head injury.
- A GCS score of 8 defines coma.
- A GCS score of 14–15 is mild.
- A GCS score of 15 is normal.

Pupillary assessment

The paramedic should continuously assess and reassess the pupils within the secondary survey as it may be indicative of rising intracranial pressure and an underlying brain injury. In trauma patients with head injury, suspect brain injury if the patient's pupils are unequal in size. Assess accordingly (PERRLA):

- Right-sided unilateral pupil dilation may be indicative of right-sided brain injury.
- Bilateral dilated pupils may be indicative of hypoxia or advanced signs of severe brain injury.
- Irregular pupils can be indicative of direct trauma to the eye.

PHYSICAL ASSESSMENT

In the trauma situation the physical assessment of the patient is of the utmost importance in providing a thorough understanding of the patient's injuries. The paramedic must ensure all injuries are identified, documented and included in the patient handover.

Creating a suitable environment

In trauma situations it is appropriate to fully expose the injured areas in order to make a thorough assessment. When the patient has multi-system trauma and is time critical, the paramedic team may decide that all clothes should be removed from the patient; in these situations paramedic should still give due consideration to the patient's privacy and dignity where possible (Department of Health, 2009).

Consent

The Health and Care Professions Council (HCPC) states that all allied health professionals, including paramedics, must ensure that they gain informed consent for any treatment they carry out. This must be documented accurately and passed on to other members of the health care team. In the trauma situation it may not always be possible to gain consent so the paramedic must ensure that they act in the patient's best interest (HCPC, 2008).

EXAMINATION: 'HEAD-TO-TOE' ASSESSMENT

In trauma situations the patient often has pain associated with their underlying injuries, therefore excellent communication skills are required from the paramedic to build an effective rapport with the patient and gain their trust. Advise the patient what you are doing and ask questions appropriately as you progress through the assessment. The paramedic should assess the patient accordingly and use the senses of *touch*, *sight* and *hearing* to gather as much information about the condition of the patient as possible. Universal precautions in the form of gloves and protective eyewear should be worn when in contact with the patient due to the possibility of contact with body fluids.

The paramedic can adopt a 'toe-to-top' assessment when treating paediatric patients as this is a less threatening approach and will help to foster a relationship of trust with the patient (see *Child Assessment, Chapter 11*).

Head

- Gently palpate and visually inspect the entirety of the head and face. Areas covered by hair are harder to assess visually therefore thorough palpation is necessary to identify underlying injuries.
- Any bruising, lacerations, abrasions, deformity and bleeding should be treated and documented. Palpate bones of the face and skull for crepitus, deviation, depression and abnormal mobility.
- Special attention should be given to the following findings:
  - 'Boggy masses' – possible fractured skull with underlying brain tissue injury
  - Cerebral spinal fluid (CSF) – a straw-coloured, oily liquid from the nose and/or ears suggests an underlying base of skull fracture

- Periorbital ecchymosis and battle signs – bilateral bruising around the orbits of the eyes and mastoid ecchymosis or bruising under the ears suggest a base of skull fracture although they may take several hours to become apparent (Salomone and Pons, 2014).

Neck

The acronym 'TWELVE' is a useful aid in assessing trauma to the neck:

- **T** – *Tracheal* deviation – is a late sign of a tension pneumothorax and not always seen.
- **W** – *Wounds* – contusions, abrasions, penetrating injuries (*entry and exit wounds*), bleeding and lacerations need to be treated and documented. The paramedic should be aware of the underlying structures in relation to the wound and have a high index of suspicion to potential complications.
- **E** – *Emphysema (surgical)* – identified on palpation as an air 'popping' sensation under the skin. This is often caused by a large transfer of energy, for example, a fall from height, RTC or a penetrating chest injury.
- **L** – *Laryngeal crepitus* – this is caused by direct trauma to the larynx and is associated with a hoarseness of voice. The paramedic should be aware this is a 'time critical' condition due to the potential deterioration of the airway.
- **V** – *Venous distension* – this is indicative of obstructive shock, for example, tension pneumothorax or cardiac tamponade.
- **E** – *Expose the thorax and Exclude injuries* (Greaves et al., 2012).

A high index of suspicion of a 'C' cervical spinal injury needs to be observed when there is a mechanism of injury present. The C spine should be palpated centrally while maintaining in-line immobilization of the neck (*see Spinal Injuries Assessment, Chapter 6*). The following may be indicative of a 'C' spine injury:

- Midline 'C' spine tenderness
- 'Bony' deformity of the spinal processes
- Neurological symptoms such as 'pins and needles'/numbness (paraesthesia), reduced power and movement of the limbs.

A 'C' spine injury cannot be excluded if any of the following are present:

- Intoxication with alcohol or drugs
- Midline 'C' spine tenderness
- Neurological deficit
- Distracting injuries
- Reduced level of consciousness.

Chest

The acronym 'FLAPS' is a useful aid in assessing trauma to the chest, and in practice is used in conjunction with the acronym 'TWELVE':

- **F** – Feel the chest (for symmetrical expansion; flail segments; rib fractures and crepitus).
- **L** – Look at the chest (for bruising; sucking wounds (*seal immediately*); and patterning on the skin caused by seatbelts and/or clothing).
- **A** – Listen to the chest (***auscultate***) (for absence of breath sounds; adventitious breath sounds; and equal bilateral air entry).
- **P** – Percuss the chest (for symmetry; hyper-resonance; and/or dullness).
- **S** – Sides (check under the sides of the chest and shoulders for deformity and/or bleeding) (Greaves et al., 2012).

The framework Inspection, Palpate, Percuss, Auscultate (IPPA) should be used by the paramedic (*see Respiratory Assessment, Chapter 2*).

Inspection

The paramedic should inspect the whole chest, including the posterior, anterior and axilla surfaces for:

- Symmetry of the thorax on inspiration/exhalation
- Chest wall markings – contusions, abrasions, penetrating injuries (entry and exit wounds), bleeding and lacerations
- Paradoxical breathing – a resultant injury of blunt trauma and indicative of a flail segment (Longmore et al., 2014)
- Penetrating objects that have remained in situ need to be left and secured to prevent excessive movement and increased damage to underlying structures.

Palpation

The paramedic should palpate the anterior, posterior and axilla chest walls of the trauma patient. In relation to the trauma patient, the following findings should be noted:

- Tenderness – bruising, contusions and fractures can be identified. The paramedic should have a high index of suspicion of possible underlying tissue injuries to the area of trauma
- Crepitus – caused by rubbing of fractured bones
- Surgical emphysema – 'popping' sensation under the skin.

Percussion

While percussion has a limited role within the trauma environment due to excessive noise and chaos that are often associated with these scenarios, in the trauma patient, percussion can be used to support the diagnosis of chest injuries:

- Hyper-resonance – indicative of a pneumothorax
- Hypo-resonance – indicative of a haemothorax or pulmonary contusions (Salomone and Pons, 2014).

Auscultation
The paramedic should perform auscultation on all trauma patients (*initially within the primary survey*). Due to the possibility of time critical injuries in trauma patients, it is sufficient to listen to the apex of the anterior chest, axilla and the bases of the posterior lungs. They should be aware of absent, reduced and added sounds in support of their diagnosis.

Sounds found on auscultation
- Stridor – high-pitched sound heard on inspiration (*obstruction due to foreign body, oedema of airway due to burns*)
- Fine crackles/coarse crackles – pulmonary contusion, aspiration of bodily fluids
- Reduced breath sounds – haemothorax
- Absent or diminished breath sounds – tension pneumothorax.

Abdomen

The paramedic should focus on detecting concealed haemorrhage in the abdominal cavity as early deaths from trauma to this region typically result from massive blood loss (Salomone and Pons, 2014). Consider a high index of suspicion in any patient who has sustained trauma to the abdomen due to the delicate and vascular nature of underlying organs. The paramedic should suspect an occult abdominal injury if there is trauma above and below this area (see *Abdominal and Gastro-intestinal Assessment, Chapter 4*).

The paramedic should focus on inspection and palpation of the abdominal region in assisting their diagnosis of injuries.

Inspection
The paramedic should expose and inspect the whole abdominal region including the anterior, flanks and posterior surfaces for:

- Abdominal wall markings – contusions, abrasions, penetrating injuries (*entry and exit wounds*), bleeding and lacerations
- Grey Turner's sign – bruising to the flanks
- Cullen's sign – bruising around the umbilicus.

Both of these signs are indicative of retroperitoneal bleeding (Salomone and Pons, 2014). Abdominal distension is a late sign that is associated with intra-abdominal bleeding and circulatory signs of shock. The peritoneal cavity can hold up to 1.5 litres of fluid before showing signs of distension, and the retroperitoneal cavity can hold 3 litres of fluid with no visible sign (Hodgetts and Turner, 2008).

Palpation
The abdomen should be split into four quadrants for palpation, and the paramedic should palpate each quadrant for:

- Tenderness – a symptom experienced due to pain on palpation
- Guarding – tensing of abdominal muscles on palpation
- Rigidity – involuntary spasm of abdominal muscles.

The presence of any one of these signs is suggestive of intra-abdominal bleeding in the trauma patient (see *Abdominal and Gastro-intestinal Assessment, Chapter 4*).

Pelvis

The pelvis is a complete ring; a fracture in one part will often result in a subsequent fracture being present within the pelvic ring. Haemorrhage in pelvic fractures occurs in 40% of pelvic trauma injuries, and is the foremost cause of death in 60% of fatal cases. Bleeding occurs usually in the retroperitoneal space, and the volume of blood relates to the degree and type of pelvic injury (Fisher et al., 2013).

The paramedic should not manually compress the pelvis to confirm a fracture but instead hold a high level of suspicion if the pelvic injury is associated with the following findings:

- Relevant mechanism of injury
- Asymmetrical alignment of the pelvis on inspection
- Pelvic and/or lower back pain
- Injuries above and below the pelvis
- Lateral displacement of both legs classically seen in an 'open book fracture'
- Bleeding per rectum (PR) or per vagina (PV), including instances of haematuria post-trauma.

Back

In the trauma situation patients who are identified with a potential SCI should be fully immobilized. The paramedic should not roll the patient to solely assess the back as the benefits of this are limited in the out-of-hospital field. However, if an opportunity arises to assess the patient's back, the paramedic should fully expose the area and inspect for:

- Contusions, abrasions, penetrating injuries (*entry and exit wounds*), bleeding and lacerations
- Paradoxical breathing – indicative of a posterior flail segment
- Vertebral bone deformity.

In addition, the following neurological signs and symptoms may be apparent in a patient with spinal injury (see *Spinal Injuries Assessment, Chapter 6*):

- Paraesthesia
- Reduced power and movement of the limbs
- Priapism.

Extremities (legs and arms)

The paramedic should expose and assess the extremities, beginning with the legs. All injuries should be documented and treated. The following assessments of each individual limb should occur:

- Inspection – areas of deformity, contusions, swelling, lacerations and pallor
- Palpation – areas of tenderness and crepitus
- Motor, sensory, circulatory (MSC) (*of all limbs*)
- Motor – ask if the patient can move their limb
- Sensory – test for sensation in the extremity of the limb
- Circulatory – assess for the presence of distal pulses and capillary bed refill (CBR)
- Blood loss – fractured limbs can cause circulatory compromise due to blood loss.

Table 7.2 highlights potential blood loss in fractures of different bones. The paramedic should be aware that an open fracture differs from a closed fracture, specifically concerning the potential blood loss which should be doubled with an open fracture.

Compartment syndrome

This is a limb-threatening injury, caused by bleeding within a contained space. This prevents blood flow to the distal tissues, causing ischaemia and necrosis. The following signs and symptoms are classed as the 'five P's' and may be associated with this condition:

Table 7.2 Potential blood loss in fractures of different bones

Bone fracture	Internal blood loss (ml)
Rib	125
Radius/ulna	250–500
Humerus	500–750
Tibia/fibula	500–1000
Femur	1000–2000

Adapted from: Salomone and Pons (2014).

- Pain
- Pulselessness
- Pallor
- Paraesthesia
- Paralysis (Greaves et al. 2012).

Penetrating trauma

Penetrating trauma creates a 'puncture' wound with potentially life-threatening implications. Injuries can range from the subtle to the obvious, therefore a high index of suspicion and a thorough patient assessment are essential in reducing patient mortality. Common penetrating injuries include:

- Stab wounds (*not necessarily from a knife*)
- Bullet or gunshot wound (GSW) (*high and/or low velocity*)
- Impalement (*fencing, railings, wooden posts*).

The mechanism of injury will provide the paramedic with valuable information concerning any possible underlying trauma to the patient. A good knowledge of human anatomy is essential in determining underlying soft tissue injuries to major organs and blood vessels.

Stab wounds and impalement injuries are localized in nature and can have a predictable injury pattern. Bullet wounds can cause unpredictable injury patterns with widespread internal trauma.

Blunt trauma

Blunt trauma involves a combination of compression, shearing and rotational forces which can cause devastating underlying soft tissue injury to the major organs and blood vessels of the body. It is the commonest form of injury, occurring from direct blows and rapid deceleration injuries (Fisher et al., 2013). Experience has shown that road traffic collisions (RTC) are one of the most common instances in which patients may receive any of these forces (NAO, 2010).

Epidemiology

Every year across England and Wales, 12,500 people die after sustaining blunt trauma injury. It is the leading cause of death among children and young adults of 44 years and under. In addition, there are many thousands who are left severely disabled for life. Already it is the commonest cause of loss of life under the age of 40 (TARN, 2015a).

Burns

Burn victims are a challenging category of patients to assess and treat due to the complexity of their injuries and associated pain. Burns can occur from thermal, chemical, electrical or flash insults and cause superficial, partial and full thickness injuries.

Elderly people

When treating elderly people who have fallen, the paramedic should have a higher index of suspicion of injuries due to chronic conditions such as arthritis and osteoporosis, for example, a fractured neck of femur (NOF), (NICE, 2013). Common signs and symptoms of a fractured NOF are:

- Hip pain radiating into the groin – be aware the elderly patient may have a higher pain threshold
- Shortening and lateral rotation of the injured extremity.

CHAPTER KEY POINTS

- The DR 'C' ABCDE framework should be used to identify life-threatening conditions affecting the trauma patient.
- If the patient has a time critical condition due to trauma, pre-alert the nearest regional trauma centre.
- If the patient does not have a time critical condition, undertake a thorough secondary survey and record findings accordingly.
- The paramedic should constantly reassess the patient to identify changes in the patient's condition and the development of life-threatening conditions.
- Definitive treatment occurs in hospital. Effective clinical interventions and history taking should occur in a timely manner in order to optimize the patient's chances of survival.

REFERENCES

Association of Ambulance Chief Executives (2013a) *UK Ambulance Services Clinical Practice Guidelines 2013 Pocket Book: Trauma – SCENE*. Bridgwater: Class Professional Publishing.

Association of Ambulance Chief Executives (2013b) *UK Ambulance Services Clinical Practice Guidelines 2013 Pocket Book: Trauma Survey*. Bridgwater: Class Professional Publishing.

Association of Ambulance Chief Executives (2013c) *UK Ambulance Services Clinical Practice Guidelines 2013 Pocket Book. Trauma Emergencies Overview (Adults): The Management of Catastrophic Haemorrhage Algorithm*. Bridgwater: Class Professional Publishing.

Association of Ambulance Chief Executives (2013d) *UK Ambulance Services Clinical Practice Guidelines 2013 Pocket Book: Intravascular Fluid Therapy (Adults): The Management of Catastrophic Haemorrhage Algorithm*. Bridgwater: Class Professional Publishing.

Association of Ambulance Chief Executives (2013e) *UK Ambulance Services Clinical Practice Guidelines 2013 Pocket Book: Trauma – ATMIST*. Bridgwater: Class Professional Publishing.

Association of Ambulance Chief Executives (2013f) *UK Ambulance Services Clinical Practice Guidelines 2013 Pocket Book: Pain Assessment Model*. Bridgwater: Class Professional Publishing.

British Thoracic Society (2015) *Emergency Oxygen Use in Adult Patients Guideline*. Available at: https://www.brit-thoracic.org.uk/searchresults/?txtSearch=2015+Oxygen+Guidelines&search= (accessed 5 June 2015).

College of Paramedics (2015) *Paramedic Post Registration: Career and Competency Framework* (3rd edn). Bridgwater: College of Paramedics.

Department of Health (2009) *Reference Guide to Consent for Examination or Treatment* (2nd edn). London: Department of Health Publications.

Fisher, J., Brown, S.N., and Cooke, M. (eds) (2013) *UK Ambulance Services Clinical Practice Guidelines 2013: Major Pelvic Trauma*. Bridgwater: Class Professional Publishing.

Greaves, I., Wright, C., Porter, K., Hodgetts, T., and Woollard, M. (2012) *Pocketbook of Emergency Care: A Quick Reference Guide for Paramedics*. Edinburgh: Saunders Elsevier.

Health and Care Professions Council (2008) *Standards of Conduct, Performance and Ethics*. London: HCPC.

Hodgetts, T., Mahoney, P., Russell, M. and Byers, M. (2006) ABC to [C]ABC: redefining the military trauma paradigm. *Emergency Medical Journal* 23: 745–6.

Hodgetts, T. and Turner, L. (2008) Civilian and military trauma care is different, in *Trauma Rules 2: Incorporating Military Trauma Rules*. Online edn. Available at: http://onlinelibrary.wiley.com/doi/10.1002/9780470757338.ch3/summary (accessed 6 June 2015).

Kodali, B.S. (2013) Capnography outside the operating rooms. *Anesthesiology* 118(1): 192–201.

Longmore, M., Wilkinson, I.B., Baldwin, A. and Wallin, E. (2014) *Oxford Handbook of Clinical Medicine* (9th edn). Oxford: Oxford University Press.

NAO (National Audit Office) (2010) *Major Trauma Care in England. Report by the Comptroller and Auditor General* HC213. London: The Stationery Office.

NCEPOD (National Confidential Enquiry into Patient Outcome and Death) (2007) *Trauma: Who Cares?* Bristol: NCEPOD.

NHS England (2010) *Trauma Centres and Systems*. Available at: http://www.nhs.uk/NHSEngland/AboutNHSservices/Emergencyandurgentcareservices/Pages/Majortraumaservices.aspx (accessed 6 June 2015).

NICE (National Institute for Health and Clinical Excellence) (2004) *Pre-Hospital Initiation of Fluid Replacement Therapy in Trauma*. TA 74. London: National Institute for Clinical Excellence.

NICE (National Institute for Health and Clinical Excellence) (2013) *Falls Assessment and Prevention of Falls in Older People*. NICE clinical guideline 161. Available at: http://www.nice.org.uk/guidance/cg161/evidence (accessed 6 June 2015).

NICE (National Institute for Health and Clinical Excellence) (2014) *Head Injury*. NICE clinical guideline 176. Available at: http://www.nice.org.uk/guidance/cg176/evidence (accessed 6 June 2015).

NICE (National Institute for Health and Clinical Excellence) (2016) *Major Trauma: Assessment and Management of Airway, Breathing and Ventilation, Circulation, Haemorrhage and Temperature Control*. Available at: https://www.nice.org.uk/guidance/indevelopment/gid-cgwave0642 (accessed 6 June 2015).

Pilbery, R. (2014) *Nancy Caroline's Emergency Care in the Streets: United Kingdom* (7th edn). Burlington, MA: Jones & Bartlett Learning.

Resuscitation Council (UK) (2011) *Advanced Life Support* (6th edn). London: The Resuscitation Council. Reprinted in 2012 (with corrections).

Salomone, J.P. and Pons, P.T. (2014) *Pre-Hospital Trauma Life Support (PHTLS)* (8th edn). Maryland Heights, MO: Mosby Elsevier.

Smith, S.F., Duell, D.J. and Martin, B.C. (2011) *Clinical Nursing Skills: Basic to Advanced Skills* (8th edn). Harlow: Pearson Education Ltd.

The Trauma Audit and Research Network (TARN) (2015a) *Trauma Care*. Available at: https://www.tarn.ac.uk/Content.aspx?ca=2&c=18 (accessed 6 June 2015).

The Trauma Audit and Research Network (TARN) (2015b) *NHS England Press Release on Major Trauma*. Available at: https://www.tarn.ac.uk/Content.aspx?c=3477 (accessed 6 June 2015).

8 Musculoskeletal assessment
Kevin Dark

In the previous decade Wardrope and English (2003) advised us that 3.5 million patients in the UK attended hospital with isolated musculoskeletal conditions; the vast majority of these conditions are self-limiting. In addition, 70%–80% of patients subjected to multi-system trauma will also have secondary musculoskeletal injuries (MSI) that represent significant socio-economic challenges for the National Health Service (Pilbery, 2014).

The Health and Safety Executive (HSE) (2015) statistics for musculoskeletal disorders (MSD) for 2013/14 in the workforce accounted for:

- 526,000 of the 1.25 million work-related illnesses
- 8.3 million working days lost (*an average of 15.9 days per MSD case*)
- Activities such as health care had higher rates of MSD compared to other occupations.

Assessment of the musculoskeletal system requires the paramedic to have a clear understanding of normal anatomy and physiology and also to have a high index of suspicion with regard to:

- Life-threatening airway, breathing and circulation (ABC) conditions that may be masked by the presence of painful MSI
- Limb-threatening conditions (*vascular occlusion, fractures, dislocation, septic arthritis, nerve damage, osteomyelitis/infection*)
- Injury/illness physiology (*fractures, strains, sprains, tendonitis, bursitis, osteoporosis, osteoarthritis, rheumatoid arthritis, gout and pathological fractures*).

When the musculoskeletal system is compromised through disease or trauma, the connective tissue and associated structures elicit signs that the paramedic will see and symptoms that the patient may feel. Injuries to bones and joints may coexist with injury to soft tissues and underlying structures organs and may be further complicated by disease. In practice, the paramedic must be able to differentiate between self-limiting conditions such as simple strains or sprains and **red flag** conditions such as 'critical skin', that

Musculoskeletal assessment

will require immediate intervention and onward referral. Therefore in practice, musculoskeletal injuries present significant challenges in terms of pain management, immobilization, moving and handling and transportation.

This chapter will examine the general assessment of musculoskeletal injuries. This chapter is not intended to give detailed anatomy or physiology. Its aim is to highlight some key assessment principles, which will help the paramedic to assess and refer the patient with MSIs safely and efficiently. In addition, it will review **red flag** conditions that are **time critical** or which require immediate intervention or referral.

Box 8.1 Key physiological aspects of the musculoskeletal system

- Muscle tissue works in conjunction with articulating joints of the skeletal system via tendons, which attach muscles to the periosteum of the bone.
- Ligaments in conjunction with muscular action provide stability to joint formations.
- Cartilage forms a cushioning membrane in place of the periosteum when joints are formed between two bones.
- Some joints have a bursa which allows for nutrition and protection of the joint capsule.
- The contractibility, extensibility and elasticity of skeletal muscle allow body movement, maintain posture, stabilize joints and generate and assist with thermostatic regulation. Skeletal muscle is encased in epimysium (there are usually many muscle fascicles that form a single muscle), and epimysium surrounds the total bundle of many fascicles, but does not allow for expansion beyond the normal limits of muscular contraction.
- In general terms, every muscle is supplied by one nerve, an artery and a vein.
- Muscular movement occurs through motor units consisting of somatic motor neurones.
- During increased muscular activity, a process called *recruitment* signals large muscle contractions as more neurones signal more muscle cells to contract. This is an 'all-or-nothing' cascade.
- The voluntary and involuntary nervous control characteristics of skeletal muscle require a continuous supply of oxygen and essential nutrients which produce metabolic waste products that need to be removed to ensure efficient muscular activity.
- The energy required for musculoskeletal function can result in significant compromise in the patient suffering from multi-system trauma. This is especially relevant in children where the paramedic needs to be aware of the effects of exhaustion.

The musculoskeletal system consists of the bones, the joints they form and the muscle groups that facilitate movement. The skeletal system consists of 206 bones. These bones are classified in terms of their function and grouped in terms of their position on the long axis of the body, axial skeleton (*skull, vertebral column, rib cage*) or the appendicular skeleton (*upper and lower limbs, shoulder bones and hip bones*) that attach to the axial skeleton. The function of the skeletal system is to do the following:

- Provide support and give protection to vital structures
- Allow body movement
- Store minerals
- Produce blood cells.

SCENE ASSESSMENT

The paramedic must use all aspects of scene assessment to build a clinical picture of the potential injury patterns that may be appropriate to the patient's presenting signs and symptoms. The mechanism of injury (MOI), direct and indirect energy patterns, age, size and co-existing morbidity will have an impact on the likelihood of the presence of MSI. The acronym ACT will assist the paramedic to consider and undertake the stages of scene assessment (Greaves et al., 2012):

A – Assess the scene
C – Communicate
T – Triage, treat and transport (*the latter if appropriate and required*)

PRIMARY SURVEY

The paramedic needs to be aware of the distracting nature of musculoskeletal injuries (MSI) and the potential to miss life-threatening airway, breathing or circulatory problems due to the presence of severe pain or dramatic nature of the injury. Often MSI will have a clear history of trauma and may lead a paramedic to move to directly assess the injury before carrying out a primary assessment. Outside of catastrophic haemorrhage, this should rarely be the case in practice.

The primary survey presents significant challenges for the paramedic as the patient may be in acute pain, which may create barriers for the initial ABC assessment. For example, is the difficulty in breathing experienced by the patient due to their perception of pain or a pulmonary embolism from a fat embolus released from an associated hip fracture?

During the primary survey, the paramedic must exclude any ABC problems before focusing on the musculoskeletal injury. Maxillofacial (*airway*) and thoracic (*breathing*) injuries may potentially require immediate assessment and

Musculoskeletal assessment

intervention. Catastrophic haemorrhage (*circulation*) should be controlled during the primary survey phase using the evidence-based 'C' ABC algorithm (Hodgetts et al., 2006) (*see Trauma Assessment, Chapter 7*).

DANGER

The majority of musculoskeletal injuries will have a history of recent trauma and an identifiable mechanism of injury (MOI). This can range from a simple mechanical fall in the home, to a sporting injury, or an injury received in a road traffic collision. The MOI should be considered by the paramedic on approach to the incident and a dynamic risk assessment should be ongoing and reviewed as the incident develops. Patients with significant MSI will have specific implied needs as a result of their injury and existing co-morbidity. Patients need to be protected from the environment to ensure that the effects of weather, traffic movement, worried relatives, young children, pets, medical paraphernalia and large equipment items do not cause further injury and increase the level of risk and danger. The lack of mobility and the onset of conditions such as hypothermia should be a prime concern for the paramedic.

> **Possible actions to be taken:**
> - Ensure personal protective equipment (PPE) in relation to the situation is worn
> - Assess the scene and ascertain actual and potential MSI
> - Ensure that patients with reduced mobility due to a MSI are protected from further injury.

RESPONSE

Patients with MSI may be in significant distress. The pain may present as aggressive behaviour as the injury dynamics affect the patient's ability to rationalize their condition. Pain relief should be instigated as soon as possible to reduce the risk of complications from serious injuries (Greaves et al., 2012).

The majority of patients with MSI will be conscious and will respond to the paramedic's approach, or to verbal commands, as higher centres in the brain are still functioning.

Eye contact and a response to verbal stimuli should be the parameter most consistent with this phase of assessment. A note of caution is suggested at this point with regard to 'lucid intervals' and the potential for patients to have concealed neurological compromise in head injuries (*see General Principles* of Assessment, Chapter 1, Neurological Assessment, Chapter 5, and Trauma Assessment. Chapter 7). Patients who are unable to respond spontaneously on approach or to verbal prompts should be considered compromised pending further assessment of primary functions.

> **Possible actions to be taken:**
> - Record the patient's level of consciousness (LOC)
> - Consider if pain is masking a more serious injury or condition
> - Administer pain relief as appropriate without delay.

AIRWAY

The patient's airway, as with any other condition, needs to be evaluated. Major injury may have caused unstable 'C' spine conditions, which may be masked by pain from distracting injuries. The paramedic needs to consider manual inline stabilization (MILS) and airway adjuncts if they suspect 'C' spine injury. Maxillofacial injuries and skull fractures may lead to significant airway compromise and reduced levels of consciousness. In addition, there is risk of nausea and vomiting as sympathetic fight or flight adrenal responses increase the risk of significant airway compromise. Outside of these specific instances, a patient with an isolated MSI should be in a position to maintain their own airway without the need for adjuncts. However, considerations need to be given to the occurrence of vasovagal episodes affecting cerebral perfusion states, which may cause the patient to become unconscious. The adoption of positional support and the introduction of the stepwise airway management are options available to the paramedic (see Respiratory Assessment, Chapter 2).

> **Possible actions to be taken:**
>
> (Consider cervical spine)
>
> - Initiate manual inline stabilization (MILS)
> - Suction
> - Airway adjuncts
> - Advanced airway techniques (see Respiratory Assessment, Chapter 2).

BREATHING

Patients with rib injuries affecting the mechanism of breathing may potentially have a time critical condition. The patient may be in significant pain and distress and this may have an effect on metabolic processes. Watch for changes in respiratory pattern and overall nature of breathing. Consider supplemental oxygen as per current guidelines (AACE, 2013). Thoracic trauma needs to be identified early and pain management options considered. The following six deadly thoracic conditions should be ruled out: aortic dissection, open pneumothorax, tension pneumothorax, massive haemothorax/haemorrhage, flail chest segment and cardiac tamponade, and need to be identified and corrected early in the primary assessment (see *Trauma Assessment, Chapter 7*).

Possible actions to be taken:

- Ensure that breathing is adequate (respirations <10 or >29 breaths per minute require ventilatory support)
- Seal chest wounds, stabilize flail segments, decompress tension pneumothoraces accordingly
- Administer oxygen appropriately to patient's injury/oxygen saturation
- Consider assisted ventilations
- Transfer to appropriate trauma unit.

CIRCULATION

During the primary survey, the paramedic will need to confirm the presence of a central pulse which is perfusing in nature, noting skin colour and temperature. Later in the secondary survey process, the paramedic is concerned with the distal nature of pulses beyond the site of injury and in comparison with uninjured limbs. Capillary bed refill times can be assessed peripherally (nail-bed) and centrally (forehead or sternum).

The presence of long-bone fractures, pelvic injuries, thoracic compromise and abdominal trauma can lead to catastrophic blood loss. Circulatory compromise leading to de-compensated shock is a life-threatening condition. Haemorrhage control (visible/concealed) and the prevention of exsanguinations from open and closed fractures should be managed appropriately.

Possible actions to be taken:

- Identify potential MSI injury (open and closed fractures)
- Estimate actual/potential blood loss; manage appropriately (see *Trauma Assessment, Chapter 7*)
- Assess and palpate limb pulses
- Pre-alert the nearest major trauma centre (if appropriate).

Table 8.1 Passive, active and resisted movements

Movement type	Physical action
Passive	The limb is at rest. There is no muscular tension. The paramedic moves limb through the range of movements consistent with joint function. *The patient does not assist.*
Active	Patient initiates muscular movement through range of movement. *The paramedic does not assist.*
Resisted	*The paramedic provides an opposing force* as the patient attempts to move limb/joint against this force.

DISABILITY

The primary assessment of disability associated with MSI compromise should include both sensory function and motor function. Sensation and power should be recorded by the paramedic and the findings noted. Check active, passive and resisted movements within the plane of a joint (see Table 8.1).

The mnemonic **SLIPDUCT** may assist the paramedic in identifying a fracture:

- **S** – **S**welling
- **L** – **L**oss of function
- **I** – **I**rregularity
- **P** – **P**ain
- **D** – **D**eformity
- **U** – **U**nnatural movement
- **C** – **C**repitus
- **T** – **T**enderness

Inspection and palpation to elicit the cardinal signs of MSI should be considered, to identify if the patient has any pain, redness, swelling, heat, and loss of normal function. The paramedic should be aware of the **red flag** 5 P's of musculoskeletal injury assessment:

- Pain
- Paraesthesia
- Paralysis
- Pallor
- Pulse.

Musculoskeletal assessment

Assess the patient's pupils, particularly if the patient has a head or maxillo-facial injury or if there is a history of unconsciousness or reduced levels of consciousness.

> **Possible actions to be taken:**
> - Record the patient's level of consciousness (LOC)
> - Record any period of unconsciousness, it may be part of the patient's lucid interval
> - Assess limb function (motor/sensory)
> - Assess for cardinal signs of MSI
> - Assess range of movement (ROM)
> - Confirm trauma history (Hx) and identify **red flag** conditions.

EXPOSE/EXAMINE/EVALUATE

The challenge for the paramedic is to ensure that they balance environmental restrictions with the need to assess injuries sustained by the patient. Issues of consent, capacity, decency and culture/religion should be considered. Where possible, assessment of MSI should occur at the level of the patient's skin. When exposing the musculoskeletal injury, consider how the environment (hypothermia) will impact on the patient. The use of a modesty blanket will aid in the retention of heat and allow for the systematic exposure/re-covering of the patient during assessment. In multi-system MSI trauma, the methodology of 'skin to scoop' can be applied.

Critical skin is a **red flag** time critical condition. It is caused by fracture or dislocation where bone or bone ends press hard against the internal surface of the skin, risking the viability of the tissue. The skin around the joint or bone appears white and under tension. This is a surgical emergency and requires urgent intervention.

In addition, open fractures and bones protruding through the skin present significant risk of secondary compromise through infection and blood loss. Stepwise haemorrhage control should include sterile dressings, tourniquets and haemostatic agents when required in support of direct and indirect pressure.

Any time critical or **red flag** conditions should be identified and managed appropriately and the patient transferred immediately to an appropriate trauma unit (see *Trauma Assessment, Chapter 7*). Alternatively, if there are no time critical problems, remain on scene and conduct a secondary survey.

> **Possible actions to be taken:**
> - Expose and examine injuries
> - Evaluate findings and if time critical, manage conditions appropriately
> - Pre-alert and transfer to the appropriate trauma unit.

SECONDARY SURVEY

Once the primary survey is completed, the paramedic should begin a secondary survey assessment. However, if during this process the patient's condition changes (*possibly due to internal bleeding from closed fractures, and hypovolaemic shock developing*), the paramedic should revert to primary assessment and evaluate the need to complete a secondary survey against the need for definitive care at an appropriate treatment centre. A secondary assessment carried out on scene needs to be justified by the paramedic and consideration to completing a secondary assessment en route should be considered where appropriate.

HISTORY

A patient with an isolated musculoskeletal injury (MSI) should have a clear history of trauma, which is consistent with the reported symptoms. Any signs or symptoms that the paramedic may elicit from the patient history should also fall within the expected injury patterns. Reported incidence of MSI without a clear mechanism of injury should be **red-flagged** and referred appropriately.

Presenting complaint

History taking should include an appropriate level of discussion regarding the reason why the paramedic has been asked to attend. Scene assessment and the MOI can and do provide additional information for the paramedic to use. The use of generalized open questions to establish the chief complaint is important. Appropriate questioning directs the paramedic to link the mechanism of injury to the condition. In addition, it allows the paramedic to focus and prioritize a review of symptoms, which in turn will help with the discovery of underlying morbidity, which may exacerbate the chief complaint. In the case of MSI, a clear history of an initiating event and a sudden change in activities of daily living (ADL) are the likely outcomes (Purcell, 2010).

History of presenting complaint

The history of MSI is the key to identifying **red flag** conditions that require further investigation. Information about the history of the presenting complaint linked to trauma will help identify key injury.

- 'I heard a crack as I twisted my ankle' (*may indicate bony or ligament injury*).
- Reports from the patient that 'Cold weather affects my joints' (*may indicate a chronic condition such as arthritis*).

During this questioning process it is important that the paramedic allows the patient time to express in their own words what happened. This is particularly important in young and older patients. A process of a summary of the history, onset and mechanism of injury can be completed by the paramedic to confirm with the patient the events leading to injury, '*Let me just confirm that ...*'

Past medical history

The patient's past medical history is significant with regard to the chief complaint. Reduced function may be directly linked to a failure of a previous condition to heal appropriately. Misdiagnosis of the chief complaint is not uncommon with an MSI and the patient may need to be assessed several times by different clinical disciplines to establish the true nature of the injury. Ascertain if the patient has been diagnosed or treated for any of the following conditions: osteoporosis, arthritis, brittle bones, anaemia, metastial tumours, and systemic infections, all of which may be related to the re-occurrence of MSI.

The paramedic will need to ask the patient about:

- Gout, arthritis, tuberculosis or cancer
- Recent blunt or penetrating trauma
- Surgery on muscles, joints or bones
- Assist devices such as frames or other mobility aids
- Changes in normal activities of daily living.

Drug/medication history

- Is the patient currently prescribed medications for any pre-existing MSI conditions? If so, ascertain what for (*osteoporosis, osteoarthritis, rheumatoid arthritis, brittle bone disease, back pain, fibromyalgia, neck pain or anaemia*). Confirm with the patient if possible, why they take each medication.
- Ascertain if the patient is prescribed steroids, diuretics or statins, as these drugs are linked to osteoporosis, pathological fractures, and muscle cramping and generalized muscular pain.

- Is the patient compliant with their medications?
- Has the patient taken any analgesics for any pain they may be suffering? If so, what time did they take the medication?
- Are they taking or undergoing any courses of complementary therapy medicines?
- If so, which therapy (*acupuncture, diets, herbal medicine, homoeopathy, massage, supplements*)?
- If conveying the patient to a treatment unit, best practice dictates that their medications should be taken with them. The paramedic should document fully any medications taken or prescribed and record the administration of any medications on scene. This is particularly relevant with regard to opiate-based analgesics.

Social/family history

- Consider the activities of daily living (ADL), ascertain what they can or what they normally do for themselves. Has this changed? And if so, how will the MSI affect them?
- Depending upon the age of the patient, ascertain if they live alone or have relatives/carers or external agency (*social services, meal deliveries, etc.*).
- Ask about hobbies and pastimes that may be a cause of injury.
- Depending on the presenting medical condition, do other members of the patient's family also suffer from the condition/illness? Familial history is often a factor in patients presenting with many autoimmune conditions, for example, brittle bone disease, osteoporosis or arthritis.

REVIEW OF SYSTEMS

Regardless of the injury or illness, a general review of systems (ROS) provides the HCP with an overall picture of the patient's health. In addition, an ROS may help establish a link to the presenting complaint. For example, a patient with diabetes can be at an increased risk of developing musculoskeletal injuries. Diabetes UK (2015) provides information about musculoskeletal conditions and diabetes, including:

- Dupuytren's contracture (*the fingers can become permanently bent down*)
- Carpal tunnel syndrome (*occurs when the median nerve becomes pressed at the wrist*)
- Tenosynovitis (*inflammation of the tenosynovium, a sheath that covers tendons*)
- Frozen shoulder (*a stiffened glenohumeral joint that has lost significant range of motion (abduction and rotation)*)

- Limited joint mobility (*a type of rheumatism that causes the joints to lose their normal flexibility, more common in the hands (diabetic cheiroarthropathy)*)
- Charcot joint (*condition affecting one or more joints, due to peripheral nerve damage*).

PHYSICAL ASSESSMENT

The physical assessment of the patient with an actual or suspected musculoskeletal injury is carried out after history taking and will include a top-to-toe survey (*in children this can be conducted toe-to-head with a view to gaining the confidence and trust of the child*) and baseline clinical observations. The review of symptoms added to the focused history will direct the paramedic to the sites of injury and facilitate the opportunity for comparison with uninjured structures or limbs.

The paramedic at this stage of assessment should be aware of the patient's normal activities of daily living (ADL). It is important for the paramedic to manage the expectations of the patient with regard to their condition. Sedentary workers may be able to function and still attend work, often with significant MSI. However, the impact of an MSI on a tradesperson may significantly impair the patient's ability to secure an income during periods of injury.

Consent for examination of the patient should follow current guidelines consistent with current practice standards (Department of Health, 2009).

It is important that the paramedic considers the need for a chaperone when examining minors or members of the opposite sex. Documentation of consent should be recorded along with any capacity statements, which may be needed in the case of refusal for examination, assessment or treatment.

Examination of musculoskeletal injuries should follow a systematic approach. The paramedic will need to negotiate with the patient to ensure that they are in the most relaxed position to carry out the physical assessment. This should include issues regarding modesty, temperature and 360-degree access to the patient where possible. Musculoskeletal injury should follow a stepwise approach and have clear goals in terms of identifying **red flag** presentations and establishing treatment goals. A suggested format for examination is:

- Joint above
- Look
- Listen
- Feel
- Move

- Function
- Nerves/blood vessels (power/sensation/vascular compromise).

The paramedic should recall the **red flag** 5 P's of musculoskeletal injury assessment:

- Pain
- Paraesthesia
- Paralysis
- Pallor
- Pulse.

And with any injury assessed, the paramedic should also have a clear understanding of the general management principles to do the following:

- Reduce pain
- Prevent further injury
- Ensure neurovascular supply distal to injury
- Reduce risk of fat embolism
- Promote recovery.

Depending on the nature of the forces applied to cause an injury, associated proximal/distal injuries may be found away from the primary site. For this reason it is good practice to assess the limb/joint above the injury. By doing this, the paramedic will limit the risk of missing an injury and also gain the patient's trust as they are likely to find no injury and this examination will not have caused any discomfort (Wardrope and English, 2003).

When the paramedic looks at the site of injury, they are evaluating for a potential spectrum of damage directly related to the mechanism of injury. This may range from complicated fractures with systemic infections to simple self-limiting strains or sprains. Identification of a fracture is important as undiagnosed breaks, chips or cracks in the continuity of a bone can have serious consequences for the patient. As previously cited, the mnemonic SLIPDUCT helps the paramedic identify fractures or create the clinical climate for a high index of suspicion. Table 8.2 provides details of the component parts of this mnemonic and identifies the significance of each finding.

Fractures that are undiagnosed and remain untreated will have a significant impact on the patient's health and limit the potential for the return of normal function. SLIPDUCT complements the joint above, look, listen, feel approach to MSI and is recommended. Differentiation between skeletal and muscular compromise can be difficult in the out-of-hospital setting as pain and swelling coexist for both injuries. Stiffness and/or weakness may provide the paramedic with evidence suggesting muscular injury but in the assessment one cannot always exclude fracture.

Table 8.2 Components of the SLIPDUCT mnemonic

Element of SLIPDUCT	Clinical findings on examination
Swelling	An inflammatory response at the site of the injury causes a vascular cascade as essential repair mechanisms are initiated. This may result in vascular compromise (*compartment syndrome*).
Loss of function	Guarding, pain and the loss of muscular conformity cause the patient to partially or totally lose limb function. Loss of function may present as reduced ROM, absent mobility, reduced sensation or unequal muscular power.
Irregularity	Muscular contraction is unresisted by broken bones causing irregularity of the bone matrix, which may be visualized or palpated.
Pain	Localized to the fracture site and backed up by a history of trauma. The patient may report hearing a crack or feeling the break at the point of impact.
Deformity	A reliable sign of a fracture. Shortening and/or rotation can also occur at the fracture site. This occurs when muscular contraction forces exceed the capacity for the fractured limb to resist the pressure. Often termed a displaced fracture, the ends of broken bones will have moved from their neutral position and may have overlapped in extreme shortening.
Unnatural movement	Paradoxical movement, e.g. flail chest, produces opposing movements which can be life threatening.
Crepitus	Not always present in fractures but occurs as the broken ends of bones articulate at the fracture site. Crepitus should not be induced but should be documented if revealed on palpation or the patient reports a 'grinding' sensation on movement.
Tenderness	The sensation of pain reduces the patient's ability to move and is a primitive protective mechanism. Pain at, above or below the fracture site is common and will require appropriate pain management with splinting and analgesia.

Table 8.3 Movements to assess the extent of MSI and loss of function

Movement type	Description
Active range	Patient moves the limb. Muscles and ligaments are stretched. The joint is in motion.
Passive range	The paramedic moves the joint, ligaments are stretched, joint is moving, muscles inactive but are stretched at the limits of range.
Resisted movement	Muscles and tendons active against an opposing force. Joint is not moving.
Stress testing	Joints are stressed to look for signs of abnormal joint mobility. Pressure is directed towards and away from the midline (common in knee examination – lateral/medial flexion, draw test).
End of range feel	Sensation felt by the paramedic at the end of range of movement. Often described as 'empty' when there is little or no resistance or 'hard' when a ligament is structurally intact.
Capsular pattern	A pattern of restricted movement in synovial joints. Used to isolate joint injury.

Adapted from: Wardrope and English (2003: 17–23).

Movement is used to assess the possible extent of MSI and loss of function (see Table 8.3). It is important as it gives the paramedic insight into the type and severity of injury.

Joint injuries often present with characteristic limitations of movement. Active and passive range of movement (ROM) directly assesses joint function. Resisted movement and stressing of joints test for muscle, tendon or ligament injury. When a muscle or tendon is damaged, the patient may feel pain on resisted movement. In addition, the patient may experience ligament tenderness when stress is applied to an injured joint. The ROM should follow physiological patterns of movement consistent with joint function. The classification of joints is dependent on the presence or absence of a space between articulating bones (*synovial cavity*), and the type of connective tissue that binds bones together. A review of joint classification is shown in Table 8.4.

Directional terms are used to describe the range of movement (ROM) for each joint type. These are used in conjunction with directional terms such as superior, inferior, lateral and medial. Table 8.5 defines them.

Table 8.4 Joint classification

Joint type	Definition	Joint example	Normal ROM
Synovial	A freely moving joint which allows for several types of movement.	Elbow, knee	Extension, flexion, abduction, adduction, circumduction
Cartilaginous	Bones are held together with cartilage. There is no synovial cavity.	Pelvis, vertebral column	Little or no movement
Fibrous	Bones held together by collagen-rich fibrous connective tissue. There is no synovial cavity.	Bones of the skull	No movement

Table 8.5 Range of movement (ROM)

Movement	Definition
Retraction	Moving backwards
Protraction	Moving forwards
Flexion	Decreasing the joint angle (bending)
Extension	Increasing the joint angle (straightening)
Circumduction	Movement in a circular pattern
Abduction	Movement away from the midline
Adduction	Movement towards the midline
Internal rotation	Turning towards the midline
External rotation	Turning away from the midline
Pronation	Turning downwards
Supination	Turning upwards
Eversion	Turning outwards
Inversion	Turning inwards

In health, joints will be able to move in various planes depending on their structure and function. When assessing for movement it is important that movement is not forced. If in doubt, splint limb/joint in position pending further expert assessment.

As a joint is taken through its ROM, crepitus or crepitations (*crunching or popping sounds*) may be felt and heard. These noises are produced by the rubbing together or grinding of bones or damaged cartilage. The combination of joint movement and palpation may elicit sounds of joint crepitus. Examples include temporomandibular (TMD) and scapulothoracic disorders and runner's knee (*patella – cartilage rub*). While, on their own, audible crepitations or popping sounds are not diagnostic of MSI, they should be considered in general terms and linked to any abnormal pathology, injury or illness. Pain, crepitations, joint 'noises' and abnormal ROM from active passive and resisted joint manipulation during assessment should be documented.

Assessment for musculoskeletal injury should be focused through history taking and will guide the paramedic to the injured area. However, in the case of nonspecific or incomplete histories, a structured head-to-toe assessment should commence.

HEAD-TO-TOE ASSESSMENT
Head, neck, jaw

- Instigate MILS if any suspicion of 'C' spine injury.
- Palpate for deformity in the cervical midline.
- Inspect the head, neck and jaw for signs of deformity, lack of symmetry, swelling and signs of trauma.
- If no suspicion of 'C' spine injury, ask the patient to turn their head from side to side.
- Check for ROM by asking the patient to touch their right ear to their right shoulder and then do the same for the left. Check for symmetry of movement.
- Ask the patient to touch their chin to their chest and then look towards the ceiling.
- With the patient's shoulders parallel, they should be able to turn their head to the left and right to achieve alignment with the shoulders.
- Palpate for clicks and observe for abnormal jaw movement at the temporomandibular joint (TMJ).
- Document all findings including pertinent negatives, e.g. no 'C' spine tenderness.

Spinal column

Rule out the need for immediate manual inline stabilization and/or immobilization from the mechanism of injury (MOI). If the patient is walking, consider if there could be an occult injury, which will require immediate immobilization. Consider the MOI and the potential arc of injuries, e.g. axial loading.

- Palpate the individual spinal processes, noting any pain, swelling or deformity (Rushforth, 2009).
- If possible, observe the patient in a standing position. Check for scoliosis (*uneven shoulder height and shoulder blade prominence*) and kyphosis (*abnormally rounded thoracic curve*).
- Ask the patient to walk away from you, to stop, to turn around and walk back towards you. Check for symmetry of movement, symmetrical gait and pedal clearance as they step.

Shoulder joint

The shoulder is the most freely moving synovial joint (*triaxial diarthrosis*). The shoulder is a ball and socket joint. When the ball (*humeral head*) sits in the socket (*glenoid cavity*), the analogy is of a golf ball sitting on a golf tee. This is known as the glenohumeral joint. Damage to the joint occurs through either blunt trauma or indirect transmission of force, such as falling onto an outstretched hand (FOOSH). Traumatic displacements are often caused by concurrent abduction, extension and external rotation of the arm. The forces involved can either cause a subluxation (*partial dislocation*) or luxation (*full dislocation*) of the shoulder joint. Due to its extreme range of movement (ROM), the shoulder is the most commonly dislocated joint as a result of trauma (Bath and Lord, 2010). As the shoulder is weakest anteriorly and posteriorly, the humerus (humeral head) tends to dislocate in a forward and downward direction. The most common form of shoulder dislocation is anterior, occurring in 95%–97% of all cases. The incidence of shoulder dislocation in 18–70-year-olds is 1.7%, with males three times more likely to suffer the injury.

The shoulders, clavicles and upper chest should be fully exposed, allowing for a visual inspection of both injured and uninjured sides from all planes.

Joint above
- Examine the neck to ensure that there is no restriction of movement or associated discomfort.
- Shoulder pain where there is no history of trauma: one should always begin with an examination of the neck to rule out a referred pathology (Purcell, 2010).

- Extension, side flexion, rotations and flexions should be pain-free for the neck to have normal pathology.
- Identify the sternoclavicular joint (SCJ) and check for any deformity as it is readily injured during trauma.

Look/Inspect
- Observe for signs of a 'step' over the acromioclavicular joint (ACJ), the sternoclavicular joint (SCJ), the scapulothoracic and sub-acromial joints.
- Check for signs of trauma, swelling, bruising, redness and fine muscle tremors.
- Check for limb symmetry and compare with uninjured side.
- Check for signs of joint wasting or previous injury/surgery.

Feel/palpation
- Gently palpate the major shoulder landmarks (ACJ, SCJ, clavicle, acromion, scapula, humeral head, upper humerus and elbow). Note any abnormalities.

Move
- Active, passive and resisted movement can be carried out to help isolate injuries.
- Synovial joints have a finite range of movement due to the design of the joint capsule.
- Observe for capsular pattern and arcs of pain. Capsular pattern refers to pain or restriction in ROM specific to injury. 'Arcs of pain' refer to the characteristic discomfort felt on moving the joint. This pain is transient depending on the ROM. The paramedic should ask, what could be causing the pain?

Nerves and vessels
- Check for axillary nerve function by checking for sensation at the top of the deltoid muscle.
- Check radial, median and ulnar nerve sensation in the hands.
- Check distal pulse at the brachial and radial arteries and compare on both limbs.
- Assess distal perfusion, limb temperature and capillary refill time (CRT).

Special tests
- *Drop arm test* – This test highlights a rotator cuff tear. The arm is abducted to 90 degrees and the patient slowly lowers the arm. Pain and/or weakness are positive findings.

- *Horizontal flexion* – This test elicits pain from an acromioclavicular sprain. The arm is abducted to 90 degrees and then the arm passes across the chest, putting the hand on the opposite shoulder. Again pain and/or weakness are a positive sign.
- *External rotation against resistance* – The patient's arm is flexed at 90 degrees at the elbow and the arm is internally rotated 20 degrees. The patient is then asked to externally rotate their arm against resistance. Weakness of fatigue is a sign of a rotator cuff tear.

Red flags

Referred pain (*myocardial infarction, pneumothorax, pneumonia, tumour, aneurysm, gall bladder infection, ruptured spleen, ectopic pregnancy*), ACJ injuries, shoulder dislocation, clavicle fractures, humeral head fracture, scapula fracture, bicep tendon rupture, scapula wing, tendonitis, impingement, capsulitis, rheumatoid arthritis, osteoarthritis.

Elbow

The elbow is a synovial hinge joint. It consists of three bones: the distal humerus, the radial head and the proximal ulna. The radial and ulnar collateral ligament connects these joints. The joint is susceptible to three types of fracture: supracondylar of the humerus, radial head fracture, and olecranon fracture. In addition, radial head dislocations, bursitis and epicondylitis (*tennis and golfer's elbow*) are common findings.

Joint above
- Examine the shoulder for any abnormal pathology or restrictions in ROM.

Look
- Assess for deformity of joint and check for obvious swelling, bruising, signs of previous injury or surgery.

Feel
- Palpate bony landmarks and feel for inflammation, heat or boggy swelling over the olecranon (*bursitis*). Support the patient's forearm so that the elbow is flexed to approximately 70 degrees. Palpate bony prominences of the elbow and record findings.

Move
- Passively flex the elbow to 90 degrees and apply a downward force to the palmar surface of the patient's hand while supporting under the

elbow. The elbow's range of movements includes flexion and extension of the elbow and pronation/supination of the forearm. Apply varus (*towards midline*) and valgus (*away from midline*) force to joint site. Note any positive findings.

Function
- Test for general function of the elbow through all planes of movement as described above.

Nerves/vascular supply
- Check for sensation around the joint and check distal pulses.

Red flags

Fractures, dislocations or suspected joint infection.

Forearm, wrist and hand

In the out-of-hospital environment, the occurrence of a fall onto an outstretched hand (FOOSH) is a common cause of injury. The nature of the fall (*mechanical or collapse*) should be investigated to rule out priority signs. Common patterns of injury of the forearm are shown in Table 8.6.

Table 8.6 Patterns of injury in the forearm

Pattern of injury	Bones
Monteggia pattern	A fracture of the ulna with associated dislocation of the proximal radius
Galeazzi pattern	A fracture of the radius with an associated dislocation of the distal ulna
Colles fracture	A fracture of the distal end of the radius, which is displaced backwards, and upwards to produce a 'dinner fork' deformity. The avulsion of the ulna styloid process also usually occurs.

Joint above
- Review the joint at the elbow and document any abnormal pathology.

Look
- Observe the forearm, wrist and hands for obvious signs of deformity, swelling, redness or loss of function.
- Observe for muscle tremors, bruising or signs of guarding from patient.

Feel
- Palpate the head of the radius when the arm is in motion. Note any crepitus.
- Palpate the scaphoid (*anatomical snuff box*).
- Systematically palpate the carpals and metacarpals of the hand and note any site-specific pain, crepitus or deformity.
- Palpate the phalanges and note any abnormal pathology.

Move
- Flex elbow to 90 degrees, extend wrist to 90 degrees. Test pronation and supination, note any pain on movement.
- Test active and passive range of movement of fingers through normal ROM.

Function
- Observe for loss of function or weakness in forearm, wrist and hand.
- Compare both limbs.

Nerves/vascular supply
- Check for sensation, distal pulses and capillary refill.
- Compare limb temperature with uninjured side.
- Note any abnormal pathology.

Red flags

Unless trauma is very minor, X-ray is indicated due to risk of permanent disability and loss of function.

Pelvis

The formation of the pelvic bones and associated structure suggests that significant trauma is required to fracture the pelvic girdle itself. A fracture of the femoral head is a more common finding. Multiple fractures of the pelvic girdle are common with significant trauma mechanisms. Suspected pelvic fractures are time critical due to the potential for catastrophic haemorrhage.

Due to the close association between the pelvis, the abdominal cavity and its organs, it is difficult to isolate pelvic pain outside of a clear trauma history. Significant trauma to the pelvis should prompt the paramedic towards analgesia, splinting and the management of internal haemorrhage (see *Trauma Assessment, Chapter 7*).

Joint above
- The pelvis articulates with the femoral head and is continuous with the vertebral column. Due to complex structures, the potential for muscle strains, ligament tears, tendon ruptures and fractures are all possibilities as the pelvis forms a large surface area for attachment to the lower limbs.
- The patient should be able to flex and extend at the hip. Rotation should be unopposed and pain-free.
- The patient should be able to carry out passive, active and resisted leg movements within their ROM, again without reporting pain.

Look
- Look for a symmetrical pelvic girdle that is continuous on light palpation. Note the presence of incontinence.
- Observe for the open 'book sign' as legs and feet externally rotate indicating pelvic fracture.
- Watch for abdominal distension and rigidity as a sign of internal haemorrhage.

Feel
- Lightly palpate the iliac crests and note any irregularity.
- **DO NOT** 'spring' the pelvis to assess. This will only increase bleeding, elicit pain and break down clot formation.

Move
- If pelvic trauma is suspected, splint and immobilize the patient using a pelvic splint at the level of the greater trochanter. A high index of suspicion of associated fractures is best practice in these circumstances.

Function
- Test for loss of power and sensation in the legs.
- Check distal pulses and capillary refill time (CRT).

Nerves/vascular supply
- Due to the nature of the pelvic anatomy, suspect neurovascular compromise in the presence of significant pelvic trauma.
- Incontinence may be a sign of nerve damage and loss of bladder control.

Knee

The knee is a complex joint which is often a source of pain and discomfort for patients. The joint suffers from injuries as a result of trauma and degenerative diseases such as arthritis. Knee pain is common among all age groups. Reports of knee pain, swelling and locking are common presentations. Ligaments, tendons, cartilage (*meniscus*) can all produce knee pain and loss of function. In extreme cases, dislocation of the knee joint can occur. The knee joint experiences significant pressure during normal ADLs. Walking up a flight of stairs increases the pressure in the knee by a factor of 4.

Joint above
- Observe the patient's quadriceps for signs of wasting and asymmetry.
- Examine the pelvis and hip joint and report any abnormal pathology.

Look
- Compare both knee joints and observe any signs of obvious inflammation.

Feel
- Palpate the bones of the knee.
- Check for signs of fluid and note any difference in joint temperature.
- Note any crepitus on movement.

Move
- Use passive, active and resisted movement to take the joint through its ROM. Note any abnormal findings.

Special tests
- *Draw test* – tests for anterior cruciate ligament stability. Knee joint is flexed to 90 degrees. The foot is isolated (*sit on it*) and the tibia is pulled anteriorly to assess excessive joint mobility.
- *Lateral stressing* – tests medial and lateral collateral ligament. Carried out on a straight leg. Pressure is applied laterally and medially against a splinted knee joint.

Function
- If possible, the patient should be observed walking, standing and sitting. If possible, ask the patient to crouch to fully assess the integrity of the joint.

Nerves/vascular supply
- Check for distal pulses, sensation and power.

🚩 Red flags
Fracture/dislocation, septic arthritis and osteomyelitis.

Ankle and foot
Ligament tears, fractures and damage to associated structures are relatively common in this area of the body. For assessment, the patient should be seated to avoid further injury or pain (Pilbery, 2014).

Joint above
- Palpate the knee and calf.
- Check for signs of inflammation behind the knee and note any swelling or pain in the calf *(deep vein thrombosis)*.

Look
- Observe for any signs of swelling, redness and/or deformity of the ankle joint.

Listen
- Note any audible noises on joint movement.

Feel
- Palpate the bones of the lower leg, ankle and foot. Include the Achilles tendon, fibula, calf, calcaneum, malleoli and 5th metatarsal.
- Note any abnormal pathology or presence of pain.
- Positive findings may require X-ray (*Ottawa ankle rules*, see Table 8.7 and Figure 8.1).

Move
- In the absence of swelling, carry out passive, active and resisted movements.

Special test
- *Simmonds' calf squeeze* – patient kneels on a chair with both feet hanging off the end. The feet should sit squarely. The calf is squeezed and the foot should flex. If the foot does not move, this is a sign of an Achilles tendon injury.

Function
- Observe for the ability to weight-bear.
- Pain may only occur on lateral or medial movement, indicating a ligament injury.

Musculoskeletal assessment

Table 8.7 Ottowa rules for X-ray of ankle and foot

Joint	Ottowa X-ray rule
Ankle	X-ray required if there is pain in the malleolar zone and any of the following: • Bone tenderness at A OR • Bone tenderness at B • Inability to weight-bear both immediately and in the minor injury unit (MIU) or emergency department (ED)
Foot	X-ray required if there any pain in the midfoot zone and any of the following: • Bone tenderness at C • Bone tenderness at D • Inability to weight-bear both immediately and in the minor injury unit (MIU) or emergency department (ED)

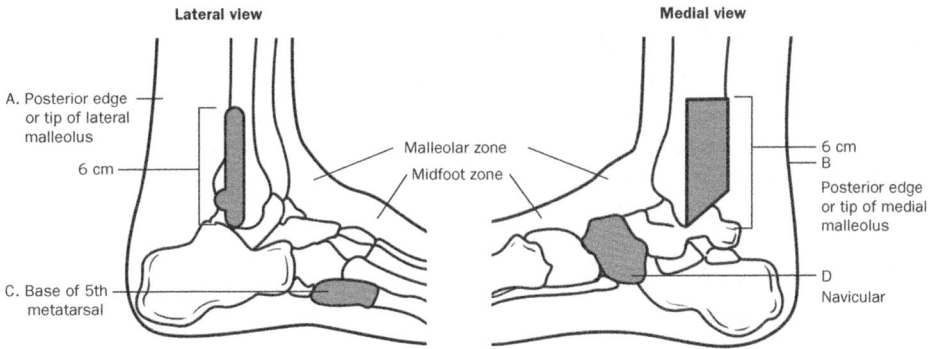

Figure 8.1 The Ottawa foot and ankle rule definitions Adapted from GP-training.net (2015)

Nerves/vascular supply
• Check distal pulses and capillary bed refill.

Red flags

The absence of distal pulses, reduced motor or sensory control. Poor perfusion (capillary refill >2 seconds).

OTHER CONSIDERATIONS

Communication

The presence of a musculoskeletal injury is often accompanied by pain. This can be a significant barrier to treatment in the young and old alike. The paramedic will need to gain the confidence of the patient by demonstrating a clear understanding of the concerns of the patient. The use of analgesia leading to effective splinting and immobilization should be incorporated as a part of the biopsychosocial model of pain management.

The paramedic will need to consider the expectations of the patient with regard to healing times and the effect that the MSI may have on their ADLs. Special consideration needs to be given when assessing patients who are cognitively impaired or unable to communicate. The use of observational pain scale such as the 'Abbey Pain scale' is recommended in instances where the patient is unable to self-report their pain. It is the responsibility of the paramedic to explore all avenues of communication (*language line, interpreters, phrase books, appropriate family members*) to ensure that every patient receives the appropriate standards of care.

Social/family/carer/guardian

When conducting a physical examination on a minor, best practice dictates that the parents/guardians are present, but in the absence of these individuals, every effort should be made to ensure the safety and well-being of the patient. Referral to welfare organizations in suspected non-accidental injury (NAI) should be initiated without delay (Fisher et al., 2013).

Ethical and legal issues

Informed consent to examine the patient should be gained and revisited throughout the assessment, and the use of chaperones considered, where appropriate. The withdrawal of consent should be noted and the assessment stopped in compliance with a consenting adult/child with capacity. Every effort should be made to ensure the safety, dignity and health of the patient without capacity who is refusing treatment. The paramedic should comply with current legislation guidelines with regard to the consent and capacity, and simultaneously be aware of the vulnerability of their patient, reporting any areas of concern via the most appropriate pathway (*social services, police*).

Destination/receiving specialist units/non-conveyance

The emergence of regional major trauma centres, minor injury units and other specialist medical facilities allows the paramedic to treat and refer MSI appropriately. Current guidelines and referral processes should be accessed by the paramedic and every effort made to ensure the patient is involved in decision-making. Non-conveyance should be followed up with appropriate referral via a clinician-to-clinician **handover** to ensure a joined-up system of care. Documentation of all findings, referrals and decision-making processes are vital to mitigate risk and protect the patient and paramedic.

CHAPTER KEY POINTS

- Musculoskeletal injuries can present significant challenges for the paramedic.
- Ensure adequate early pain relief and assess for effect.
- Remember the joint above, look, listen, feel, move, function approach to assessment.
- Clear histories of MOI should be consistent with injuries sustained.
- Watch for **red flag** conditions and inconsistent history.
- Consider and use appropriate referral to trauma units, minor injury units, or general practitioner.
- If in doubt, refer patient for further assessment and tests.

REFERENCES

Association of Ambulance Chief Executives (2013) *UK Ambulance Services Clinical Practice Guidelines 2013 Pocket Book: Oxygen*. Bridgwater: Class Professional Publishing.

Bath, T. and Lord, B. (2010) The risk/benefit of paramedic initiated shoulder reduction, *Journal of Paramedic Practice*, 1(6).

Department of Health (2009) *Reference Guide to Consent for Examination or Treatment* (2nd edn). London: Department of Health.

Diabetes UK (2015) *Muscular Conditions*. Available at. http://www.diabetes.org.uk/Guide-to-diabetes/What-is-diabetes/Related-conditions/ (accessed 13 May 2015).

Fisher, J., Brown, S.N. and Cooke, M. (eds) (2013) *UK Ambulance Services Clinical Practice Guidelines 2013: Safeguarding Children*. Bridgwater: Class Professional Publishing.

GP-training.net (2015) *Ottowa Ankle and Foot Rules*. Available at: http://www.gp-training.net/rheum/ottawa.htm (accessed 11 May 2015).

Greaves, I., Wright, C., Porter, K., Hodgetts, T. and Woollard, M. (2012) *Pocket Book of Emergency Care: A Quick Reference Guide for Paramedics*. Edinburgh: Saunders Elsevier.

Health and Safety Executive (HSE) (2015) Musculoskeletal Disorders (MSD) in Great Britain. Available at: http://www.hse.gov.uk/statistics/causdis/musculoskeletal/index.htm (accessed 11 May 2015).

Hodgetts, T., Mahoney, P., Russell, M. and Byers, M. (2006) ABC to [C]ABC: redefining the military trauma paradigm. *Emergency Medical Journal* 23: 745–6.

Pilbery, R. (2014) *Nancy Caroline's Emergency Care in the Streets: United Kingdom* (7th edn). Burlington, VA: Jones & Bartlett Learning.

Purcell, D. (2010) *Minor Injuries: A Clinical Guide* (2nd edn). Edinburgh: Churchill Livingstone Elsevier.

Rushforth, H. (2009) *Assessment Made Incredibly Easy.* (UK edn). Philadelphia, PA: Lippincott Williams & Wilkins.

Wardrope, J. and English, B. (2003) *Musculoskeletal Problems in Emergency Medicine.* Oxford: Oxford University Press.

9 Assessment of minor injuries
Marlon Steill

INTRODUCTION

In order to assess minor injuries in the out-of-hospital environment, the paramedic should have a clear understanding regarding the number of decisions that must be taken in order that the patient receives the right treatment and advice without delay. To inform decision-making with patients with minor injuries, paramedics should familiarize themselves with local policies on treatment and discharge. Part of the referral process should include an understanding of what treatment the patient will receive if the paramedic decides to refer. Patients should also be given analgesia, where not contra-indicated, at the earliest opportunity. With minor injuries, analgesia such as ibuprofen and paracetamol are the recommended frontline treatments. By administering analgesia at the earliest opportunity, the degree of pain felt by the patient will be reduced and will allow a more in-depth examination of the injury. This is particularly pertinent for injuries to joints.

Patients may be examined before being referred back to their GP or community nurse. A visit to the emergency department (ED) may be avoided with careful examination of a minor injury. The paramedic can arrange referral to a community service without the need for attendance at the emergency department.

The paramedic, before embarking on assessment, must exclude any potential life-threatening or life-changing conditions for the patient. Once you have excluded the possibility that any such condition is present, the paramedic should consider **red flags** which may not be immediately observable or information obtained from the patient history. Red flags serve as a trigger to refer the patient to a more experienced paramedic or health professional for review and investigation. If the patient does not trigger any **red flags**, then a paramedic may continue to assess the patient with view to not conveying to the ED or urgent care centre.

This overview of minor injuries covers the following areas:
- Head injury and neck pain
- Facial injuries
- Upper and lower limb injuries
- Wounds.

HEAD INJURY: BACKGROUND

Head injuries are common presentations in the out-of-hospital setting. It is estimated that 1.4 million people attend the ED in the United Kingdom as result of a head injury per year. Of this number, 40,000 patients are thought to have sustained fractures to the skull or received damage to the brain (NICE, 2014a) (see *Trauma Assessment, Chapter 7*).

Patients who experience a minor head injury are unlikely to experience serious pathology. Recent studies estimate that 85% of patients deemed to have minor head injury make a full recovery. This leaves 15% of patients who develop symptoms that result in life-threatening or life-changing outcomes (Headway, 2012). Head injury assessment should focus on differentiating between minor, moderate and severe head injuries, how to evaluate your patients' cognitive and physiological function, and, if referring, understanding the reason for referral and the nature of your intervention.

The paramedic should employ an appropriate framework to gain a history of events. A common error is to assume the language the patient uses corresponds to physical symptoms. It is important to clarify what they mean, for example when discussing pain. Patients should rate their pain, but also describe the type. Another example is when patients complain of feeling unwell. This may mean nauseous, but a vague description such as feeling unwell can easily be misinterpreted by the paramedic and ascribed to a sign or symptom not present. The history will give you clues as to potential seriousness of the patient's condition.

Mechanism of injury (MOI)

Patients may present with seemingly minor injuries, however, a significant mechanism of injury should alert the paramedic to the potential for a serious underlying condition.

In addition to falls, road traffic collisions, blunt trauma and sport injuries, consider incidents where safeguarding is an issue, e.g. domestic violence, and whether a weapon has been used. It is important that the mechanism of injury is documented.

Assessment of minor injuries

Head injury red flags

The following are considered **red flag** in relation to patients with head injuries:

- Unconsciousness or loss of consciousness (LOC) since the injury
- Any focal neurological deficit since the injury
- Any seizure (*'convulsion' or 'fit'*) since the head injury
- High-energy head injury (*blow to the head, fall*)
- Amnesia of events before or after the injury
- Persistent headache since the injury
- Any vomiting episodes since the injury
- Any previous brain surgery
- Any history of bleeding or clotting disorders
- Current anti-coagulant therapy such as Warfarin
- Current drug or alcohol intoxication
- If the paramedic obtains a history where there are safeguarding concerns (*possible non-accidental injury (NAI) or a vulnerable person is affected*)
- Irritability or altered behaviour (*'easily distracted', 'not themselves', 'no concentration', 'no interest in things around them'*), particularly in infants and children younger than 5 years
- Continuing concern by the professional about the diagnosis
- Suspicion of a skull fracture or penetrating head injury
- No one is able to observe the injured person at home
- Continuing concern by the injured person or their family or carer about the diagnosis
- Some patients may present with a pre-existing condition which may make it more difficult to assess, for example, patients with dementia, underlying chronic neurological disorders or learning disabilities.

Treatment of wounds and bruising in head injuries

Head injury wounds may be treated as long as they are minor and do not require referral. Factors which affect the treatment of wounds and may require referral are:

- Potential fractures and injury to the underlying structures in face and head, e.g. tendons and muscles
- If the injury is as a result of an assault
- The risk of infection to the patient
- Wounds which are around the eyes, nose and mouth (*may require referral to a plastic surgeon to reduce scarring. Keloid scarring occurs in population groups with darker skin.*)
- Foreign bodies. It is possible the wound may contain gravel and grit. If the wound cannot be treated at the location due to the presence of

dirt and grit, the patient may be referred. When the patient's skin re-grows over the wound, there is a risk of tattooing.
- Wounds should be cleaned and irrigated as far as possible. Puncture wounds should be explored. Assume a foreign body is still in situ if the laceration has occurred as the result of broken glass.
- Test sensation around wound (*loss of sensation indicates possible vascular or neurological injury*) (Purcell, 2013a).

FRAMEWORK FOR ASSESSING PAIN IN PATIENTS

The SOCRATES framework can be used to assess pain (AACE, 2013):

S – Site. Where exactly is the pain? Or the maximal site of the pain?
O – Onset. When did the pain start, and was it sudden or gradual? Include also whether if it is progressive or regressive.
C – Character. What does the pain feel like?
R – Radiate. Does the pain go anywhere else?
A – Associated symptoms. Is it associated with any other symptoms? For example, nausea and/or vomiting.
T – Time/duration. Does the pain follow any pattern?
E – Exacerbating/relieving factors. Does anything make the pain better or worse?
S – Severity. Obtain an initial pain score (*0 = no pain, 10 = worst pain ever*).

The patient should also be examined for the following ailments using the JACCOL process:

J – Jaundice
A – Anaemia
C – Clubbing
C – Cyanosis
O – Oedema
L – Lymphadenopathy

The presence of any of these symptoms indicates that the patient may require referral and a more detailed examination.

NECK PAIN AND COMMON CAUSES

A patient may present with a stiff neck in the morning or neck stiffness over a number of days. The most common cause is acute torticollis. This condition also known as wry neck is usually self-limiting and resolves in a number of days, though occasionally longer. The recommended treatment for this condition is gentle exercise and analgesia.

The causes of neck pain can include:

- Poor posture
- Neck strain
- Sporting and occupational activities, e.g. sitting at a desk for long periods
- Cancer
- Cervical spondylosis
- Cervical inter-vertebral disc lesions and prolapse
- Infection, e.g. osteomyelitis
- Osteoarthritis, osteoporosis, fibromyalgia
- Rheumatoid arthritis
- Scoliosis and kyphosis
- Trauma
- Torticollis (acute neck spasm).

Neck examination

History should establish the chain of events which have led to the patient presenting.

- What is the mechanism of injury?
- What was the patient's activity at the time of the injury or onset of pain?
- Patient's level of alcohol consumption?
- The number of pillows that the patient uses to sleep.
- Has there been any history of recent illness, for example, vomiting, fever or rash?
- Have there been any symptoms such as shortness of breath, headache, palpitations, and/or earache?
- It is important to avoid leading questions when talking to your patient.
- Has the patient noticed any new swelling around the neck?
- Use the SOCRATES framework to assess any pain in the patient's neck.
- Be sure to obtain past medical and family history.

The process of examination follows: LOOK, FEEL and MOVE.

- LOOK; Check the site of injury for any abnormalities as listed above.
- FEEL: Palpate the neck to feel for any swelling, deformities and pain. (Think JACCOL here and check lymph nodes and oedema during neck examination.)

- MOVE: consists of three elements:
  - Active: is what the patient can do for themselves. How much degree of movement do they have before it is uncomfortable or painful? How does this compare to normal movements?
  - Passive: the paramedic moves the affected joint carefully in order to establish the degree to which muscles are involved in the presenting complaint.
  - Resisted: the patient moves the affected limb/joint against resistance. The paramedic provides the resistance in order to elicit the power remaining within the muscles.

Reference to these three movements will be abbreviated to APR in other parts of this chapter (see *Musculoskeletal Assessment, Chapter 8*) (Bickley, 2013; Purcell, 2013b).

The paramedic needs to clearly understand what the local pathway is for the management of head and neck injuries. Finally, ensure the patient receives the right aftercare. Are you able to administer or prescribe analgesia, antibiotics and order interventions? If you are unable to do this, then the patient needs referral to a senior paramedic or health professional.

UPPER LIMB INJURY

This section covers injuries to the shoulders, arms and wrists. Paramedics should familiarize themselves with the anatomy of the upper limbs. During the history taking, **red flags** should be seen as reason for referral to a more senior and experienced paramedic or health professional.

Shoulder joint

The shoulder joint (see *Musculoskeletal Assessment, Chapter 8*) is akin to a 'golf ball on a golf tee' and consists of:

- Glenohumeral joint
- Acromioclavicular joint (ACJ)
- Scapula and posterior chest wall.

This joint is held together by ligaments and a web of muscles.

Look

- Expose both shoulders.
- Compare sides, noting: swelling? Discoloration? Deformity? Atrophy?
- Remember: problems elsewhere (e.g. neck, abdomen) can cause referred pain.

Feel

Identify and palpate each of the bony surface landmarks:

- Acromion
- Clavicle
- Humerus
- Scapula
- Assess neurovascular status.

Move

- Compare affected and unaffected side.
- Normal range of movements for shoulder joint APR are: flexion, extension, internal, external rotation, and adduction/abduction.

Shoulder dislocation: management strategies

Look and Feel assessment ONLY. The patient may present with the following:

- Classic step deformity
- Severe pain, 10/10
- Check neurovascular status. Regimental badge sign may be present (*loss of sensation in the deltoid muscle of the affected limb*).
- Check peripheral pulses
- Patient should be referred for X-ray
- Management should include immobilization or self-splinting.

Red flags

Referred pain (*aneurysm, gall bladder infection, ruptured spleen, ectopic pregnancy, myocardial infarction, pneumothorax, pneumonia, tumour*), ACJ injuries, clavicle fractures, humeral head fracture, scapula fracture, shoulder dislocation, bicep tendon rupture, scapula wing, tendonitis, impingement, capsulitis, rheumatoid arthritis, osteoarthritis.

Elbow

The elbow is a hinge and pivot joint and consists of humerus, ulna and radius. The normal elbow examination is:

- Clear joints above and below/shoulder wrist and hand
- Look
- Feel
- Move.

Normal range of movements of the elbow is active, passive, resisted:
- Pronation/flexion
- Supination/extension.

Common conditions are:
- Olecranon bursitis
- Septic joint
    - Consider with any entry point/wound
    - Staphylococcus aureus likely pathogen
    - Refer if cellulitis – may need IV antibiotics
- Non-septic joint
    - Causes include trauma/overuse
- Systemic conditions: rheumatoid arthritis, gout.

For gout, use simple PRICE advice:

P – Protection
R – Rest
I – Ice (10–20 minutes every 2 hours for 72 hours) (no direct contact with skin)
C – Compression (if significant swelling)
E – Elevation

Advice on what to do if things go wrong and how to look after the limb and the type of analgesia needed are given in Clinical Knowledge Summaries (2012).

Red flags

Fractures, dislocations or suspected joint infection.

Wrist and hand injuries

Common ED/out-of-hospital presentation. Significant risk to function following injury – be aware of litigation risk!

Key points
- Injuries may involve multiple structures.
- Injuries can also involve bones, tendon, muscles, nerves, vessels.
- Wrist/hand: Look.
- Wrist/hand: Feel.
- Normal range of movements for wrist and hand active, passive, resistance:
    - Extension and flexion of the radius and ulna

- Common injury caused by FOOSH (fallen on outstretched hand)
  - Dorsal displacement of distal fragment (dinner fork deformity) – with or without ulna fracture
  - May not always be clinically obvious
  - Low index of suspicion in any patient with bony tenderness – increased risk with age
  - Consider falls aetiology and future falls risk
  - Consider scaphoid fractures. Theses fractures are often missed. Important to remember the scaphoid bone does not have its own blood supply
  - May not be apparent on initial X-ray
  - Risk to long-term function in the use of the affected hand.

Red flags

Unless trauma is very minor, X-ray is indicated due to risk of permanent disability and loss of function.

Knee

The knee is composed of the femur and proximal tibia. It is a hinge joint, stabilized with muscles, ligaments, tendons and menisci which are situated below the patella. The patella is a sesamoid bone that protects and supports movement.

Normal range of movements for the knee
- Passive extension
- Extensor mechanism
- Active, passive, resisted flexion
- Passive lateral rotation of the tibia
- Passive medial rotation of the tibia
- Medial collateral ligament
- Lateral collateral ligament
- Anterior cruciate drawer
- Posterior cruciate ligament.

The MOI is important – will give clues to type of injury, such as a direct blow, or varus/valgus force (inversion/extension of knee). Imaging in knee injuries is rarely required for most injuries.

Ottawa X-ray rules: determines the need for X-rays, proven sensitive for fracture. Example:
- Age >55 years
- Tenderness head of fibula

- Isolated patellar tenderness
- Inability to flex knee 90 degrees
- Inability to bear weight.

Consider septic arthritis when examining a knee, especially those which are warm to touch.

Risk factors are:

- Age >80 years
- Diabetes mellitus
- Rheumatoid arthritis
- Prosthetic joint
- Recent joint surgery
- Skin infection, cutaneous ulcers
- IV drug abuse, alcoholism
- Previous intra-articular corticosteroid injection
- Open fractures (Rossi and Margheritini, 2014)

Assess range of movement of knee and compare good limb to injured limbs to test medial and lateral ligaments, posterior and anterior ligaments and palpate below the patella to assess damage to the meniscus.

Ankle and foot

Ankle injury often presents as result of an inversion or eversion movement of the ankle, resulting in stretching of ligaments causing damage to the surrounding tissue. The ligaments which can be damaged in ankle sprains are the calcaneo fibular ligament and the anterior talofibular ligaments. It is important to understand the functional impairment following injury.

Normal range of movements for ankle and foot:

- Active/resisted
- Dorsi-flexion
- Plantar flexion of the ankle
- Inversion
- Eversion.

The Simmonds test is an examination that is used to test for the tear of the Achilles tendon. The test is performed with the patient lying face down with feet hanging off the edge of the bed. The calf of the affected limb is squeezed. The test is positive if there is no movement of the foot (normally plantar flexion), indicating there may be damage to the Achilles tendon (see *Table 8.7, Ottowa ankle & foot X-ray rules*, and *Figure 8.1, Musculoskeletal Assessment, Chapter 8*).

Assessment of ankle sprains

Ankle injuries are extremely common but many features on history and physical examination are unreliable. Treatment for ligament injuries should include dynamic splinting and RICE:

    R – Rest
    I – Ice
    C – Compression
    E – Elevation

Assessment: Mechanism of injury (MOI)

- Can you tell me (show me) what exactly happened?
- Inversion/eversion/twisting forces/direct blow
- Fall from height/diffuse blunt forces – consider additional injuries
- What are the symptoms?
- Why are you presenting today?
- Have you seen anyone else about this injury?
- Consider alternative causes
- NAI/non-injury pathologies
- Use SOCRATES history to establish pattern of any pain experienced.

Additional pain concerns are:

- Not affected by movement or at night
- Sudden onset – non-trauma
- Severe – no relief with opiates
- Extremes of age
- Limb weakness/paraesthesia.

Additional questions on:

- Weight loss and anorexia
- Patient history of cancer
- Steroid use
- Systemic symptoms.

Red flags

The absence of distal pulses, reduced motor or sensory control. Poor perfusion (capillary refill >2 seconds).

Strain

The stretching or tearing of muscle or tendon (*fibrous cord of tissue that connects muscles to bones*).

Sprain

The stretching or tearing of ligaments (*tough bands of fibrous tissue that connect one bone to another*). Very common presentations in ankle injuries and sports, can lead to instability and re-injury of muscle or joint. They need careful assessment and physiotherapy/guided self-management.

There are three grades of sprain:

- Grade I: is the stretching of ligaments associated with swelling around the joint depending on the mechanism of injury.
- Grade II: is the partial tearing of ligaments.
- Grade III: is defined as the stretching or tearing of muscle or tendon (fibrous cord of tissue that connects muscles to bones).

WOUNDS

All wounds contain a degree of bacteria on their surface. The source of this bacteria may be the patient themselves or from the environment. The presence of bacteria or micro-organisms is a natural phenomenon on the skin and does not mean that an open wound is infected.

The degree and type of wound can be classified depending upon the severity and level of colonization. Therefore, the paramedic must understand how to identify, assess and manage wounds and understand the factors that will influence the recovery of the patient.

There are a number of factors any paramedic should consider before beginning to treat wounds in primary care:

- Are you able to competently identify this type of wound?
- Does this patient have a care plan that covers the treatment of the wound?
- Do you have access to a suitable tool or treatment framework to assess this patient's wound?
- Are you up to date in your education on how to treat and dress wounds?
- What type of dressing would be needed to treat this wound?
- Are you able to refer the patient to the correct health care professional if required?
- Are you able to provide the right aftercare advice to the patient, if you are not conveying to minor injury unit/hospital (Andrews, 2013)?

Wound classification

The normal wound healing process consists of four stages which overlap: (1) initial coagulation leads to an inflammatory phase; (2) tissue granulation is tissue formation aided by white blood cells neutrophils, and including platelets; (3) the presence of blood vessels produces the granular appearance; and (4) the final stage of healing takes between 1 to 2 weeks with the granulated tissue being remodelled, with eventual formation of a cellular scar.

Acute injuries are classified by the degree of trauma experienced by the body's tissues:

- *Incision injuries*: typically involves broken glass, sharp metals, covering a small surface area. Presentation may involve exposure of the deep tendons or underlying tissue, nerves and tendons of the affected limb. Distal neurovascular status in arms and hands (radial, median and ulna nerves) and in the tibial, common fibular, medial plantar nerve, lateral plantar nerve, plantar digital nerves and calcaneal branches of the tibial and sural nerve, and musculo-tendonous function should be tested, and one should consider the likelihood of foreign bodies in the wound (Bowen and Slaven, 2014).
- *Laceration injuries*: can be caused by a punch to the face, or blunt impact to pre-tibial skin. Laceration wounds cover a wider area due to the nature of MOI and the wound may be contused. The impact causes the tissue to split. Common presentations are split lips and cuts to eyebrows.
- *Abrasion injuries*: are the result of falls or low intensity skid. The loss of tissue on the affected body part is varied in terms of the surface area and the depth of the abrasion. Careful examination should exclude the possibility of an underlying de-gloving injury. Abrasions present with dirt, grit and other foreign bodies. These wounds must be cleaned and irrigated thoroughly to minimize the risk of infection and to avoid tattooing where the skin heals over the grit and dirt (Barnard and Allison, 2009).

History taking

When ascertaining the history surrounding the wound, ascertain and address the following;

- Is this wound acute or chronic?
- How was the wound caused?
- Are any foreign bodies present in the tissues?
- How many layers of tissue involvement are there?

- How deep is the wound and which tissues are involved?
- Is the wound producing fluid?
- Is the fluid blood, serum or exudate?
- Is the patient in any pain?
- What are the characteristics of the pain?

Where possible, all wounds should be cleaned, irrigated (with normal saline) and closed. This gives the patient a greater chance to avoid infection and complications as a result of the injury.

Check capillary refill distal to injury to assess the extent to which arteries may be damaged.

Contra-indications to closure of a laceration in the community setting is where there is a high risk of a wound developing an infection, such as a human or animal bite. The patient should be considered for prophylactic antibiotics. The paramedic should be aware of the local guidelines on the treatment and closure of wounds which are over 6 hours old. In such cases, it is probable that the wound edges may have begun the healing process, so closing the wound will be of limited use. In such cases, referral to health care professionals who have wound expertise is necessary.

Possible actions to be taken:

- Ascertain the classification of the wound
- Where possible clean, irrigate (*with normal saline*) and close all wounds
- Check distal capillary refill distal to the wound for circulation damage
- Be aware of local guidelines regarding treatment/closure of wounds >6 hours old.

Acute wound types

Knuckle, fingers or hand (including bites)

Patients involved in a fight may present with a puncture wound over the exposed metacarpo-phalangeal (MCP) joints or proximal inter-phalangeal (PIP) joint of the dominant hand, where the hand comes into contact with their opponent's teeth.

These groups of patients should be referred for radiography to exclude fractures and the possibility of any foreign bodies. Wounds caused as the result of bite marks are highly susceptible to infection due to the likely presence of oral bacteria.

Pre-tibial lacerations

Older patients develop 'thin skin' which renders them more susceptible to pre-tibial wounds and exacerbates the damage sustained (Cornforth, 2013). The majority of patients who experience pre-tibial lacerations that require hospital treatment are elderly (Demidova-Rice et al., 2012). A significant number of these patients have underlying conditions which may have contributed to the injury being sustained, or as a result of a fall (NICE, 2013).

Consider any co-morbidities which may be present when formulating your treatment plan and medication prescribed, for example, anti-coagulants which may hinder wound healing. Skin flaps can be treated in the out-of-hospital setting with irrigation and providing the sides of the wound can be opposed. Any skin flaps should be assessed for tissue viability.

Continuance of the management of pre-tibial wounds should be the responsibility of community services.

Aftercare ensures patients who are vulnerable, especially the older patient, or those with long-term conditions do not go on to develop a decline in health. Pre-tibial injuries are associated with patients who are often dependent, and require a high level of support in the community. The relationship between injury and level of care required is unclear though it is possible pre-tibial lacerations (often the result of a fall) may lead to loss of confidence and a decline in mobility (McClelland et al., 2012).

Assessment of chronic wounds

Acute injuries generally have positive outcomes without the need for any significant interventions. Chronic wounds, however, require frequent monitoring and interventions to promote recovery. The inability of chronic wounds to heal is caused by both cellular and molecular abnormalities occurring within the wound bed (Demidova-Rice et al., 2012).

Chronic wounds may be caused by:

- Infection
- Ischemia
- Radiation poisoning wounds
- Surgery.

Chronic wounds are graded, and the most common type of chronic wounds are ulcers (see Table 9.1).

Table 9.1 Grading of chronic wounds

Grade	Characteristics of wound
Grade 1	The initial stage of wound infection begins with the inflammatory stage. The patient's skin may present erythematic, swelling, oedema, pain around the wound (*or referred pain*), exudate, and potential peri-wound maceration.
Grade 2	Characterized by partial thickness skin loss or damage involving the dermis and/or dermis capsule.
Grade 3	Wounds that have begun to necrotize and become infected may demonstrate the following; necrotic tissue may present alongside healthy tissue. Tissue starts out as white in colour, diffuse, which covers the wound. As the tissue continues to deteriorate, the colour changes to yellow before going brown and black. The wound itself dehydrates as it changes from a mucus texture before hardening when turning black.
Grade 4	Patient experiences full thickness skin loss with extensive damage and tissue death involving underlying tendons, bones and joint capsule.

Compromised wound healing

The patient may give a history of a healing over a long period of time, and changes in the character of the pain. The patient may report swelling around the wound, increased exudates, or increased malodour.

Wounds which may be septic and lead to a systemic infection may have the following characteristics/patient symptoms; tachycardia, high temperature or hypothermia, inflammation around the wound, and spreading erythema. When assessing the wound, carefully make note of the borders of the wound so any spread of erythema can be noted. When examining the patient, the paramedic may also discover lymphadenopathy and lethargy. It is important to consider that patients who present with such symptoms may have wounds which lead to sepsis, osteomyelitis and cellulitis.

Patients should be referred to hospital for intravenous antibiotics ensuring precautions are taken to prevent the spread of the infection. If possible, identify the most likely sources of the infection. Chronic wounds are also susceptible to abscess formation. Abscesses can be identified by swelling and/or oedema

Assessment of minor injuries

around the site of the wound, and erythema with tenderness around the site of the wound. Infected wounds emit heat which can be felt. Abscess formation is accompanied by purulent discharge, malodour and dehiscence and patients may exhibit systemic symptoms (Tickle, 2013).

Factors to consider which influence wound recovery

This is not a definitive list of factors that may influence the healing of a wound, but should serve as triggers for the paramedic to consider the care the patient may need in order to recover fully.

Diabetes and associated neuropathy; wounds as a result of recent surgery; patient with neurological deficit or spinal injury; burns (Mudge and Orsted, 2010). Consider patients with chronic obstructive pulmonary disease (COPD); anaemia; thrombocytopenia; congestive cardiac failure (CCF); excessive exudate; human immunodeficiency virus (HIV); rheumatoid arthritis; tumours and cancers; radiotherapy and chemotherapy; dehydration; vitamin deficiency; steroids; anti-coagulants and anti-platelets; and reduced renal function (Stechmiller, 2010).

Patients who have a poor dietary intake, are less mobile and are dehydrated have an increased risk of infection. Smokers experience a delay in the healing process, as smoking reduces white cell activity and hence prolongs the inflammation around the wound. The process of epithelization is also delayed (Jones, 2012).

Documentation

It is important that clinical findings are recorded accurately. Consider the use of jargon and acronyms/mnemonics as patients and others who are non-medically trained may need to view the notes. Ensure that you record:

- Date of assessment
- The numbers of wounds present
- Clear identification of the type of wound and the location
- The duration of the wound
- The grade and classification of wound
- The type of tissue involvement, for example, is the injury near a bone or is bone exposed? Is the wound in close proximity to a stoma or fistula? Is there leakage?
- An estimate of the total percentage area covered by the wound. The condition of the surrounding skin and tissue should be assessed, type and level of pain the patient is experiencing, assess the smell of the

wound. Document the spread of erythema, and whether there has been a deterioration or improvement.
- Level of malodour and exudates/pus
- Wound colour
- Patient's pain score
- If it is necessary to refer the patient, be sure to note any concerns of the patient or carer.
- All interventions undertaken/types of dressings. Have you recorded all the care you have undertaken? Ensure that any wound assessment framework used is recorded.
- Patient allergies or skin sensitivities
- Patient medical history
- Your plan for the patient.

Taking photographs of wounds has become common practice in primary and out-of-hospital care. Other health professionals can view injuries without the need to immediately remove dressings. You need to be aware of any local policy that exists for the recording of patients' conditions and injuries using recording equipment, and where this information is digitally stored, and who has access to this information. Consent must be obtained from the patient, or family member or guardian. This must adhere strictly to Caldecott guidance regarding information sharing and governance (Department of Health, 2009, 2013).

Ensure the equipment you use is able to take pictures with sufficient quality to take close-ups. Ensure that the pictures maintain patient confidentiality and that the pictures can not identify patients from limbs, e.g. tattoos may be present or there may be items in the home environment which could identify the patient.

Wounds should be photographed against a dark background. You will find the flash from the camera is absorbed and will serve as a contrast to the wound itself. Include a measurement scale in the photograph. If the patient's condition allows, take subsequent photographs from the same position, distance and angle, using the same camera settings.

Ensure that the photographs are stored securely and are not published without the patient's permission.

When to refer

When considering which patients with a minor injury can be safely referred to a general practitioner, a nurse practitioner or other health care professional, a number of factors need to be taken into consideration.

If the mechanisms of injury or **red flags** do not trigger referral, the paramedic should consider:

- Activities of daily living
- The function of the affected limb
- Environmental considerations
- Interventions required
- Aftercare.

Consider the example of a 65-year-old female who has fallen and sustained a laceration to her forehead. There are no triggers from mechanism of injury or **red flags**. Using the above categories:

- Is the patient able to perform normal tasks?
- Can they mobilize as normal, make themselves a drink or prepare a meal?
- Is the home environment safe?
- Will the patient need to walk up and down stairs to use the toilet/bathroom?
- What interventions can you do at home or in the community, e.g. dressings/steri-strip wound? What will the hospital do if you refer, e.g. CT scan or observation?

CONCLUSION

Correctly diagnosing and treating wounds is a clinical skill that requires frequent observation of a range of wounds and their treatments to gain a deep understanding of the clinical signs and symptoms that accompany each presentation.

The skills required are understanding of the key stages in the healing process, underlying medical conditions and medication which will affect the healing process, and conditions which may mask the signs and symptoms of systemic illness.

Paramedics should also have a good appreciation of the different types of dressings and the situations when these should be applied. The National Institute for Health and Care Excellence provide guidance on the dressings applicable for acute and chronic wounds (NICE, 2014b).

The best outcomes are obtained for the patient with early detection of wounds which may present as chronic wounds. Patients with acute injuries require prompt assessment to ensure they are treated correctly and referred if required to the correct facility, e.g. plastic surgery units or maxilla-facial departments.

CHAPTER KEY POINTS

- First, the paramedic must exclude any potential life-threatening or life-changing conditions for the patient.
- The paramedic should then consider **red flags** that may not be immediately obvious, so detailed verbal and visual history taking is essential.
- Record and document findings, treatment and management accordingly.
- Always consider analgesia as a frontline treatment.
- The paramedic should be familiar with local policies/procedures/referral pathways, in order that the patient receives the best and most appropriate care possible.
- Minor injuries are capable of being assessed and managed without the need to transfer to an Emergency Department. Refer to a specialist or advanced paramedic or appropriate health professional as required.

REFERENCES

Andrews, H. (2013) Wound care checklists: role and wound assessment. *British Journal of Healthcare Assistants* 7(1): 8–9.

Association of Ambulance Chief Executives (2013) *UK Ambulance Services Clinical Practice Guidelines 2013 Pocket Book: Pain Assessment Model*. Bridgwater: Class Professional Publishing.

Barnard, A. and Allison, K. (2009) The classification and principles of management of wounds in trauma. *Trauma* 11(3): 163–76.

Bickley, L.S. (2013) *Bates' Pocket Guide to Physical Examination and History Taking* (7th edn). Philadelphia, PA: Lippincott Williams & Wilkins.

Bowen, T.W. and Slaven, M.E. (2014) Evidence-based management of acute hand injuries in the emergency department. *Emergency Medicine Practice* 16(12). Available at: http://www.slremeducation.org/wp-content/uploads/2015/02/1214-Hand-Injuries.pdf (accessed 13 June 2015).

Clinical Knowledge Summaries (2012) Sprains and strains. Available at: http://cks.nice.org.uk/sprains-and-strains#!topicsummary (accessed 8 March 2015).

Cornforth, A. (2013) Holistic wound assessment in primary care. *British Journal of Community Nursing* 18(12): S28–34.

Department of Health (2009) *Reference Guide to Consent for Examination or Treatment* (2nd edn). London: Department of Health.

Department of Health (2013) *Information: To Share or Not to Share? The Information Governance Review*. Available at: https://www.gov.uk/government/uploads/system/uploads/attachment_data/file/192572/2900774_InfoGovernance_accv2.pdf (accessed 13 June 2015).

Demidova-Rice, T.N., Hamblin, M.R. and Herman, I.M. (2012) Acute and impaired wound healing: pathophysiology and current methods for drug delivery, Part 1. *Advanced Skin Wound Care* 25(7): 304–14.

Headway, The Brain Injury Association (2012) *Key Facts and Statistics: Traumatic Brain Injury*. Available at: www.headway.org.uk/key-factsand-statistics.aspx (accessed 10 February 2015).

Jones, J. (2012) Examining the multifactorial nature of wound infection. *Wounds Essentials* 2: 90–7.

McClelland, H., Stephenson, J., Ousey, K., Gillibrand, W. and Underwood, P. (2012) Wound healing in pre-tibial injuries: an observation study. *International Wound Journal* 9(3): 303–10.

Mudge, E. and Orsted, H. (2010) Wound infection and pain management made easy. *Wounds International* 1(3). Available at: http://tinyurl.com/md8bhq7 (accessed 12 June 2015).

NICE (National Institute for Health and Clinical Excellence) (2013) *Falls: Assessment and Prevention of Falls in Older People*. NICE clinical guidance 161. Available at: http://www.nice.org.uk/guidance/cg161/evidence (accessed 20 June 2015).

NICE (National Institute for Health and Clinical Excellence) (2014a) *Head Injury: Triage, Assessment, Investigation and Early Management of Head Injury in Infants, Children and Adults*. NICE clinical guidance 176. London: NICE.

NICE (National Institute for Health and Clinical Excellence) (2014b) *The Debrisoft Monofilament Debridement Pad for Use in Acute or Chronic Wounds*. MTG17. Available at: http://www.nice.org.uk/guidance/mtg17 (accessed 20 June 2015).

Purcell, D. (2013a) Minor wounds and burns. In: *Minor Injuries: A Clinical Guide* (2nd edn). London: Churchill Livingston.

Purcell, D. (2013b) The neck and upper limbs. In: *Minor Injuries: A Clinical Guide* (2nd edn). London: Churchill Livingston.

Rossi, R. and Margheritini, F. (2014) *Acute Medial and Posteromedial Injury in Knee Ligament Injuries: Extra-articular Surgical Techniques*. London: Springer.

Stechmiller, J.K. (2010) Understanding the role of nutrition and wound healing. *Nutritional Clinical Practice* 25(1): 61–8.

Tickle, J. (2013) Wound infection: a clinician's guide to assessment and management. *British Journal of Community Nursing* Suppl. S16: S18–22.

10 Minor ailments
Rob Slee

According to NHS Choices (2015), annually around 50 million patients visit their GPs on account of coughs, cold and other minor ailments, despite many pharmacists being able to give advice and treatment on a 'walk-in' basis. For the most part, these cases are relatively straightforward, requiring only simple treatment or advice, and they now are part of the ever changing role of paramedics, who are now delivering treatments previously only performed by a doctor.

Paramedics are already working in Urgent & Emergency Care Centres (UECCs), Walk in Centres (WICs) and Minor Injury Units (MIUs) as well as in GP surgeries, prisons and offshore and remote locations. The future will provide a paramedic equipped with suitable education and training with increasing opportunities to practise and develop outside of the emergency ambulance environment in more of an urgent and unscheduled care arena (College of Paramedics, 2015).

The aim of this chapter is to consider some of the more common minor illness presentations that paramedics may encounter, it is not intended to give detailed anatomy or physiology. Its purpose is to highlight some key assessment principles, which will aid the paramedic to assess and refer the patient with a minor ailment safely and efficiently.

In terms of treatment with the use of antibiotics, legislation restricts the administration (by some practitioners) to Patient Group Directives (PGDs) though the recent Keogh Report has given clear direction for extending paramedic education/training to include prescribing in the foreseeable future (NHS England, 2013).

EAR, NOSE AND THROAT (ENT)

Most patients complaining of an ENT problem who present in the out-of-hospital arena have only minor ailments. The danger is that something that seems simple at first can become life threatening, requiring immediate attention (Carter and Laird, 2005). Identifying any life-threatening priorities such as full or partial obstruction of the airway (A), difficulty in breathing (B), or circulatory collapse (C) must be identified within the **primary survey**, and the respective element dealt with before proceeding to the next.

The difficulty then arises in recognizing those patients who, while they are not displaying any physical signs that are potentially significant, as they are in the early stages, still have the potential to deteriorate quickly, and, as suggested by Carter and Laird (2005), any patients cleared on the primary survey must have a thorough history undertaken, to identify the issues and focus the examination on the corresponding systems.

Basic anatomy

The ear is made up of three compartments:

1. The external ear comprising the pinna or auricle (which is mainly cartilage) and the ear canal. Behind and below the ear canal lies the mastoid part of the temporal bone, the lowest part of the mastoid process is palpable.
2. The middle ear contains the tympanic membrane or eardrum, an air-filled cavity that contains the ossicles; malleolus (hammer), incus (anvil) and stapes (stirrup), three tiny bones that transmit sound. The middle ear is connected to the nasopharynx via the Eustachian tube.
3. The inner ear contains the semi-circular canals and the cochlea which are unobservable under direct examination.

It is advisable to refer to a good anatomy and physiology text to familiarize oneself with the structure and functions of the ear, however, Figure 10.1 presents the ear compartments.

Ear examination/problems

Hearing loss is described by Knudson (2013) as a disturbance or break within the complex path of sound waves that are converted to electrical impulses which are transmitted to the brain and interpreted as sound. Knudson identifies also that hearing loss can be divided into three categories:

1. Conductive hearing loss (CHL) caused by a blockage of the ear canal, tympanic membrane impairment or middle ear impedance such as an effusion.
2. Sensorineural hearing loss (SHL) due to impaired function of the inner ear or cochlea, damage to the eighth cranial nerve or central nervous system.
3. Mixed Hearing Loss (MHL), a combination of both of the above.

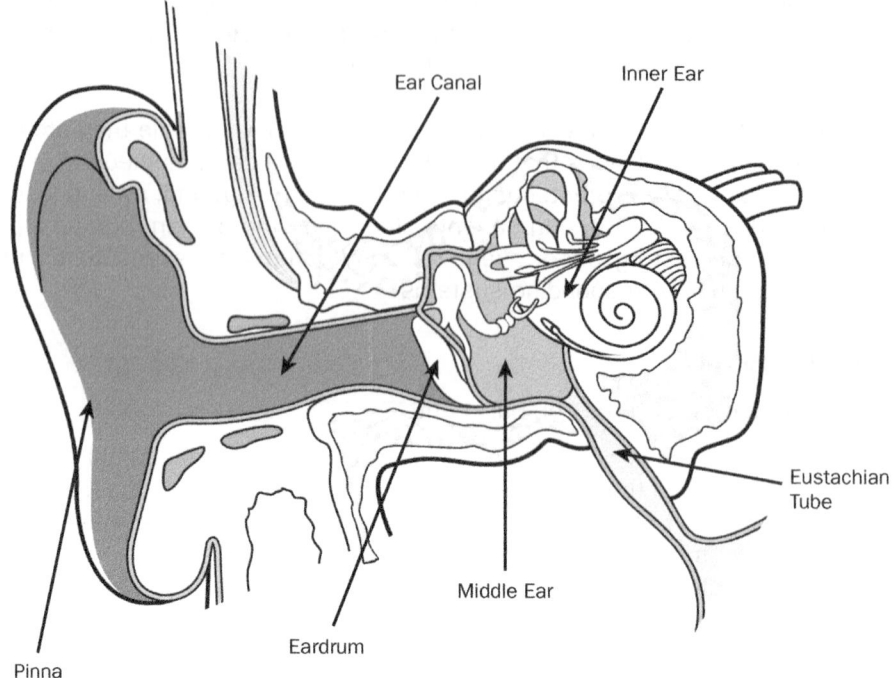

Figure 10.1 Ear: outer, middle and inner ear compartments

History

Use of the modified SOCRATES format is useful to follow with any ear complaints, and the history of symptoms such as a cold, a sore throat, coryzal symptoms, previous ear complaints, for instance due to swimming or flying, and use of cotton buds should be established. If there is any history of trauma, refer the patient to an appropriate place of care.

- **S** – Site. Where exactly is the pain or symptoms?
- **O** – Onset. What were they doing when the pain or symptoms started?
- **C** – Character. What does the pain feel like? Is it associated with coryzal symptoms?
- **R** – Radiate. Is the pain referred or is there redness around the ear?
- **A** – Associated symptoms. Is it associated with any activities, such as swimming, diving, flying?
- **T** – Time/duration. How long have they had the pain or loss of hearing?
- **E** – Exacerbating/relieving factors. Have they had previous ear infections?
- **S** – Severity. Obtain an initial pain score (0 = *no pain*, 10 = *worst pain ever*).

Examination

Ideally a thorough examination should involve the use of an otoscope, but it is recommended that education/training and simulated practice should be undertaken prior to using this equipment on a patient.

However, there are other techniques that can be considered, that, while they are not diagnostic, may help in formulating a differential diagnosis when combined with the patient history.

- Look at both ears (*non-affected first*) to identify the normal anatomy compared to the other side and any previous wounds or scars
- Check for any inflammation or discharge (*if the latter, how much, and is it offensive?*)
- Unilateral or bilateral associated pain?
- Press on the tragus: pain identifies either otitis externa or a furnacle (*an infection of a hair follicle in the outer ear canal*).

Possible ear conditions

Otitis media

This is the term given to generalized inflammation of the inner ear associated with an effusion which is usually preceded by an upper respiratory tract infection (URTI) with the accumulation of fluid in the middle ear, resulting in hearing loss. Often the symptoms are fairly rapid and the patient will be complaining of pain and discomfort, a discharge of mucus with a pungent smell may also be present, indicating perforation of the tympanic membrane. This is a common condition mainly among children and caused by both **viruses** and bacteria (NICE, 2015a).

Symptoms may include:

- Pain
- Fever
- Hearing loss (*rarely mastoiditis*)
- Facial nerve paralysis
- Tinnitus.

On examination, the tympanic membrane may appear yellow, cloudy or most commonly very red and often bulging.

Management

Current guidance (NICE, 2015a) advises that paracetamol and non-steroidal anti-inflammatory drugs (NSAIDs) such as ibuprofen are the most common treatment to deal with the pain and fever. Antibiotic treatment is not usually required unless the patient is presenting systemically unwell or has had symptoms more than four days without improvement. First line recommended treatment is a five-day course of Amoxicillin or, if allergic or sensitive, Clarithromycin/Erythromycin can be used.

Otitis externa

This is described as an infection of the sub-dermis and skin of the external ear canal which is often narrowed due to swelling (Bickley and Szilagyi, 2012). It can be acute, lasting up to three weeks, or chronic, lasting longer than three weeks. It is normally due to the persistent infection results in the thickening of the skin and a loss of the normal skin structure and reduced earwax production.

Slightly more common in women than men, common causes include excessive moisture and small trauma, with complications including abscess or tympanic membrane inflammation.

Uncomplicated symptoms tend to present as pain, itching, hearing loss and occasionally discharge. Kauffman (2013) suggests that palpation prior to the use of an otoscope (*if educated/trained*) will identify the need to exercise caution.

The use of paracetamol or a NSAID such as ibuprofen for symptomatic relief of pain and consideration of a topical application to treat the infection is recommended.

Any complicated presentations or persistent symptoms should be referred for specialist advice or follow-up.

EPISTAXIS

Nosebleeds are a common presentation to both emergency and unscheduled care services, but still require careful assessment and management. For some patients, nosebleeds can be very distressing, especially if it is a first presentation or has been bleeding for some time.

Management

Any patients deemed **time critical** on primary survey or history should be managed appropriately. Posterior bleeds tend to present from both nostrils and be profuse in flow. These patients should be transferred to an ED, especially when basic measures fail to stop the bleeding.

For all non-time critical patients, current guidance from NICE (2015b) advocates the following:

- Lean the patient forward to decrease nasopharynx blood flow, pinch the soft cartilaginous part of the nose firmly for at least 10 minutes, telling the patient to breathe only through their mouth.
- Should this be sufficient, self-care advice to avoid repetition can be considered, including avoidance of alcohol and hot drinks, lying flat, avoiding heavy lifting or strenuous exercise, blowing or picking the nose.
- Should the bleeding not arrest after 10–15 minutes, consideration should be given to transport the patient to facilities that can offer nasal cautery if the bleeding point can be observed or nasal packing if the bleeding point is not visible.

Possible actions to be taken:

- Sit patient up and ask them to lean forward
- Pinch the soft cartilaginous aspect of the nose for a minimum of 10 minutes (*telling the patient to breathe only through their mouth*)
- If bleeding has not arrested after 10–15 minutes, consider the need to transfer to an appropriate facility
- Reassure patient and relatives throughout.

SORE THROAT

Often patients complain of having a sore throat, but in principle it is a symptom that results from the upper respiratory tract becoming inflamed which incorporates the regions of the larynx, pharynx, tonsils and occasionally the epiglottis (Sambrook, 2013).

Presentations will vary and history is again key to identifying the problem:

- Painful swallowing
- Fever
- Severity and duration of symptoms
- Breathing difficulties
- Coryzal symptoms.

Examination can be undertaken using a tongue depressor and pen torch, but if stridor or epiglottitis is suspected, then this should be avoided, and for some patients this procedure is uncomfortable and may cause them to gag, so appropriate patient positioning should be used. The examination may reveal redness of the tonsils and pharynx, plus swelling of the tonsils, and possible exudate, palpation may reveal swelling of the cervical glands.

A useful tool for identifying the likelihood of a sore throat being due to a bacterial infection is the Centor criteria:

- Tonsillar exudate
- Tender anterior cervical adenopathy
- Temperature >38°C (100.5°F)
- Absence of cough.

It is suggested that the presence of three or more of the above is a positive predictive value of up to 60%. However, patients who present without three or four of the above imply there is an 80% possibility of it being a viral infection.

Management may or may not require the administration of antibiotics according to current guidance for this and other respiratory tract infections (NICE, 2008), however, NICE (2012) recommend ibuprofen 400mg three times daily (TDS) for the relief of pain, fever or headache. For those patients who are unable to take ibuprofen, paracetamol 1g four times a day (QDS) is recommended as an alternative.

TONSILLITIS

This is described as inflammation of the tonsils due to infection. It is identified as being an extremely common condition, more often in children of the 5–10 age group and the 15–25 age group of young adults (Tidy, 2014). Signs may include:

- Reddening of the pharynx
- Swollen inflamed tonsils, which may have white flecks of pus (*or yellow exudate*) visible
- Possibility of a raised temperature >37°C
- Swollen localized lymph glands
- Acute onset with abdominal pain, dysphagia and/or headache (*consider streptococcal tonsillitis*).

Symptoms may include:

- Changes or loss of voice
- Abdominal pain (*in small children*)
- Headache
- Pain on swallowing
- Severe pain in throat which lasts for >48 hrs
- In certain occasions, the pain may be referred to the ears.

Similar to sore throats, the management of tonsillitis may or may not require the administration of antibiotics, according to current guidance for this and other respiratory tract infections (NICE, 2008).

QUINSY (PERI-TONSILLAR ABSCESS)

Quinsy is defined as an 'Acute inflammation of the tonsils and the surrounding tissue, often leading to the formation of an abscess' (American Heritage®, 2011). It occurs as a complication of tonsillitis, resulting in peritonsillar abscess, wherein pus becomes entrapped between the tonsillar capsule and the lateral wall of the pharynx. Galioto (2008) suggests it is 'the most common deep infection of the head and neck', identifying that it primarily (but not exclusively) affects young adults, and therefore prompt recognition and intervention are important.

Red flag signs and symptoms may include:

- Swollen (*enlarged*) tonsil
- Red swollen soft palate (*with uvula deviated away from the affected tonsil*)
- Trismus (*clenching of the teeth due to spasm of the masticatory muscles, resulting in difficulty in opening the mouth*)
- Drooling
- Muffled voice
- Offensive breath
- Swollen localized lymph glands
- Swelling on affected side of face.

Other symptoms may include:

- Severe sore throat (worse on side of infection)
- Otalgia (earache on affected side)
- Fever – temperature >37.8°C (100°F)
- General malaise
- Headache
- Dysphagia (difficulty in swallowing).

Paramedics should consider the need to arrange transfer to an emergency department for those patients presenting with a quinsy/peri-tonsillar abscess, due to the risk of airway compromise or rupture of the abscess (NICE, 2012).

DERMATOLOGY

Of all the body's organs the largest and arguably the most important is the skin, and in dermatological terms includes hair, nails, mouth, mucous membranes, and genitalia, with one third of the UK population believed to have a problem with their skin at any one time, with a variety of dermatology conditions (Watkins, 2013a, 2013b, 2013c, 2013d, 2013e, 2013f, 2014).

In effect, the range of different dermatological conditions is vast, and the presentation is not to be under-estimated, for while some may be fairly innocuous in terms of presentation, they can be life threatening, and a good basic knowledge of the skin's anatomy and physiology and thorough history taking are paramount when assessing such complaints, to understand which layer of the dermis may be affected, and which conditions require referral onwards.

In terms of history taking, Watkins (2013a) suggests that the use of a body chart (Figure 10.2) is a useful tool to demonstrate sites and distribution patterns of any rashes, lesions (single or multiple) or bites (animal, human or insect), with the colour, shape and size all being documented, using simple basic terminology, and in association with common objects that other health care professionals can relate to.

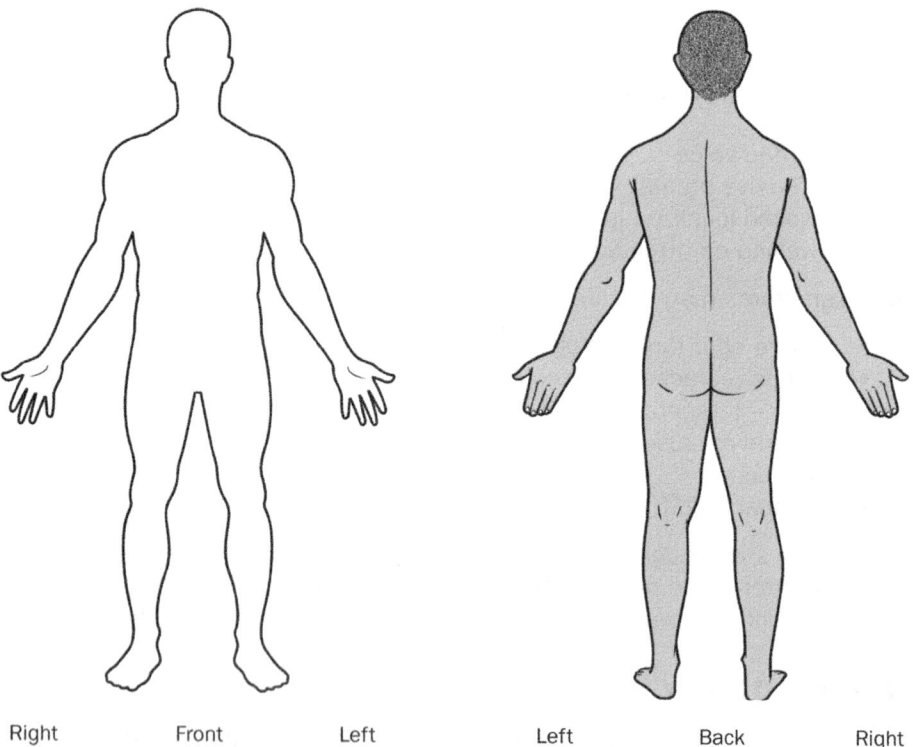

Right   Front   Left   Left   Back   Right

Figure 10.2 Body chart

Assessment of minor ailments

Example: The patient has a single lesion, grey/brown in colour on the dorsal aspect of his left hand about the size of a 50 pence piece.

Use of the SOCRATES framework will help guide the paramedic when taking the history:

- **S** – Site. Where exactly is the site of the problem?
- **O** – Onset. When did the problem start?
- **C** – Character. What was the cause of the injury/problem?
- **R** – Radiate. Is any relief found by the application of warmth, cold compress, etc.?
- **A** – Associated symptoms. Is it associated with any aggravating factors? Have they used any treatments, such as over-the-counter creams/herbal applications?
- **T** – Time/duration. How long have they had the pain?
- **E** – Exacerbating/relieving factors. What pattern does pain follow over 24 hours? Specific condition-related questions, e.g. swelling.
- **S** – Severity. Obtain an initial pain score (*0 = no pain, 10 = worst pain ever*).

CELLULITIS

Various micro-organisms that happily coexist with each other survive without issue to the host until a break in the skin occurs and causes an invasion, more commonly known as an infection which is bacterial in origin; one such infection is known as cellulitis (Morris et al., 2014). This is a painful condition that will affect a patient's well-being if left untreated, and quick diagnosis and following treatment has been shown to improve recovery time and decrease the likelihood of more serious complications arising (Nazarko, 2012).

Such a condition will require treatment with antibiotics, especially with associated malaise, and if the infection is no longer localizing. The paramedic should be considering admission to hospital for intravenous antibiotics and blood cultures. See Table 10.1 regarding diagnosed cellulitis that may be treated in the community setting by a community nurse in an advanced role.

Table 10.1 Cellulitis classifications and treatments

Diagnosed cellulitis			
Grade I	**Grade II**	**Grade III**	**Grade IV**
Home oral antibiotic therapy unless contra indicated	Consider non-acute IV therapy	Admit to acute bed	Admit to acute bed and seek specialist advice urgently

SEPTIC ARTHRITIS

This is described as an inflammation of a joint (*natural or prosthetic*) due to bacterial invasion, of which the most common involved is the knee (50%), then the hip (20%), the shoulder (8%), the ankle (7%), and then wrists (7%), and can be seen at any age, including infants. It can be acute or chronic, however, the prompt diagnosis and resulting treatment will significantly reduce both morbidity and mortality of patients presenting with this condition.

Septic arthritis in children occurs most often in the under-3 age group, and can be easily missed due to the absence of localizing signs, or be confused with other conditions such as trauma or transient synovitis. The hip and knee joint are most frequently affected, figures suggesting a third of cases.

 Red flags the child may present with fever, pain in the affected joint, or an unwillingness to move or use the joint (*e.g. if the hip is affected, then they may have a limp, or alternatively refuse to weight bear*). Between the ages of 3 and adolescence, it tends to be uncommon, after which it may redevelop (Tidy, 2013).

Risk factors

These include suppression of the immune system through other infections, chronic illness, diseases or medications, sickle cell disease, artificial joint implants, rheumatoid arthritis, or recent joint investigative procedures or surgery. Signs and symptoms may include:

- Pain with active or passive movement of the joint
- Pain in prosthetic joint (*may be due to an abscess, or loosening of the implant*)
- Swelling, and tenderness of the joint
- Joint feels warm to touch
- Effusion
- Fever and rigors (*attacks of shivering*)
- Chest wall pain (*if the acromioclavicular, sternoclavicular, sternocostal or manubrosternal joints are affected*)
- Hypotension, prostration or vomiting due to bacteraemia (*occurs when the bacterium from the source of infection spreads to a joint via the bloodstream or if the site of injury is directly over the joint, mainly through penetration or surgical procedures*).

Treatment

The only reliable way of diagnosing this condition is through aspiration of the affected joint and sending the fluid for culture, along with blood cultures and

X-ray imaging. Prior to the results of the cultures, commencement of a broad spectrum antibiotic through an intravenous route for up to three weeks may be needed and as such, any patient should be referred directly to the ED for further investigation and treatment.

GOUT

Gout is a type of arthritis which causes painful inflammation in joints. Overall in the UK it is estimated that 1 in 70 adults has gout, with symptoms occurring in males after 30 years of age and women after 60 years of age. Gout attacks occur when blood levels of uric acid levels become too high, causing small crystals of uric acid to form. Uric acid is a waste product normally excreted in urine, but in some people the levels build up, and these sharp grit-like crystals collect typically in joints such as the first metatarsophalangeal joint (the big toe), resulting in pain, inflammation and swelling. While any joint can be affected, lower limbs are more commonly involved.

Mild attacks may only last up to 48 hours while more severe ones can peak early on but take anywhere between seven and ten days for the symptoms to fully subside.

Causes for the build-up of uric acid may include:

- Excessive use of alcohol
- Sugar-sweetened soft drinks (not artificial sweeteners)
- Fructose rich juices
- Medications including Bendroflumethiazide, and high doses of aspirin
- Hypertension
- Diabetes mellitus
- Vascular disease
- Obesity.

Treatment

According to Knott (2013), a brief course of anti-inflammatory medications such as diclofenac, naproxen or indometacin (which can be obtained via a GP prescription) will help to resolve the pain, along with elevation of the affected limb, use of ice packs (avoiding direct contact with skin) for about 20 minutes at a time. NICE (2013) undertook studies of other medicines for the treatment of gout, however, specialists advised that it was important to ensure that standard treatments for gout, including NSAIDs, colchicine and corticosteroids are used before canakinumab is considered.

GASTROENTERITIS

A common presentation in primary care. Care should be taken with the very young and very old, and those with other underlying chronic conditions such as diabetes, due to the risk of dehydration. NICE has produced guidance on diarrhoea and vomiting caused by gastroenteritis in children <5 years of age (NICE, 2009), and has also produced advice on medication used to treat the symptoms of gastroenteritis (NICE, 2014), and this is available to paramedics (AACE, 2013). Consideration is needed of patients who are taking strong medications such as digoxin, which can lead to changes in toxicity levels.

Undertaking an abdominal examination (*observing hand hygiene*) (see *Abdominal and Gastro-Intestinal Assessment, Chapter 4*) with any patient presenting with these symptoms is a must, as conditions such as appendicitis can begin with gastroenteritis-like symptoms.

According to Clinical Knowledge Summaries (2013), most acute episodes in adults are mainly due to infection and the incubation periods for this illness can vary between one and ten days depending upon the underlying bacteria or virus, and, if the presenting patient was known to have eaten with a group, the time between each becoming ill will help identify the incubation period.

However, it is important to identify any patients who may have recently travelled abroad, had contact with sources of enteric infection (*such as farm visits*), have been prescribed any new drugs, or who are undergoing aggressive radiotherapy treatment. The paramedic should be aware of any local guidelines for referral and treatment for these incidences.

Norovirus is also very prevalent at certain times of the year and the paramedic should be aware of local policies.

Differential diagnosis:

- Norovirus
- Rotavirus
- Salmonella
- E-coli
- Campylobacter
- Listeria
- Cholera.

Red flag symptoms:
- Blood in stools
- Persistent vomiting

- Weight loss
- Watery high volume diarrhoea (*increased risk of dehydration*)
- Recent hospital or antibiotic treatment
- Nocturnal disturbances (*most likely organic in cause*).

General assessment and treatment

- Identify the frequency and severity of symptoms.
- Attempt to identify the underlying cause.
- Treat nausea and vomiting with anti-emetic drug (*unless contra-indicated*).
- Treat dehydration with IV fluids.

ACUTE DIARRHOEA

Acute diarrhoea is classed as being of sudden onset but lasting less than four weeks and the most common cause is infection of the gut, either from the presence of food that is infected, or from close contact and poor hygiene, resulting in the pathogen easily being spread from one person to another.

Symptoms can range from mild stomach discomfort with few episodes of loose stools to watery stools and cramping-style abdominal pains that pass after each bowel movement, but lasts for several days. The main danger is the patient suffering from dehydration, which is not quickly reversed with oral hydration.

Red flags include the very young and very old, pregnant women, and those unable to replace the lost fluids. Symptoms include:

- Headache
- Dry mouth and tongue
- Reduced urine output
- Lethargy
- Light-headedness
- Muscle cramps.

Severe symptoms include:

- Tachycardia
- Confusion
- Reduced level of consciousness.

General assessment and treatment

- Identify the frequency and severity of symptoms.
- Attempt to identify the underlying cause.

- Treat nausea and vomiting with anti-emetic drug (*unless contraindicated*).
- Treat dehydration with IV fluids.

URINARY TRACT INFECTION (UTI)

Organs involved in the urinary system include the kidneys, the bladder and the urethra, and the range of problems can be from simple asymptomatic to potential life-threatening systemic illness. Females are more prone than males to developing a urinary tract infection, with risk factors including sexual intercourse, history of UTIs, pregnancy, the diaphragm contraceptive and immunosuppression.

CYSTITIS

Symptoms include:

- Frequency, urgency, dysuria, haematuria, nocturia, burning and discomfort.
- Urine may be cloudy and smelly.
- Low grade fever.

PYELONEPHRITIS

May be classified in several ways: acute, chronic, complicated or uncomplicated. Onset is usually fairly rapid and the patient presents with pyrexia, tachycardia, pain and tenderness in the loin, suprapubic, back and flank either unilaterally or bilaterally, nausea and vomiting.

Investigations

Urinalysis

Urine volume	Normal measurement
Neonate	2–4 ml/kg/hour
Child:	Depending on age, 600–1000 ml in 24 hrs
Adult	Average output 800–2500 ml in 24 hrs
Specific gravity	1002 and 1040 (specific gravity of urine indicates the quantity of dissolved substances present)
Normal pH value	4.3–8 (Skinner, 2005)

Urine dipsticks should not be relied upon solely to confirm or exclude a UTI as a diagnosis.

When obtaining a urine sample, explanation should be given to the patient regarding what is required in terms of a mid-stream urine (MSU) and a suitable sterile container should be provided.

Other investigations are:

- *Nitrites*: The majority of urinary pathogens reduce nitrate to nitrite. A positive test suggests bacteria indicative of UTI. A negative result, however, does not rule out a UTI, due to the pathogen involved not being able to produce the nitrite in time, such as with cystitis where urination is frequent, allowing less time for the enzyme to act.
- *Leucocytes*: The marker for leucocytes is leucocyte esterase. A positive test suggests a UTI due to the specimen containing pyuria. However, this substance is not always found in patients with a UTI, and a negative test does not rule out infection, this makes the test insensitive.
- *Blood*: The presence or absence of blood in urine is a poor indicator in the diagnosis of a UTI, in uncomplicated cystitis, haematuria is not uncommon, and resolves well with simple treatment.
- *Protein*: A UTI will cause proteinuria.
- *Ketones*: The urine should test negative for ketones (ketone bodies appear in urine when the body's production of ketones exceeds their use).
- *Specific gravity*: Requires a urinometer to assess and the normal range is 1002 and 1040.
- *pH*: Various factors can influence the urine pH, such as time of day, and consumption of food or fluids, but normal range should be 4.3 to 8.0, with an average of about 6.0.

CONSTIPATION

Constipation is a common condition and is defined as infrequent bowel actions of three times a week or less, that often includes the requirement of straining to pass hard or pellet-like stools, which at times may include pain or incomplete evacuation. While constipation affects all ages, it is more common among elderly patients with poor diets and fluid intakes and in children, affecting 5%–30% of the child population (NICE, 2010).

History taking to identify any causative conditions or red flags is essential and should cover the areas of fluid and food intake, mobility, normal frequency, stool consistency and drugs (*including over-the-counter medication*). Other considerations include the presence of any blood or mucus in the stools, or episodes of diarrhoea between constipation. Females have higher reported incidences of constipation than males.

Causes of constipation include:

- Depression or anxiety
- Ignoring the urge to pass stools
- Low calorific intake
- Poor fibre diet (not enough cereals, fruit and vegetables)
- Polypharmacy
- Physical and sexual abuse
- Insufficient fluid intake
- Changes in lifestyle (changing eating habits).

In adults, constipation can often be relieved by:

- Drinking more water
- Undertaking more exercise
- Including more fibre in the diet.

Red flag symptoms:
- New onset in an elderly patient
- Unexplained anaemia
- Rectal bleeding
- Family history of bowel cancer or inflammatory bowel disease
- Tenesmus (*painful spasm of the anal sphincter accompanied by an urgent need to evacuate the bowel or bladder, and involuntary straining that results in the passing of little or no matter*)
- Weight loss.

Pathophysiology

Constipation may be due to a patient having normal stools but poor muscle tone in response to faecal matter, or stools that are hard and impacted but normal muscle tone.

To assist and increase the knowledge and understanding of constipation, paramedics should read Appendix G: 'Bristol Stool Form Scale' (NICE, 2010) which explains the seven types of stool, available at: http://www.nice.org.uk/guidance/cg99/evidence

CHAPTER KEY POINTS

- Minor ailments are capable of being assessed and managed without the need to transfer to an ED.
- Understand the local policies for referring to GP services, Community Nurses, Specialist/Advanced Paramedics, Walk-In Centres, Minor Injury Units, and Urgent Care Centres.

- Undertake a complete history and examination of the minor ailment.
- Record and document findings, treatment, management accordingly.
- Manage **red flag** symptoms appropriately.
- Refer the patient to a senior paramedic or health professional as required.

REFERENCES

American Heritage (2011) *Dictionary of the English Language* (5th edn). Boston: Houghton Mifflin Harcourt.

Association of Ambulance Chief Executives (2013) *UK Ambulance Services Clinical Practice Guidelines 2013 Pocket Book: Ondansetron*. Bridgwater: Class Professional Publishing.

Bickley, L.S. and Szilagyi, P.G. (2012) *Bates' Guide to Physical Examination and History Taking* (11th edn). Philadelphia, PA: Lippincott Williams & Wilkins.

Carter, S. and Laird, C. (2005) Assessment and care of ENT problems. *Emergency Medical Journal* 22: 128–39. doi: 10.1136/emj.2004.021642.

Clinical Knowledge Summaries (2013) Diarrhoea – adult's assessment – Scenario: Assessment of acute diarrhoea (<4 weeks). Available at: http://cks.nice.org.uk/diarrhoea-adults-assessment#!scenario (accessed 23 June 2015).

College of Paramedics (2015) *Paramedic Post Registration: Career Framework* (3rd edn). Bridgwater: College of Paramedics.

Galioto, N.J. (2008) Peritonsillar abscess. *American Academy of Family Physicians* 7(2): 199–202. Available at. http://www.aafp.org/afp/2008/0115/p199.html (accessed 22 June 2015).

Kauffman, M. (2013) *History and Physical Examination: A Common Sense Approach*. Burlington, VA: Jones and Bartlett Publishers.

Knott, L. (2013) *Gout*. Available at: http://patient.info/health/gout-leaflet (accessed 2 June 2015).

Knudson, M.P. (2013) Hearing loss. In Paulman, P.M., Paulman, A.A., Harrison, J.D., Laeth, N., and Kimberley J. (eds) *Taylor's Differential Diagnosis Manual* (3rd edn). Philadelphia, PA: Lippincott Williams and Wilkins.

Morris, F., Wardrope, J. and Ramlakhan, S. (2014) *Minor Injury and Minor Illness at a Glance*. Chichester: John Wiley and Sons Ltd.

Nazarko, L. (2012) An evidence-based approach to diagnosis and management of cellulitis. *British Journal of Community Nursing* 17(1): 6–12.

NHS Choices (2015) *GP Attendances – Minor Illness*. Available at: http://www.nhs.uk/NHSEngland/keoghreview/Documents/UECR.Ph1ReAport.FV.pdf (accessed 29 May 2015).

NHS England (2013) *High Quality Care for All, Now and for Future Generations: Transforming Urgent and Emergency Care Services in England – Urgent and Emergency Care Review End of Phase 1 Report*. Leeds: Urgent and Emergency Care Review Team.

NICE (National Institute for Health and Care Excellence) (2008) *Respiratory Tract Infections – Antibiotic Prescribing. Prescribing of Antibiotics for Self-Limiting Respiratory Tract Infections in Adults and Children in Primary Care*. NICE clinical guidance 69. Available at: http://www.nice.org.uk/guidance/cg69/evidence (accessed 22 June 2015).

NICE (National Institute for Health and Care Excellence) (2009) *Diarrhoea and Vomiting Caused by Gastroenteritis: Diagnosis, Assessment and Management in Children Younger Than 5 Years*. NICE clinical guidance 84. Available at: http://www.nice.org.uk/guidance/cg84/evidence (accessed 23 June 2015).

NICE (National Institute for Health and Care Excellence) (2010) *Constipation in Children And Young People: Diagnosis and Management of Idiopathic Childhood Constipation in Primary and Secondary Care*. NICE clinical guidance 99. Available at: http://www.nice.org.uk/guidance/cg99/evidence (accessed 23 June 2015).

NICE (National Institute for Health and Care Excellence) (2012) *Sore Throat: Acute*. available at: http://cks.nice.org.uk/sore-throat-acute#!scenario (accessed 20 June 2015).

NICE (National Institute for Health and Care Excellence) (2013) *Gouty Arthritis: Canakinumab*. NICE advice ESNM23. Available at: https://www.nice.org.uk/advice/esnm23/chapter/Key-points-from-the-evidence (accessed 23 June 2015).

NICE (National Institute for Health and Care Excellence) (2014) *Management of Vomiting in Children and Young People with Gastroenteritis: Ondansetron*. NICE advice ESUOM34. Available at: https://www.nice.org.uk/advice/esuom34/chapter/Key-points-from-the-evidence (accessed 23 June 2015).

NICE (National Institute for Health and Care Excellence) (2015a) *Acute Otitis Media*. Available at: http://cks.nice.org.uk/otitis-media-acute#!topicsummary (accessed 20 June 2015).

NICE (National Institute for Health and Care Excellence) (2015b) Epistaxis (nosebleeds). Available at: http://cks.nice.org.uk/epistaxis-nosebleeds#!scenario (accessed 20 June 2015).

Sambrook, J. (2013) Sore throat. Available at: http://patient.info/doctor/sore-throat-pro (accessed 22 June 2015).

Skinner, S. (2005) *Understanding Clinical Investigations: A Quick Reference Manual* (2nd edn). London: Elsevier.

Tidy, C. (2013) Septic arthritis. Available at: http://patient.info/doctor/septic-arthritis-pro (accessed 22 June 2015).

Tidy, C. (2014) Tonsillitis. Available at: http://patient.info/doctor/tonsillitis-pro (accessed 22 June 2015).

Watkins, J. (2013a) Skin rashes, part 1: Skin structure and taking a dermatological history. *Nursing Practice* 24(1): 30–3.

Watkins, J. (2013b) Skin rashes, part 2: Distribution and different types of rashes. *Nursing Practice* 24(3): 124–7.

Watkins, J. (2013c) Skin rashes, part 3: Localized rashes. *Nursing Practice* 24(5): 235–41.

Watkins, J. (2013d) Diagnosing rashes, part 4: Generalized rashes with fever. *Nursing Practice* 24(7): 335–41.

Watkins, J. (2013e) Diagnosing rashes, part 5: Itchy rashes. *Nursing Practice* 24(9): 438–44.

Watkins, J. (2013f) Diagnosing rashes, part 6: Itchy rashes in specific conditions. *Nursing Practice* 24(11): 556–61.

Watkins, J. (2014) Diagnosing rashes, part 7: Purpuric rashes. *Nursing Practice* 25(1): 23–8.

11 Child assessment
Denise Aspland

This chapter will provide an overview of the principles of assessment of the child. It will follow a **DR ABCDE** approach in the **primary survey** and will identify aspects of paediatrics to consider within the secondary survey. The primary survey, when followed in a structured manner, will identify areas of concern. As with adults, these problems should be treated as they are found and the primary survey used as an on-going tool. For the purpose of clarification of ages, an infant is a child aged 1 month to 1 year, and a child is between 1 year and puberty (Resuscitation Council (UK), 2010).

SCENE ASSESSMENT

The scene assessment involving children can and does include injuries and trauma. The leading cause of death after the first year of life is through injury and this is responsible for 31%–58% of death in the over-1s (Wolfe et al., 2014). The most significant of these injuries are head related trauma predominantly through road traffic collisions (TARN, 2012). Alternatively the child may have become unwell and the parent/guardian/carer has called the 999 emergency ambulance service. Assessing the scene of a child who came off their skateboard in a skate-park area would potentially raise different problems to being called to an infant who has become unwell over a period of hours or days.

Is your experience of paediatrics sufficient to assess and make an appropriate management decision? Do you understand normal paediatric parameters for vital signs? When assessing any ill child but especially the under-5-year-olds, it is vital that a full set of observations are recorded on the child. This should include: respiratory rate and SpO_2 saturations, heart rate, capillary refill time (CRT) and temperature as well as looking at the effort, efficacy and effects of breathing and overall colour of the child.

Table 11.1 defines normal paediatric values. The paramedic should take every opportunity to familiarize themselves with the well child to fully appreciate abnormal findings.

Table 11.1 Normal paediatric values

Age (years)	Heart rate (bpm)	Respiratory rate (RR)	Blood pressure mmHg (Systolic BP = 80 + (age × 2))
<1	110–160	30–40	70–90
2–5	95–140	23–30	80–100
5–12	80–120	20–25	90–110
>12	60–100	15–20	100–120

Advanced Life Support Group (2011).

PRIMARY SURVEY

The primary survey of the child continues to use the DR ABCDE framework. An emergency call to an unwell child can differ from one call to another and situations will vary considerably upon arrival. Often the child will be accompanied by an assortment of relatives and carers with different degrees of composure and offering different levels of assistance. It is imperative that the child remains as your main focus throughout your assessment, but it is also important to mention here that the composed and calm carer will be invaluable to your assessment and management of the child. Communication with carers throughout, particularly in the younger child and infant, will enhance your knowledge of the child and the history surrounding the illness. It is also helpful to note that, when dealing with children, first impressions are important.

DANGER

Children do not appreciate or see danger in the same way as adults. The child who enters the building site or derelict building and subsequently injures themselves will pose added problems to the attending paramedic. Entering unfamiliar territory possesses various potential hazards. Therefore, every paramedic should be aware of the precautions to be taken upon entering property and each scene should be assessed for danger.

- Ensure that the scene/site is secure before entering, if appropriate, request emergency rescue services.
- Ensure personal protective equipment (PPE) is worn, especially due to the potential of contact with body fluids.
- Ensure dogs are removed from the working areas as they may see you as a threat when dealing with the child.

> **Possible actions to be taken:**
> - Ensure the scene/site is secure before entering
> - Wear PPE as appropriate
> - Request dogs to be removed from scene.

RESPONSE

A child who is alert and aware of their surroundings will inevitably react to a stranger entering their environment. They may well become distressed and upset upon examination. Stranger anxiety is part of paediatric development and first manifests around 7–9 months of age. This advances at a second level around 18 months when children develop separation anxiety. This is all part of the normal cognitive development of the child and it is important to recognize this and assess each situation on an individual basis. (For more information on normal child development, see Whitnell, 2012.) Steps should be taken to calm and reassure in order to avoid a screaming and unco-operative child. However, as this anxiety is a normal process, this may not always be successful. It should be noted that a distressed child will have altered vital signs that may impair your assessment and may require reassessment at a later stage.

A rapid assessment tool used in paediatrics to assess the level of consciousness is AVPU:

$\quad$ **A** – Alert (Glasgow Coma Score, GCS = 15)
$\quad$ **V** – Voice, responds to voice commence (GCS = 13)
$\quad$ **P** – Pain, responds to painful stimuli (GCS = 8)
$\quad$ **U** – Unconscious (GCS = 3)

A child who is P or U on AVPU needs immediate airway management as they are at significant risk of airway compromise, due to loss of gag reflex and risk of aspiration and this should be managed appropriately.

When assessing the child:
- Refer to the child by their first name rather than he, she or baby.
- Assess a small child on the parent's/carer's lap or at least with them nearby (separation anxiety).
- With toddlers, kneel down to their level.

Some children, however, may be extremely delighted to see you and be more than willing to allow assessment with the hope of a ride in an ambulance!

> **Possible actions to be taken:**
> - Assess and record the patient's level of consciousness (AVPU)
> - Refer to the child by name, and approach them at their level
> - Calmly and confidently approach the child.

AIRWAY

A child's airway has significant anatomical and physiological differences to that of an adult and will change with age. Each age will present with a different set of problems at each stage of childhood; these can and may include:

- Nasal breathers below 2 months of age
- Occipital cervical flexion
- Small face – large head
- Anterior larynx
- Short trachea
- Large floppy tongue.

An important aspect of the narrow airway in children is that airway resistance is significantly increased. Small changes in the airway diameter will therefore increase airway resistance and even a small amount of oedema from illness such as croup will significantly increase the work of breathing for a child and lead to fatigue and potential respiratory failure.

Due to anatomical differences, airway positioning alters with development. In an infant, a neutral position needs to be maintained while a younger child requires a 'sniffing' position and the older child requires a full head tilt to maintain a good open airway. In the absence of trauma and to obtain an open airway, a head tilt/chin lift manoeuvre may need to be applied. When performing a chin lift, care should be given to finger positioning, so as not to press on the soft tissue and occlude the airway further. Fingers should be placed on the bony prominences of the mandible. Due to a large occiput, large tongue and narrow trachea, the airway may occlude fairly easily in an unwell and collapsed child.

When assessing the child's airway, consider:

- Does the child have a patent airway? If not patent, is the airway compromised?
- Do you need to re-position the airway?
- Does the child need advanced airway support and/or ventilation?

Due to the complex differences in the child's airway, intubation and advanced airway management should only be performed by a skilled and competent paramedic. A short narrow trachea, posterior placed epiglottis and narrowing at the cricoid ring make intubation extremely difficult and can cause significant oedema and further compromise to the airway if not performed correctly. Correct airway positioning, an oropharyngeal airway or bag-valve-mask ventilation with high flow oxygen will be adequate in a compromised airway until further expertise can be sought.

Possible actions to be taken:
- Open the child's mouth and remove any visible obstruction. Do not perform a blind finger sweep
- Consider gentle suction and airway adjuncts if appropriate
- If epiglottitis is possible, then exercise extreme caution so as not to cause further harm
- If head tilt and chin lift have not opened the airway, try the jaw thrust method
- Stepwise airway management if appropriate and trained (see Respiratory Assessment, Chapter 2).

BREATHING

This element of the primary survey is paramount in assisting the paramedic to recognize a sick child. It may appear complex but it is essential to obtain a good clear assessment to determine how unwell the child is. To obtain a thorough breathing assessment, the child's chest should be fully exposed during examination. The child with any respiratory distress or failure should be treated with caution and urgency as there is a high risk of rapid deterioration.

In paediatrics; Effort, Efficacy and the Effects of inadequate breathing should be assessed.

Effort
- What is the child's respiratory rate and how does it compare to normal values?
- An increased RR (*at rest*) may be an indication of respiratory compromise or a metabolic acidosis.
- A decreased RR may indicate exhaustion, neurological impairment or a sign of peri-arrest.

Examine the chest and ascertain if there is evidence of increased work of breathing. Is there evidence of any of the following?

- Intercostal recession (*in drawing is seen between the ribs*)
- Subcostal recession (*in drawing occurs at the costal margins where the diaphragm attaches*)
- Sternal recession (*in small babies even the sternum may be drawn in*)
- Tracheal tug
- Head bobbing in infants (*due to the sternocleidomastoid accessory muscle being used*)
- Nasal flaring (*indicates significant respiratory distress*)
- Positioning of the child. (Older children will present in the tripod position, sitting leaning forward with hands supported on the knees, to optimize ventilation and lung expansion. This is classic in the child with asthma who has significant respiratory distress).
- See-saw abdominal breathing.

If the child is demonstrating multiple respiratory signs, there is a greater risk of respiratory compromise and potential respiratory failure and arrest and prompt intervention may be required.

- Are there added noises and if so, are they inspiratory or expiratory?
- Is the chest silent? (A pre-terminal sign and needs immediate management.) Are there any added specific noises? If so, are they inspiratory or expiratory?
- Snoring (stertor) (upper airways). May be present if there is an obstruction in the pharynx (possibly due to swollen inflamed tonsils).
- Stridor (upper airways). May indicate tracheal or laryngeal obstruction and will be heard on inspiration (consider epiglottitis).
- Grunting in infants. This sound is produced when exhaled air goes against a partially closed glottis. It is an attempt to prevent airway collapse by producing positive end-expiratory pressure. It is a sign of severe respiratory distress (ALSG, 2011).

Efficacy

How efficient is the breathing?

- What are the child's oxygen saturations? Although this gives a baseline, oxygen saturations are unreliable in the acutely ill child due to peripheral shutdown. In air <95% considered abnormal, <85% potentially life-threatening) (ALSG, 2011).
- O_2 saturations should be used in correlation with other respiratory signs.
- Observe the chest for degree of expansion. This can indicate how much air is being inspired/expired.

- Are the movements deep and sighing (*signs of metabolic acidosis*), quick and shallow (*respiratory distress*) or slow and shallow (*exhaustion*)?

Effects of respiratory inadequacy

Respiratory distress, if left untreated, will rapidly result in respiratory failure which in turn will result in a hypoxic child. Some 60% of paediatric cardiac arrests are caused by prolonged hypoxia and the survival rates from arrest are poor, with figures less than 20% with out-of-hospital arrests significantly lower (Scholefield et al., 2012).

Hypoxia in a child can be appreciated by assessing the following:

- Heart rate
- Mental status
- Skin colour
- Cyanosis
- Central cyanosis in a child is a late sign of respiratory failure and a clear indicator of peri-arrest.

It should be noted that there may be certain situations where there is little or no evidence of increased work of breathing but the child may still be in significant respiratory failure.

These exceptions are:

- A child with cerebral depression caused by such conditions as raised intra-cranial pressure (ICP), poisoning or infection. This is due to an alteration in the respiratory drive.
- A child with known neuromuscular disease such as muscular dystrophy.
- Prolonged respiratory distress leading to exhaustion and a decrease in respiratory effort.

If the child is showing signs of respiratory compromise, all possible attempts should be made to minimize further distress to the child. This can exacerbate the problem and send respiratory distress into respiratory failure and arrest. If appropriate, keep main carers close by to familiarize and settle the infant/child.

In the injured child, any signs of rib fractures should be taken seriously. Children with rib fractures have a high mortality rate of around 42% (Furhman and Zimmerman, 2011). Ribs in small children are soft and pliable due to decreased calcium formation and the chest wall having a higher elasticity. Therefore a significant level of force will have occurred to cause fractures and will undoubtedly have caused underlying injury to the lungs.

Possible actions to be taken:

- Ensure adequate oxygenation
- Ascertain the child's SpO_2 levels and administer oxygen accordingly
- Children with sickle cell disease, suspected carbon monoxide poisoning or cardiac disease should be administered high flow oxygen despite the SpO_2 reading
- Assess the effort, efficacy and effects of their breathing
- Consider assisted ventilation if the child is hypoxic with SpO_2 <90% or the RR is less than half or more than three times their normal rate or if chest expansion is inadequate
- If required, implement Basic Life Support (Child) (AACE, 2013a).

CIRCULATION

Assessment of the circulatory system should be quick but thorough. Alongside airway and breathing assessment, it can assist the paramedic in ascertaining the severity of the child's illness/injury. A child will compensate well in shock and will have a relatively normal blood pressure even though they may be acutely unwell. Obtaining a blood pressure (BP) early will provide a baseline for assessment. Children have superior compensatory mechanisms and will maintain their blood pressure for relatively long periods. A dropping BP or hypotension in a child is pre-terminal sign.

- What is the child's pulse rate and how does this compare to normal values?
- Initially, a child's pulse rate will rise in shock due to the catecholamine release.
- Tachycardia occurs, but in severe hypoxia the pulse rate and strength will fall pre-empting cardio-respiratory arrest (asystole).
- A child has superior compensatory mechanisms and will maintain a tachycardia for a prolonged period of time before decompensating.
- A rapidly failing pulse rate or a significant bradycardia is a pre-terminal sign and may indicate raised intracranial pressure or decompensatory shock and is therefore a clinical emergency.
- In an infant the pulse rate should be felt at the brachial or femoral arteries.
- In a child and an older child, carotid or femoral pulses may be sought.
- What is the child's blood pressure?
- The correct-sized blood pressure cuff must be used to obtain an accurate reading.

Table 11.2 Systolic blood pressure by age

Age (years)	Systolic BP (mmHg)	
	50th centile	5th centile
<1	80–90	65–75
1–2	85–95	70–75
2–5	85–100	70–80
5–12	90–110	80–90
>12	100–120	90–105

ALSG (2011).

- Incorrect BP cuff-sizing will give a false reading, too large will lower the blood pressure and too small will give an artificially high blood pressure.

Peripheral and central pulses can be checked and compared. An absent peripheral pulse and a weak central pulse indicate severe shock and significant hypotension (see Table 11.2).

- How does the child look?
- Examine the child's skin colour, looking for pallor, mottling and peripheral shutdown.
- Skin colour – due to the catecholamine release caused by hypoxia, vasoconstriction occurs and the child appears pale and mottled (catecholamines include dopamine, epinephrine (adrenaline), and norepinephirine (noradrenaline) and are produced by the adrenal glands when the patient is under physical or emotional stress (Tortora and Derrickson, 2012)).
- Check the child's central capillary refill (CRT).

The CRT can be achieved by pressing on the sternum for 5 seconds. The capillary refill should be less than 2 seconds. This examination should not be used in isolation but with other circulatory assessment checks. This clinical assessment is particularly useful in septic shock where the child is likely to have warm peripheries and look comparatively well, but have a prolonged central capillary refill. This is due to a relatively normal cardiac output (*usually bounding on palpation*) but poor tissue perfusion due to abnormal distribution of blood in the circulatory system.

If there are signs of hypovolaemic shock which is thought to be due to blood loss, you need to look for where the child is bleeding. These are anatomical and general areas to examine for blood loss in the hypovolaemic child. To remember these, think; **'Floor plus 4 more'**.

- Floor – at the scene of the incident or from external haemorrhage
- Chest
- Abdomen
- Pelvis
- Long bones.

If the patient is an infant, do they have abnormal fontanelles? There are two fontanelles, anterior and posterior. The fontanelles should feel firm and very slightly concave to the touch (see Figure 11.1).

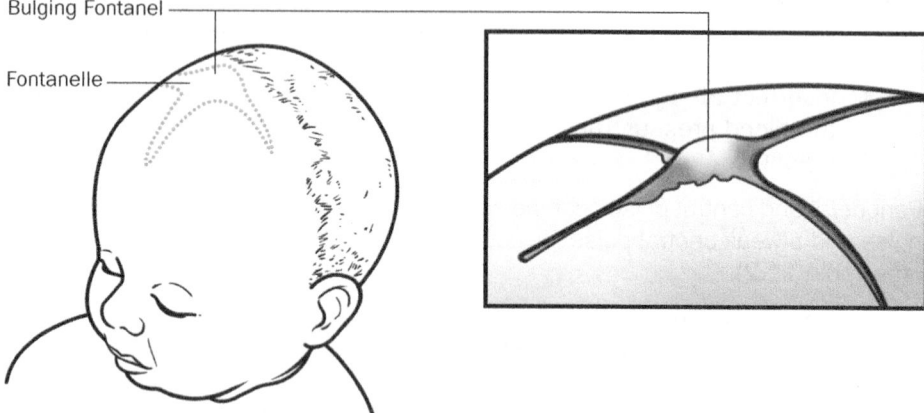

Figure 11.1 Normal and bulging fontanelles

The anterior fontanelle closes around 18 months of age and is the fontanelle used for assessment. By examining the fontanelle, the following assessment can be made:

- A tense bulging fontanelle will indicate raised intra-cranial pressure (ICP).
- A markedly sunken, depressed fontanelle will indicate dehydration.
- Note – fontanelles will bulge in the crying infant.

It is important to be aware of the child who may be septic with raised inter-cranial pressure, for example, a child with meningococcal sepsis. In these cases the vital signs may look fairly normal as the raised BP and bradycardia from the Cushing's triad may counteract the tachycardia and hypotension from septic shock. These children will present as looking acutely unwell and usually in a collapsed condition. Consider alternative indicators to assess the severity of the illness.

> **Possible actions to be taken:**
> - Assess the child's pulse, is it tachycardic or bradycardic? (*manage accordingly*)
> - Assess the child's skin colour
> - Ascertain the signs of circulatory inadequacy early
> - Assess and record the blood pressure (remember that hypotension is a late pre-terminal sign in the child)
> - Manage haemorrhage accordingly (AACE, 2013b)
> - Manage catastrophic haemorrhage accordingly (AACE, 2013c)
> - Manage shock accordingly (AACE, 2013d)
> - Pre-alert the receiving paediatric unit.

DISABILITY

Assessment of the disability element will give an indication of potential central neurological failure. The assessment should include level of consciousness, pupils, posturing and blood glucose levels. There is a modified Glasgow Coma Scale for children that can be used in the **secondary survey** to give a more comprehensive assessment of level of consciousness and should be used in conjunction with the National Institute for Health and Care Excellence (NICE) guideline on *Head Injury: Triage, Assessment, Investigation and Early Management of Head Injury in Children, Young People and Adults* (NICE, 2014a).

Level of consciousness

- To assess the level of consciousness in paediatrics a quick neurological assessment for the primary survey is obtained through AVPU. When assessing painful stimuli in the child up to the age of 7, or, for those who are unable to communicate their pain, consider using the Face, Legs, Activity, Cry, Consolability, or FLACC Scale (AACE, 2013e) or alternatively use the Wong-Baker FACES Pain Rating Scale (AACE, 2013f).
- Mental status – a child may show signs of agitation or drowsiness and an infant may appear floppy (hypotonic) or irritable, and a high-pitched cry (cerebral cry) may indicate raised ICP.

Pupils

Assessment of pupillary response:

- Assess the pupils and ascertain if they are: Pupils Equal and Round; React to Light and Accommodation (PERRLA).
- Are they unequal or dilated?

- Non-reacting pupils may indicate significant neurological impairment due to pressure on the optic nerve.
- Pupillary size and reactivity may be indicative of certain drugs/or poisons. Sympathetic responses during seizures may cause pupillary dilation (Devinsky, 2004).

Posture

- Posture – what is the child's posture?
- Is there decorticate posture (flexed arm/clenched fists/extended legs)?
- Is there decerebrate posture (extended arms/extended legs) (see *Neurological Assessment, Chapter 5*)?

Either of these positions is indicative of significant neurological impairment. Caution should be given as these postures may be mistaken for the tonic phase of a convulsion.

A clear clinical sign that a child is suffering from a serious illness is that they will become hypotonic and listless.

If the evidence suggests the child has any form of febrile illness, then use the NICE Traffic Light tool to assess: Colour, Activity, Respiratory, Hydration and Other (AACE, 2013g, 2013h, 2013i).

Blood glucose level

- What is the child's blood sugar?
- In a child who is lethargic, floppy or unresponsive, a blood sugar level must be obtained. This is particularly significant in the child who is fitting.
- The paramedic should consider the Airway, Breathing, Circulation, DEFG, use the phrase '**D**on't **E**ver **F**orget **G**lucose'.
- Due to poor fat reserves and an increased metabolic rate exacerbated by illness, the child will use up their glucose reserves rapidly. Therefore, the child is at increased risk of hypoglycaemia. A blood glucose of 3 mmols is classified as 'hypoglycaemia' in a child and may result in seizures if not treated (ALSG, 2011).

Possible actions to be taken:

- Assess and record the child's LOC (*AVPU*)
- Assess and document the size and equality of pupils (*PERRLA*)
- Assess and record abnormal postures
- Monitor and record blood glucose levels (*manage accordingly*).

EXPOSE/EXAMINE/EVALUATE

Undress the child, having obtained the appropriate consent (College of Emergency Medicine, 2013). By exposing and examining the child, the paramedic will obtain further clues to the child's illness. Observe for signs of rashes, unexplained bruising and general skin colour.

What does the rash look like?

- Is there purpura? Appearance of red or purple discolorations on the skin that do not blanch on applying pressure, caused by bleeding underneath the skin and measure 3–10 mm.
- Are there petechiae? (*pinpoint, flat, round, red spots under the skin surface caused by bleeding into the skin*); petechiae are red because they contain blood that has leaked from the capillaries into the skin. They are quite tiny (less than 3 mm in diameter), and do not blanch when pressed.
- Is there urticaria? (*commonly referred to as hives*) It appears as raised, well-circumscribed areas of erythema and oedema involving the dermis and epidermis that are very pruritic (*intense sensation of itching*), otherwise it has a distinctive appearance, and it blanches completely with pressure. If consistent with small blisters, consider Varicella Zoster Virus (*chickenpox*).
- Is there erythema? (*redness of the skin caused by dilation and congestion of the capillaries, often a sign of inflammation or infection*).

Rashes and marks can change rapidly in an unwell child; the paramedic should remember that a few spots of petechiae on initial assessment can rapidly develop into widespread purpura in the case of sepsis.

Consider:

- If there is a non-blanching rash in an unwell child, meningococcal septicaemia must be assumed. If a glass tumbler is pressed firmly against a purpuric rash, the rash will not fade, and the rash remains visible through the glass.
- A non-blanching rash is indicative of meningococcal septicaemia but it is not a fool-proof technique (there may be NO rash); up to 30% of cases start with a blanching pink rash which fades with pressure and then becomes purpuric.
- Meningococcal septicaemia is a medical emergency where the earliest administration of benzyl penicillin may save life and reduce morbidity; the septicaemia patient needs immediate benzyl penicillin en route to hospital (AACE, 2013j). Further information regarding signs and symptoms of meningococcal sepsis can be found at http://www.meningitis.org/

Document carefully any marks found on the child. Bruising noted on assessment may be indicative of sepsis but may also indicate non-accidental injury (NAI) and so therefore documentation is paramount (comply with local and/or national procedures).

- Is there any unexplained bruising?

Most unwell children will have or have had a raised temperature at some point during their illness. However, in septic shock the child may be normal-thermic or even hypothermic and therefore the absence of raised temperature does not rule out serious illness. Cold sepsis is a late sign and indicative of critical illness and irreversible septic shock.

- Does the child have a temperature?

A child with an underdeveloped hypothalamus (premature or underdeveloped neonate) will have difficulty maintaining haemoregulation. Caution should be given to prolonged exposure as the child will use further energy reserves in an attempt to keep warm. This in turn may exacerbate potential hypoglycaemia as previously mentioned. If a child is pyrexial (temperature >38.5°C) and symptomatic, then measures should be taken, as per local procedures and NICE (2014b) guidelines, to reduce temperature. It is important to note, however, that a raised temperature is a natural response to infection and is present to prevent bacteria multiplication, and consideration to this should be given prior to administration of medication.

Rapid, thorough assessment of the child's primary survey, performed in a structured manner, will identify problems and provide the paramedic with an indication of the severity of the illness or injury. A useful acronym to identify and evaluate pre-terminal signs in a child is **BECHS**:

B – Bradycardia
E – Exhaustion
C – Central cyanosis
H – Hypotension
S – Silent chest

A child who is unwell and presenting with any of the above symptoms should be considered by the paramedic as time critical (ALSG, 2011).

Possible actions to be taken:

- Expose patient and examine (*remember appropriate consent*)
- Observe for rashes (*especially those that do not fade under pressure*)

- Assess by pressing a glass against the skin (*if present consider bacterial meningitis, manage appropriately*)
- Examine the patient for bruising (*is it due to illness, normal for age or an NAI?*)
- Assess the child's temperature (*hypothermic, normal-thermic, pyrexia or hyperpyrexia?*)
- Evaluate – if time critical, transfer to the appropriate treatment unit or centre
- Alternatively undertake a secondary survey.

SECONDARY SURVEY

Once the primary survey is complete and in the absence of any life-threatening problems the paramedic needs to gain further information in order to deal with the child's condition. Caring for a child has multiple areas for consideration; a specific area to be considered is the *age* of the patient. Other areas that are appropriate to the on-going assessment of the patient would be the ethical and legal aspects. All of these need to be addressed while performing a secondary survey and obtaining a comprehensive history and physical examination to ascertain and detect if there are any less immediate threats to the patient (AAP-ACEP, 2012).

History

Presenting complaint
The paramedic needs to clearly identify the reasons why the parent, carer or patient (child) has requested their attendance. This may be due to the exacerbation of an existing medical condition (asthma, epilepsy, diabetes), or it may be that the child has become unwell and is presenting with symptoms of specific condition (appendicitis, croup, viral illness). Alternatively the patient may have suffered a trauma injury and the paramedic will need to ascertain the mechanism of injury (MOI) (Bledsoe et al., 2014) and injury severity score (ISS) to measure the overall severity of the injured child (TARN, 2012).

- What is the presenting complaint?
- What is the age of the patient? (Infants and small children may require you to address your questions to the parent/carer.)
- What is the nature of the presenting complaint (illness or injury)?
- If illness, does it affect a specific system (abdominal pain, chest)?
- If an injury, does it affect a specific limb (arm or leg)?

What is the history of the presenting complaint? The history of the presenting complaint for an infant who has diarrhoea and vomiting (D & V), may have an entirely different diagnosis to a 7-year-old child who is complaining of abdominal pain, and will require the paramedic to assess accordingly:

- PC: 7 ♀ C/O Abdominal pain
- HPC: Call received at approximately 21.30 hrs. Child's mother states that her little girl went to bed as usual at 7.30 pm. At 9.15 pm she awoke crying saying her 'tummy' hurt her because she could not go to the toilet.

Child

- Exactly where is the pain? (Ask the patient to point to the location.)
- Implement the SOCRATES framework to assist in gaining a more through impression of the presenting complaint (see *General Principles of Assessment*, Chapter 1).
- If constipated, consider treatment in accordance with NICE guidelines (NICE, 2010).

Infant

- When was the onset of the vomiting and/or diarrhoea? And what is the frequency? What is the colour of the vomit? Is it bilious in nature?
- The amount of oral fluid intake since symptoms commenced?
- The total number of wet nappies during the previous eight hours?
- When did they last urinate or have a wet nappy?

Possible actions to be taken:

- Ascertain the blood glucose level of any child who presents with a history of vomiting, diarrhoea and poor oral fluid intake
- Ascertain degree of dehydration according to NICE guidelines (NICE, 2009a) and consider shock.

Past medical history

When ascertaining a child's past medical history, depending upon their age, this may need to incorporate information regarding their gestation/birth period, then any childhood illnesses and/or injuries since birth. For the infant/younger child, consider their birth and development history.

Birth history

- Did the child have a difficult neonatal period?
- Were there special care needs at birth?
- Was the child premature?

These elements can potentially impact on respiratory or neurological systems and the child may have known pre-existing conditions arising from birth complications.

Development history

- How is the child developing according to childhood milestones?
- Is this impacting on their current health?

These are particularly helpful questions in the under-2-year-olds, or if the child has a known developmental condition. It will help ascertain the 'norm' for the child and assist with the child's assessment. For example, a child with cerebral palsy may normally have poor muscle tone and be hypotonic, and so therefore, in isolation, this is not an unduly concerning aspect of the disability assessment of the primary survey. Alternatively, the paramedic can obtain a focused paediatric history by using a modified version of the **SAMPILE** framework (see Table 11.3).

Table 11.3 Modified SAMPILE framework

S – Signs/symptoms	Onset and nature of the symptoms of pain or fever?
	Are they age-appropriate-related signs of distress?
A – Allergies	Any known drug reactions or allergies (food or drugs)?
M – medications	Exact name/s and dosages of prescribed drugs (GP/doctor/hospital)
	Exact name and dosages of any non-prescribed (over-the-counter (OTC) drugs) (purchased and administered by parent/carer/guardian, etc.)
	What was the time and amount of the last dose?
	The time and dose of any analgesics/antipyretics (paracetamol, ibuprofen, etc.)
P – Past medical problems	History of gestation, labour and delivery?
	Any previous illness or injuries
I – Immunizations	HIB, MMR, etc. (check their immunization record book)
L – Last food or liquid	The time of the child's last food or drink?
	For infants, this could be breast or bottle
E – Events leading to the injury and/or illness incident	Ascertain what were the key events leading to this. Any history of fever?

Drug/medication history

This provides the paramedic with an opportunity to obtain specific information regarding the actual (intended) and potential (non-intentional/accidental) administration of the child's drugs/medications.

- Is the child on any current prescribed or over-the-counter medication? If so, when was it last given?
- If poisoning is suspected, did the child have access to other medications in the house?

Immunizations and contact with infectious diseases

- Is the child up to date with their vaccinations or have they been in contact with any infectious diseases?
- Do the child's symptoms correlate to any signs and symptoms of infectious disease?

Family history

Always ask about the health of the rest of the family. The child may have an inherited disorder or may well have been in contact with an infection or ill member of the family who may have contributed to the current problem. Children under the age of one are considerably more at risk from death and over half of deaths in childhood occur during the first year of a child's life, and are strongly influenced by pre-term delivery and low birth weight (Wolfe et al., 2014).

Social history

- Who are the child's main carers and who has parental responsibility?
- Who does the child live with?
- Gaining an understanding of these aspects may help to determine the possibility of a non-accidental injury (NAI) or a child in need.

EXAMINATION

Use the 'toe-to-head' structure when undertaking a physical examination of the infants, toddlers and pre-school patients, and the opposite 'head-to-toe' structure for the older child.

Incorporating this arrangement into your approach will help to gain the child's trust and co-operation, and increase the accuracy of the physical findings obtained. When doing so, remember to obtain the assistance of the parent/carer in the examination process. Explain to the child and parent/carer what you are about to do, leaving the more unpleasant tasks until last. The examination should include the following:

- General observations (*clothing, if wet or soiled, remove*). If the child has vomited or does vomit, note the presence of bile or blood. Bile suggests an obstruction; blood suggests trauma or GI bleeding.
- Skin (*inspect for rashes, bite marks, burns, abnormal bruising*)
- Head (*infants 0-18 months, assess the anterior fontanelle*). Bulging and non-pulsatile may indicate IC bleeding, meningitis or encephalitis. Sunken anterior fontanelle indicates dehydration. Look for bruising, swelling and haematomas.
- Eyes (PERRLA)
- Nose (*assess for obstructions, foreign bodies, rhinorrhoea*)
- Ears (*presence of discharge or pus, otorrhoea - infection or perforation*)
- Mouth (*if a stridor is present, epiglottis?*) Breath smell, sweet suggests acidosis, drooling suggests upper airway infection or partial obstruction.
- Neck (*ensure trachea is midline, auscultate over midline of trachea, ascertain if wheezing and stridor are present*)
- Chest (*assess for bruising, rashes, tenderness, auscultate*)
- Back (*assess for bruising, rashes, tenderness, deformity, auscultate*)
- Pelvis (*assess and consider instability*)
- Extremities (*assess for symmetry, compare limbs for colour, warmth, size and tenderness*)
- Neurological – conduct a cranial nerve evaluation:
  - Ask them to open and close their eyes
  - Ask them to smile
  - Ask them to stick out their tongue
  - If co-operative, hold an object in front of their eyes
  - Assess and track eye movement: upwards, downwards, left and right
  - Assess gross motor function
  - Ask them to lift their arms and legs
  - Ask them to shrug their shoulders
  - Ask them to push against resistance (use your hand)
  - Ask them to squeeze your hands
  - If old enough and no injury, ask them to walk (assess gait, balance) (AAP-ACEP, 2012).

Consent to treatment

It is also vital to determine who at the scene gives consent to care. There are many legal papers regarding children's consent and the subject is not as straightforward as it may seem. Due to the complexity of the subject, further information can be found in the Mental Capacity Act (Department of Health, 2005) and the Department of Health's *Reference Guide to Consent for Examination or Treatment* (Department of Health, 2009).

Guidance provided by the General Medical Council (GMC, 2007) states that children and young people should be involved as much as possible in decisions about their care, even when they are not able to make a decision on their own.

Ideally, in order to assist with consent of treatment, an adult with parental responsibility should be present (DH, 2009; NHS UK, 2011). Once again, this is an area of complexity. Further guidance on persons who may have parental responsibility can be found in the Children Act, 1989 (Department of Health, 2009).

Paramedics should remember that children who are deemed competent either by Gillick competence or Fraser guidelines cannot have their consent decision overruled by someone with parental responsibility, unless this specifically relates to their refusal of life-saving treatment. In any emergency situation where you believe it is in the best interests of the child, treatment must be given to the best of your ability in order to prevent further complications, whether consent is given or not. This must be fully documented and recorded and also witnessed by colleagues. Paramedics should familiarize themselves with internal policies surrounding this area.

Safeguarding children

The National Society for the Prevention of Cruelty to Children (NSPCC) reported that in 2012, 44 children aged under 15 died as a result of assault or undetermined intent across the UK. They further advised that studies have indicated that the number of child deaths where abuse or neglect is suspected as a factor is higher than shown in the mortality figures (NSPCC, 2014).

Safeguarding children is a vast topic and extremely important for the paramedic when dealing with children and their families. There are numerous guidelines and legislative literature pertaining to this subject and it is the paramedic's responsibility to ensure that they are up to date and familiar with safeguarding policies within their area of professional practice. Further guidance can be found at:

- *When to Suspect Child Maltreatment* (NICE, 2009b)
- *Working Together to Safeguard Children* (HM Government, 2013)
- *Safeguarding Children and Young People* (Royal College of Paediatrics and Child Health, 2014).

Child assessment

When attending a sick or injured child, child protection should always be present in the paramedic's thought process. Child abuse may present in many ways but the four classifications are as follows (NSPCC, 2014):

- Physical
- Emotional
- Neglect
- Sexual.

Although abuse is not always apparent and evident, there are some helpful indicators or **red flags**:

- Late presentation
- History does not correlate with injury/illness
- Concern for the child by the carer may be either indifferent and off-hand or may present as over the top and/or angry
- The history is inconsistent with each telling.
- The child does not interact with the carer or appears frightened of the carer or indeed may be over-familiar with the paramedic.

The term 'Toxic Trio' has been used to describe high risk factors for those children who have been identified as being particularly at risk because: (1) they are victims of domestic violence; (2) they have parents with *mental health issues*; and (3) they have parents who also suffer with *substance abuse* (DH, 2012).

Attention should be given to the child's surroundings while at the scene and impressions conveyed to the appropriate professionals if concerns are present. There are seven golden rules for sharing information which can help the paramedic in their decision process for referral.

1. Remember that the Data Protection Act is not a barrier to sharing information.
2. Be open and honest with the person.
3. Seek advice if you are in any doubt.
4. Share with consent where appropriate.
5. Consider safety and well-being.
6. Necessary, proportionate, relevant, accurate, timely and secure information.
7. Keep a record.

Further explanation on these rules can be found in *Information Sharing: Guidance for Practitioners and Managers* (HM Government, 2009) and *Working Together to Safeguard Children* (HM Government 2013). Information regarding the requirements of responsibility for health professionals can also be found in the Royal College of Paediatrics and Child Health (2014) publication.

If non-accidental injury (NAI) or abuse is suspected by the paramedic, then good documentation and communication with other agencies are paramount. Policy guidelines should be followed and the paramedic involved should be at the forefront of this process. It is good practice to complete all documentation at the time of the incident as errors may occur if written in retrospect. In all cases, the primary and secondary surveys should be completed appropriately with the findings recorded.

OTHER CONSIDERATIONS
Communication

Remember that some patients may not yet even have learned how to talk, therefore ensure communication with relatives and carers throughout; particularly if the patient is a younger child or infant, it will enable you to enhance your knowledge of the child and the history surrounding the illness. Involve children and young people as much as possible in decisions about their care, even when they are not able to make decisions on their own, and ensure you obtain the appropriate consent.

Destination/receiving specialist units/non-conveyance

Convey the patient to the appropriate unit of care. The National Institute for Health and Care Excellence (NICE) offers guidance in the following areas relevant to out-of-hospital practice;

- *Diarrhoea and Vomiting in Children under 5* (NICE, 2009a)
- *Neonatal Jaundice* (NICE 2010)
- *Quality Standard for Asthma* (NICE 2013)
- *Constipation in Children and Young People* (NICE, 2010)
- *Feverish Illness in Children* (NICE, 2014a)
- *Head Injury: Triage* (NICE, 2014b)
- *Gastro-Oesophogeal Reflux Disease* (NICE, 2015a).

Further guidance regarding children and young people is available at: https://www.nice.org.uk/guidance/population-groups/children-and-young-people

Social/family/carer

In the majority of situations, an appropriate member of the patient's family will be present, and able to provide the history. Ascertain the relationship of the adults present at the incident to the patient. Remember you may on occasions have to convey a patient whose relatives are not with you; use teachers and/or police officers as chaperones.

Ethical and legal

Consider and obtain the appropriate level of consent to treatment ideally from an adult with parental responsibility if the circumstances dictate. The paramedic may also, in certain situations, need to consider the possibility of NAI, completing all relevant documentation, ensuring that this is passed to the appropriate agencies.

COMMON CONDITIONS AFFECTING PAEDIATRIC PATIENTS

Asthma

Asthma is a chronic inflammatory disease of the airways, associated with widespread, variable outflow obstruction which may reverse either spontaneously or with medication. The underlying inflammation is associated with bronchial hyper-responsiveness or airway hyper-reactivity to a variety of stimuli, such as environmental allergens and irritants.

Currently, 5.4 million people are receiving treatment for asthma, 1.1 million of whom are children. Asthma is the cause of death for three people every single day, however, as many as 90% of these deaths are preventable (Asthma UK, 2014).

Signs and symptoms
- Cough
- Difficulty breathing
- Chest tightness
- Wheeze
- Increased Respiratory Effort.

Laryngo-tracheo-bronchiolitis (croup)

Croup is a condition which results from the inflammation or irritation of the larynx and trachea and bronchial passageways, due to viral infection. It is more prevalent in infants and children between 3 months to 3 years old, the majority of whom are males, but may also occur at any age, but is most common in 18-month-olds.

Croup is more prevalent during the late autumn and winter months and usually lasts for about five days; the symptoms are more severe at night, and worse during the first two nights.

Signs and symptoms
- Sore throat
- Mild cold (with low grade fever)

- Runny nose
- Loss of appetite
- Cough.

Over a period of one to two days the characteristic signs and symptoms of croup develop:

- Bark-like cough
- Hoarse or croaky voice
- Dyspnoea
- Stridor.

Assess the severity of the croup score and identify if Mild (1–2), Moderate (3–4), or Severe (5–6) (AACE, 2013k).

Measles (rubeola)

Measles is an infection of the respiratory system caused by a virus, it is highly contagious and is spread by respiration (either contact with fluids from the infected person or airborne). The incubation period of the infection has an average of 4 days (range 6–19 days). The infections period lasts from 2–4 days prior until 2–5 days following the onset of the rash (i.e. 4–9 days infectivity in total.

Measles remains one of the leading causes of death. In 2013, globally, there were 145,700 measles deaths, which equates to 400 deaths per day, or more than 1 death per hour (16 per day) (WHO, 2015).

Signs and symptoms
- Fever (*Over 4 days, may reach 40°C*)
- Cough
- Coryza (*runny nose*)
- Conjunctivitis (*red eyes*)
- Erythematous (*red*) rash (*begins several days after the fever starts*)
- It starts on head before spreading to cover most of the body (*often causing itching*)
- The rash is said to 'stain' (*changing red to dark brown before disappearing*).

Bronchiolitis

This illness is the most common severe lower respiratory infection in children under the age of 18 months and is most prevalent in the winter months. Up to 80% of cases are caused by the Respiratory Syncytial Virus (RSV). NICE has published the guideline, *Bronchiolitis: Diagnosis and Management in Children* (NICE, 2015b).

Signs and symptoms
- Coryza symptoms (cold)
- Fever
- Wheeze
- Recession
- Cough
- Fatigue leading to poor feeding.

Gastroenteritis

Children may present to the health care services with a sudden onset of abdominal cramps and diarrhoea with or without vomiting. Symptoms usually resolve without treatment, over a matter of days but young children and particularly infants are more at risk of complications such as dehydration and low blood glucose and in extreme circumstance, shock.

Signs and symptoms
- Sudden onset of diarrhoea
- +/− vomiting
- Possible fever, if bacterial
- Dehydration (refer to D&V in children, for severity of dehydration) (NICE, 2009a).

CHAPTER KEY POINTS
- Always follow a structured approach to the primary survey.
- Ensure consent is obtained appropriate to the child and the situation.
- Fully assess each area of the primary survey.
- Manage identified problems as they are found
- Complete a structured secondary survey (history, physical examination and vital signs).
- Be aware of the normal values for each stage of childhood.
- Involve carers as much as is reasonable in order to pacify the child.
- Have a clear understanding of child safeguarding policies and procedures.
- Always document clearly your management and interaction with the child.

REFERENCES

Advanced Life Support Group (2011) *Advanced Paediatric Life Support: The Practical Approach* (5th edn). London: Blackwell Publishing.

American Academy of Pediatrics (AAP) and American College of Emergency Physicians (ACEP) (2012) *APLS: The Pediatric Emergency Medicine Resource* (5th edn). Burlington, VA: Jones & Bartlett Learning.

Association of Ambulance Chief Executives (2013a) *UK Ambulance Services Clinical Practice Guidelines 2013 Pocket Book: Basic Life Support (Child)*. Bridgwater: Class Professional Publishing.

Association of Ambulance Chief Executives (2013b) *UK Ambulance Services Clinical Practice Guidelines 2013 Pocket Book: Trauma Emergencies Overview (Children). The Management of Haemorrhage Algorithm*. Bridgwater: Class Professional Publishing.

Association of Ambulance Chief Executives (2013c) *UK Ambulance Services Clinical Practice Guidelines 2013 Pocket Book: Trauma Emergencies Overview (Children): The Management of Catastrophic Haemorrhage Algorithm*. Bridgwater: Class Professional Publishing.

Association of Ambulance Chief Executives (2013d) *UK Ambulance Services Clinical Practice Guidelines 2013 Pocket Book: Intravascular Fluid Therapy (Children)*. Bridgwater: Class Professional Publishing.

Association of Ambulance Chief Executives (2013e) *UK Ambulance Services Clinical Practice Guidelines 2013 Pocket Book: The FLACC Scale*. Bridgwater: Class Professional Publishing.

Association of Ambulance Chief Executives (2013f) *UK Ambulance Services Clinical Practice Guidelines 2013 Pocket Book: Wong-Baker FACES Pain Rating Scale*. Bridgwater: Class Professional Publishing.

Association of Ambulance Chief Executives (2013g) *UK Ambulance Services Clinical Practice Guidelines 2013 Pocket Book: GREEN: NICE 'Traffic Lights' Clinical Assessment Tool for Febrile Illness in Children*. Bridgwater: Class Professional Publishing.

Association of Ambulance Chief Executives (2013h) *UK Ambulance Services Clinical Practice Guidelines 2013 Pocket Book: AMBER: NICE 'Traffic Lights' Clinical Assessment Tool for Febrile Illness in Children*. Bridgwater: Class Professional Publishing.

Association of Ambulance Chief Executives (2013i) *UK Ambulance Services Clinical Practice Guidelines 2013 Pocket Book: RED: NICE 'Traffic Lights' Clinical Assessment Tool for Febrile Illness in Children*. Bridgwater: Class Professional Publishing.

Association of Ambulance Chief Executives (2013j) *UK Ambulance Services Clinical Practice Guidelines 2013 Pocket Book: Meningococcal Meningitis and Septicaemia*. Bridgwater: Class Professional Publishing.

Association of Ambulance Chief Executives (2013k) *UK Ambulance Services Clinical Practice Guidelines 2013 Pocket Book: Modified Taussig Croup Score*. Bridgwater: Class Professional Publishing.

Asthma UK (2014) *Asthma Facts and FAQ's*. Available at. http://www.asthma.org.uk/asthma-facts-and-statistics (accessed 24 November 2014).

Bledsoe, B.E. Porter, R.S. and Cherry, R.A. (2014) *Paramedic Care: Principles & Practice*, vol. 5, *Trauma* (4th edn). Harlow, Essex: Pearson Education Limited.

College of Emergency Medicine (2013) *Consent, Capacity and Restraint of Adults, Adolescents and Children in Emergency Departments*. Available at. http://www.collemergencymed.ac.uk/Shop-Floor/Clinical%20Guidelines/College%20Guidelines/ (accessed 24 November 2014).

Department of Health (2005) *Mental Capacity Act*. London: The Stationery Office.

Department of Health (2009) *Reference Guide to Consent for Examination or Treatment* (2nd edn). London: Department of Health.

Department of Health (2012) *Health Visiting and School Nursing Programmes: Supporting Implementation of the New Service Model No. 5: Domestic Violence and Abuse – Professional Guidance.* Available at: https://www.gov.uk/government/uploads/system/uploads/attachment_data/file/211018/9576-TSO-Health_Visiting_Domestic_Violence_A3_Posters_WEB.pdf

Devinsky, O. (2004) *Effects of Seizures on Autonomic and Cardiovascular Function.* Available at: http://www.ncbi.nlm.nih.gov/pmc/articles/PMC531654/ (accessed 24 November 2014).

Furhman, B.P. and Zimmerman, J. (2011) *Pediatric Critical Care* (4th edn). Philadelphia Elsevier Mosby.

General Medical Council (2007) *0–18 years: Guidance for All Doctors.* Available at: www.gmc-uk.org/guidance (accessed 23 Feb. 2015).

HM Government (2009) *Information Sharing: Guidance for Practitioners and Managers.* Available at: http://webarchive.nationalarchives.gov.uk/20100623194820/publications.everychildmatters.gov.uk/eorderingdownload/00807-2008bkt-en-march09.pdf (accessed 21 November 2014).

HM Government (2013) *Working Together to Safeguard Children. A Guide to Inter-Agency Working to Safeguard and Promote the Welfare of Children.* Available at: https://www.gov.uk/government/uploads/system/uploads/attachment_data/file/281368/Working_together_to_safeguard_children.pdf (accessed 21 November 2014).

NHS UK (2011) *Does My Child have the Right to Refuce Treatment?* Available at: http: www.nhs.uk/chq/pages/900.apx?categoryid=26&subcategoryid=66 (accessed 30 December 2015).

NICE (National Institute for Health and Care Excellence) (2009a) *Diarrhoea and Vomiting Caused by Gastroenteritis Diagnosis, Assessment and Management in Children Younger than 5 Years.* NICE clinical guideline 84. Available at: http://www.nice.org.uk/guidance/cg84/evidence (accessed 23 February 2015).

NICE (National Institute for Health and Care Excellence) (2009b). *When to Suspect Child Maltreatment.* Updated February 2014. Available at: http://www.nice.org.uk/guidance/cg89/evidence (accessed 23 February 2015).

NICE (National Institute for Health and Care Excellence) (2010) *Constipation in Children and Young People Diagnosis and Management of Idiopathic Childhood Constipation in Primary and Secondary.* NICE clinical guideline 99. Available at: http://www.nice.org.uk/guidance/cg99/evidence (accessed 23 February 2015).

NICE (National Institute for Health and Care Excellence) (2014a) *Head Injury: Triage, Assessment, Investigation and Early Management of Head Injury in Children, Young People and Adults.* NICE clinical guideline 176. Available at: http://www.nice.org.uk/guidance/cg176 (accessed 22 February 2015).

NICE (National Institute for Health and Care Excellence) (2014b) *Feverish Illness in Children.* NICE quality standard 64. Available at: https://www.nice.org.uk/guidance/qs64 (accessed 24 February 2015).

NICE (National Institute for Health and Care Excellence) (2015a) *Gastro-Oesophogeal Reflux Disease: Recognition, Diagnosis and Management in Children and Young People.* NICE guideline 1. Available at. https://www.nice.org.uk/guidance/ng1 (accessed 24 February 2015).

NICE (National Institute for Health and Care Excellence) (2015b) *Bronchiolitis: Diagnosis and Management of Bronchiolitis in Children.* NICE guideline 9. Available at: http://www.nice.org.uk/guidance/NG9/evidence (accessed 6 June 2015).

National Society for the Prevention of Cruelty to Children (NSPCC) (2014) *How Safe Are Our Children? 2014.* Available at: https://nspcc.org.uk/preventing-abuse/research-and-resources/how-safe-are-our-children-2014/ (accessed 23 February 2015).

Resuscitation Council UK (2010) *Resuscitation Guidelines 2010: Chapter 9. Paediatric Basic Life Support.* Available at: http://www.resus.org.uk/pages/guide.htm (accessed 22 February 2015).

Royal College of Paediatrics and Child Health (2014) *Safeguarding Children and Young People: Roles and Competences for Health Care Staff. Intercollegiate Document* (3rd edn). London: Royal College of Paediatrics and Child Health.

Scholefield, B., Raman, S., Hussey, A., Haigh, F., Kanthimathinathan, H.K., Skellet, S., Peters, M., Duncan, H., and Morris, K. (2012) 152 predictive factors for survival after paediatric out-of-hospital cardiac arrest: a UK multicentre cohort study. *Archives of Disease in Childhood.* Available at: http://adc.bmj.com/content/97/Suppl_2/A43.2.full.pdf+html?sid=7db45d4d-fb31-4118-9b68-6898bc4cc136 (accessed 22 February 2015).

The Children Act (1989) Available at: http://www.legislation.gov.uk/ukpga/1989/41/contents/enacted (accessed 23 February 2015).

TARN (The Trauma Audit & Research Network) (2012) England and Wales: Severe Injury in Children 2012. Available at. https://www.tarn.ac.uk (accessed 22 February 2015).

Tortora, G.J. and Derrickson, B.H. (2012) *Essentials of Anatomy and Physiology*: International Student Version (9th edn). Singapore: John Wiley & Sons, Ltd.

Whitnell, J. (2012) Developmental psychology and safeguarding children. In A.Y. Blaber (ed.) *Foundations for Paramedic Practice: A Theoretical Perspective* (2nd edn). Maidenhead: McGraw-Hill.

WHO (World Health Organization) (2015) Measles. Available at: http://www.who.int/mediacentre/factsheets/fs286/en/ (accessed 24 February 2015).

Wolfe, E., Macfarlane, A., Donkin, A., Marmot, M. and Viner, R. (2014) *Why Children Die: Death in Infants, Children and Young People in the UK, Part A.* On Behalf of: Royal College of Paediatrics and Child Health, National Children's Bureau, British Association for Child and Adolescent Public Health. London: Royal College of Paediatrics and Child Health.

Useful website

www.meningitis.org

12 Older person assessment
David Kerr

The UK population is projected to reach 73.3 million by mid-2037. Of these, the number continuing to age, with the number of people aged 80 and over is expected to more than double to 6 million in the same period (ONS, 2013). This increase has been attributed to improvements in medical treatment, housing, living standards and nutrition. In the past 25 years the expected years of good or fairly good health, and the expected years without a limiting illness or disability have increased for both men and women. However, they have not increased at the same rate as overall life expectancy. The conclusion drawn from this is that the paramedic will encounter increasing numbers of older people presenting with poorer health with limiting illness and/or disability.

This chapter will provide an overview of the clinical skills required for an effective assessment of the older patient in the out-of-hospital environment. It will identify areas of key importance and discuss the considerations required to aid the assessment process.

SCENE ASSESSMENT

When called to the aid of an older person, numerous clues can be gained by a thorough scene assessment as you approach the patient. As a person ages, their thermoregulation becomes less efficient, making them prone to hypothermia especially if they have a poor diet.

If the patient is outdoors, take account of:
- The weather, especially the ambient temperature
- Clothing that the patient is wearing
- Due to poor thermoregulation and loss of subcutaneous body fat, do not be surprised if the older patient is wearing many layers of clothing even in weather that you might consider quite mild.

If the patient is indoors observe:
- The general state of the house and its garden. Signs of neglect of a person's dwelling can indicate general neglect of the person themselves

either through the person's inability to cope or from a general lack of support for that person.
- Observe the general condition of the house and the ambient temperature. Many older people resist having the heating at a high enough temperature during cold weather for fear of being unable to pay the fuel bill.
- Clues such as handrails, walking frames and commodes can provide an insight into the patient's general mobility.

Support can take many forms, including friends, neighbours and relatives as well as the more formal social services such as home helps or carers. Many older people choose to live in communities with others of a similar age. These can range from sheltered accommodation with a warden, where the resident retains their privacy and independence, to nursing/care homes, where the person is looked after by a team of nurses and carers. As with the domestic dwelling, it is worth noting the general condition of the facilities and the other residents, as people in these facilities are vulnerable and can suffer from neglect, even if unintentional.

Remember, as a pre- and out-of-hospital practitioner, you are ideally placed to identify potentially vulnerable adults and alert the appropriate authorities.

Depending on any specific information and the circumstances of the incident, whether it is winter or summer, it may be appropriate to use blankets for warmth and/or to maintain the patient's dignity.

PRIMARY SURVEY

Remember that the older patient has a lifetime of knowledge and experience behind them and deserves the honour of being treated with respect. The purpose of the primary survey is to rapidly assess and identify potentially life-threatening conditions that require prompt intervention by the paramedic. Certain conditions are more prevalent in the older population. It is worth remembering that the unwell or traumatized older person may have more than one complaint at the same time. The primary survey provides the opportunity to assess whether the patient is ill, injured or both. The paramedic should bear in mind that with the older person an underlying medical condition may be the cause of the events leading to an injury, or conversely that trauma could exacerbate an existing medical condition.

DANGER

On approaching the patient, consider if there is any danger to yourself, colleagues, the patient and bystanders (if present) in this order. Consider the cause of the incident (*fall, road traffic collision, epistaxis*), and identify actual or potential risks. Once you are satisfied the scene is safe, approach the patient in a friendly yet respectful manner.

Older person assessment

Possible actions to be taken:

- Ensure safety of self, colleague(s), and patient
- Wear appropriate personal protective equipment (PPE) (gloves and/or high visibility jacket).

RESPONSE

Using the AVPU scale to assess the patient's response gives an early indication of the mental state of the older patient. Ageing by itself does not cause mental status changes so NEVER accept confusion as *normal* (Snyder, 2016). In the conscious older patient who may suffer from an underlying dementia or delirium, the possibility of an inaccurate assessment of their current state compared with what is normal for them could arise.

Possible actions to be taken:

- Assess and record the patient's level of consciousness (AVPU)
- Remember that older patients may have existing conditions which may cause an inaccurate assessment of their **level of consciousness (LOC).**

AIRWAY

When assessing the older patient's airway, especially in the unconscious patient, check for false teeth (*dentures*). If the patient has kyphosis (*posterior curvature of the spine*), this may give the paramedic airway management problems (Snyder, 2016).

Possible actions to be taken:

- Assess airway and consider the need for dentures to be removed or left in situ
- If obstructed, manage by using stepwise airway management (see *Respiratory Assessment, Chapter 2*)
- If the patient has kyphosis, consider the need to pad the gaps under the head and neck, if in the supine position
- Ensure airway is patent and secure before proceeding to next element.

BREATHING

Many older people suffer from chronic obstructive pulmonary disease (COPD) (National Clinical Guideline Centre, 2010), or other long-term conditions, of which the symptoms may be displayed in the respiratory system, such as left ventricular failure (see *Cardiovascular Assessment, Chapter 3*). As a consequence of these conditions the patient may present with new symptoms or an exacerbation of an existing condition.

- Do they have any shortness of breath, difficulty in breathing (dyspnoea)? If so is the dyspnoea normal for them?
- Do they have a chronic respiratory condition? If so, ask them if there any associated signs or symptoms.
- Are these new or old?

Possible actions to be taken:

- Assess breathing and ensure that the rate and rhythm is adequate
- Assess the patient's oxygen saturation (SpO_2) level
- Maintain an oxygen saturation of 88%–92% for those with COPD (British Thoracic Society, 2015)
- Ensure the patient is not hypoxic
- Administer oxygen appropriate to patient's illness/injury.

CIRCULATION

Assess the patient's circulation, initially checking the pulse for rate, rhythm and volume. The pulse can provide an early indication of the need for further investigation, and is the easiest and least intrusive to initially assess and it also helps to begin the process of physical contact that will be necessary to fully assess the older patient. Assess whether the rhythm is regular or irregular; in the irregular pulse, consider arrhythmias as they are common in the otherwise asymptomatic elderly patient. Orthostatic (*postural*) hypotension is common in the elderly, and is defined as a drop in blood pressure (usually >20/10 mmHg) within 3 minutes of standing.

- If an injury, is there any obvious external haemorrhage?
- Assess the patient's pulse (*regular or irregular*).
- Does the problem occur when the patient stands? (*orthostatic or postural hypotension*)
- Assess the blood pressure (*if normally hypertensive, and reading is within normal adult parameters, consider internal haemorrhage*).
- Ascertain if the patient takes medications for circulatory/cardiac conditions.

- If so, ascertain what they are (*antihypertensives, anticoagulants or glycosides*).

Possible actions to be taken:

- If applicable, control external haemorrhage (see *Trauma Assessment, Chapter 7*)
- Assess the patient's pulse, if appropriate, obtain an ECG trace and manage accordingly
- Ascertain if the problem occurs on standing (*consider orthostatic (postural) hypotension*)
- Obtain and record the blood pressure (consider internal haemorrhage, manage accordingly) (see *Trauma Assessment, Chapter 7*)
- Ascertain if the patient takes medications for any circulatory/cardiac conditions.

DISABILITY

Having assessed the patient's initial response on your approach to them, take time now to reassess their mental status (AVPU). The older person has an increased risk of a stroke or transient ischaemic attack; undertake a FAST assessment. Check their pupils for equality, reactivity and accommodation (PERRLA), bearing in mind the possibility of the patient having existing conditions, such as cataracts, blindness or even a glass eye. Remember that the older patient will have differing metabolic needs. Ensure that their blood glucose levels are assessed as part of this element.

Possible actions to be taken:

- Reassess and record the patient's LOC
- Assess and document size and equality of the patient's pupils (PERRLA) (*consider cataracts, blindness and/or glass eyes*)
- Obtain and record blood glucose levels (manage accordingly, IV glucose (10%) or appropriate drink or food if conscious)
- Undertake a Face, Arms, Speech Test (FAST) (NCCfCC 2008; Fisher et al., 2013; NHS UK, 2015)
- If positive, pre-alert and transfer to a hyper-acute stroke unit (HASU).

EXPOSE/EXAMINE/EVALUATE

Exposing the older patient, whether it is to assess an injury or to begin a more detailed secondary survey, can bring its own challenges as many older patients are often very modest and therefore uncomfortable at being exposed, especially by someone they have just met! Explain to the patient exactly what you need to do, and why, and obtain consent. Examine the patient accordingly: the presence of a scar on the median thoracic wall may indicate previous heart (cardiac) or thoracic surgery. Where possible, protect their privacy by only exposing where necessary and covering them with appropriate blankets. With respect to the environment, the blankets may help maintain the patient's temperature loss, as their thermoregulatory function is often impaired due to loss of fat reserves, thinning skin and slowing metabolism (Snyder, 2016).

Possible actions to be taken:

- Expose the patient's affected areas
- Examine and ascertain if there is an existing condition (*evidence of median cardiac scars or thoracic injuries, glyceryl trinitrate GTN patches, implantable cardioverter defibrillator ICD*)
- Remember patient dignity and consider the environment (*possible hypothermia*)
- Evaluate – transfer patient to an appropriate unit or move onto secondary survey.

SECONDARY SURVEY

The older patient often has more than one complaint and these can be a combination of chronic problems, such as arthritis or chronic obstructive pulmonary disease (COPD), and acute problems, such as sudden chest pain or a fall. Also, there could be an exacerbation of a chronic problem such as COPD due to an acute chest infection. Therefore, careful patient questioning will be required to identify the problems and their priority for assessment and treatment. Remember to consider the following:

- Give elderly patients time to respond to your questions.
- Speak slowly and clearly but do not shout or raise your voice.
- Visual cues may be important, so make sure your face is well lit.
- If they wear glasses, make sure they put them on (Bickley and Szilagyi, 2012).

Ideally, you want to obtain the history of the chief complaint from the patient, but there are times when the patient will be incapable of answering your questions, such as when suffering from an altered mental status or unconsciousness, and you must rely on the patient's carer.

Presenting complaint

Asking an older patient 'What is wrong?' often results in a lengthy and wide-ranging answer, therefore, it is important that you get the patient to focus on what their current most important problem is. This is best achieved by asking questions such as 'What made you call us today?' or 'What is different about what is bothering you today?' If the reason for attendance was a fall, ascertain if it occurred due to trauma or was due to an underlying medical condition.

Ask yourself the following questions:
- Did the patient really trip, or fall?
- Is there a medical reason for the fall?
- Dizziness (*may be suggestive of orthostatic (postural) hypotension*)
- Palpitations (*may be suggestive of cardiac arrhythmias*)
- Is there an environmental hazard that caused the fall? (*loose handrails or carpets*)

Common complaints in the older patient include:
- Shortness of breath
- Chest pain
- Altered mental status
- Abdominal pain
- Dizziness or weakness
- Fever
- Trauma
- Falls
- Generalized pain
- Nausea, vomiting and diarrhoea (Snyder, 2016).

History of presenting complaint

While the history of the presenting complaint is concerned with the events leading up to the emergency call (presenting complaint), the paramedic will need to consider the fact that the patient may not be able to recall events. The patient who has fainted (syncope) may not even be aware that they had passed out prior to the fall. In situations where the incident has occurred in a public place, or the patient lives alone, then information concerning what occurred may have to be obtained from bystanders, the carer or relatives. The SAMPLE framework will assist the paramedic to structure the investigation into the events preceding the history of the presenting complaint, and the SOCRATES framework should be used in assessing pain that the patient presents with (see *General Principles of Assessment, Chapter 1*). Consider the following:

- Ask the patient, 'What is the last thing you can remember?'
- If applicable, ascertain history of the presenting complaint from bystanders, carer or relatives.
- Does the information provided correlate with the mechanism of injury?
- If concerned, question patient regarding specific causes (*dyspnoea, chest pain, dizziness, loss of balance, etc.*).

Past medical history

A lot of information can be gleaned from the answer to questions regarding an older patient's past medical history but care must be taken to keep the conversation focused on relevant information. The fact your patient broke their wrist falling from a tree at the age of 10 probably has no bearing on their current complaint! Try and keep your questions open. Asking a patient if they suffer from cardiac problems might get the answer 'no', even though they have such medication as GTN, digoxin, aspirin and frusemide. When questioned further, the patient may well consider themselves free of cardiac problems because they take that medication. Consider asking the following:

- Can you tell me about your past medical history?
- Do you have any other medical conditions?
- Do you have diabetes? If so, what type, I or II?
- Do you suffer with a breathing problem? If so, is it a long-term condition (*COPD, emphysema or chronic bronchitis*)?
- Do you have a problem with your heart (*hypertension, angina, LVF, RVF, CCF*)?
- Have you ever been hospitalized or had any operations? If so, what for?

Drug/medication history

This is a vital aspect of the older patient's history and consideration must be given to the normal parameters of drug pharmacology (absorption, distribution, metabolism, excretion and tissue sensitivity). Renal function declines with increasing age and will therefore affect the 'pharmacokinetics' of various drugs, specifically those that are predominantly eliminated by the kidney. Excretion of these drugs will occur more slowly, resulting in their half-lives (*duration of action*) being prolonged, and they can accumulate to a higher (potentially toxic) concentration even in a well state. Consider the patient's overall hydration (Kane et al., 2013). Older people use more prescription medicines than younger people and therefore there is an increased chance of them experiencing side-effects. Older people also tend to use more over-the-counter medications, including herbal remedies, so it is important to ask about these as well (Snyder, 2016). Remember that the older patient with chronic conditions will often have a repeat prescription list which is useful in ascertaining the patient's medication especially if the patient is confused or forgetful. However, it is important to check that the patient is adhering to their medication regimen. It is also worth checking if the patient is taking any prescription medication not prescribed specifically for them (e.g. a spouse's sleeping tablets) (Pilbery, 2014).

Social/family medical history

When asking about the social aspect of the older patient's history, include asking about their activities of daily living (ADLs) and how these have changed over time. Bickley and Szilagyi (2012) tell us there are two standard categories of assessment: physical ADLs and instrumental ADLs (see Table 12.1), and the paramedic should assess whether the patient can carry out these activities independently, with some help, or is entirely dependent.

Table 12.1 Activities of daily living (ADL)

Physical ADL	Instrumental ADL
Bathing	Using the telephone
Dressing	Shopping
Toileting	Preparing food
Transfers	Housekeeping
Continence	Laundry
Feeding	Transportation
Managing money	Taking medicine

Other aspects of the older patient's social history include their diet, exercise, sources of stress, especially bereavements, leisure activities, alcohol and drug use. Check for non-adherence to dietary regimens such as diabetic diets causing hyperglycaemia and restricting salt intake which can worsen congestive heart failure (Snyder, 2016). It is likely that today an older person will have smoked at some point in their life, so try and ascertain how much they smoked and for how long. For cigarettes this is often reported as pack years (number of packs smoked per day × number of years smoking). If they have given up, ascertain how long ago. Alcohol use is on the rise in the older population with a smaller amount using illegal drugs. This can often be in response to a life-changing event such as loss of a spouse, declining health or low self-esteem (Pilbery, 2014).

Social exclusion is defined as being cut off from the mainstream of society, and is described as being unable to access things in life that most people take for granted, such as a properly equipped, well-maintained home, close friends and regular company, stimulating activity and easy access to important services like GPs, shops and post offices. Ascertain if the patient lives alone, their marital status, occupation, living in social housing (rented) or if they are homeowners, and if possible their financial position; evidence has shown how the older person is, and feels, excluded due to these (see Table 12.2).

Table 12.2 Social exclusion in later life

	Vulnerable to social exclusion
Age and gender	Older people >75 years are more vulnerable to social exclusion
	Women >75 yrs are more vulnerable to social exclusion than men
Occupational status	Older people with routine or manual rather than managerial or professional occupations are more at risk of social exclusion. The differences are most marked in the 50–64 and 65–74 age groups.
Marital status	Older people who have never married are more likely to be socially excluded than those who have been married, or are widows
Ethnicity	Older ethnic minorities suffer higher rates of social exclusion than older white people
Long-term illness/ disability	Older people with long-term illness/disability are at higher risk of social exclusion than older people in good health
Depression	The more socially excluded the older person is, the more likely they are likely to suffer from depression

Age Concern (2009).

When asking about the older patient's family medical history, you are trying to ascertain a genetic link for common familial diseases, such as cancer, cardiovascular diseases, respiratory diseases and neurological diseases, so ask about the health and, where appropriate, cause of death of grandparents, parents, siblings, children and grandchildren.

REVIEW OF SYSTEMS AND VITAL SIGNS

This section will review the systems and associated vital signs of the older patient highlighting the most common conditions, illnesses and injuries that you may find.

Respiratory system

Older people have decreased ability to clear secretions, as well as decreased cough and gag reflexes, making aspiration and obstruction more likely. Complaining of shortness of breath is common among older people with the potential causes being the only symptom of a heart attack, COPD, congestive heart disease (*all cause wheezing*) or other medical reasons such as pain, bleeding or medication interactions (Snyder, 2016). Consider the following when undertaking the review of the following systems and vital signs:

- Normal range for respiratory rate, character and work of breathing for the older patient is the same as for the younger patient (12–20 breaths per minute).
- Chest stiffness could make it more difficult to assess chest rise.
- Loss of elasticity of the lungs and a decrease in the size and strength of the respiratory muscles.
- The above changes cause decreased vital capacity (50% by age 75) and increased residual volume, leading to a progressive decline in the proportion of air usefully used in gas exchange.
- Musculoskeletal changes such as kyphosis (*curvature of spine*) can also impact on respiratory function. The older patient also has a declining partial pressure of oxygen ($pO_2 = 100 - age/3$).
- Dulling of the respiratory drive due to decreased sensitivity to arterial blood gas changes causes older patients to have a slower reaction to hypoxaemia and hypercarbia (Pilbery, 2014).

Oxygen saturation (SpO_2)
- Due to the increased incidence of COPD in older people, the oxygen saturation levels can be lower. Aim for a target saturation of 94%–98% in the acutely unwell patient or where there is a risk of the patient having a hypoxic drive, a target range of 88%–92% should be aimed for (British Thoracic Society, 2015).
- There may be difficulty in gaining an accurate SpO_2 due to poor peripheral circulation. If in doubt, do not withhold oxygen but monitor the patient closely for changes in breathing rate and level of consciousness. When assessing the respiratory system of the older patient, ascertain whether the presentation is an existing chronic problem, a worsening of the chronic problem, or a new problem.

Cardiovascular system

Pulse
- The ageing heart is less responsive to nervous stimulation which can lead to a lower heart rate and weaker pulses.
- Always check pulses bilaterally to exclude obstruction rather than a reduced heart function.
- Peripheral pulses can be difficult to find due to vascular changes and poor circulation.
- Palpate the carotid pulse gently to avoid dislodging a thrombus. Alternatively, use a stethoscope to listen to the apical heartbeat (Snyder, 2016).

One third of patients around 60 years old, and over half who reach 85 years, have had an aortic systolic murmur heard on examination due to a process of fibrosis and calcification known as aortic sclerosis. A similar process affects the mitral valve approximately a decade later leading to a systolic murmur of mitral regurgitation which cannot be discounted due to the extra load placed on the heart by the leaking mitral valve.

- If auscultating the middle or upper carotid arteries and turbulence (*known as a bruit*) is heard, it can suggest, but not prove, a partial arterial obstruction secondary to atherosclerosis (Bickley and Szilagyi, 2012).
- When assessing the older patient's heart rate and character, remember to take account of any medication the patient takes, especially beta-blockers. A normal response to shock is a rise in heart rate which beta-blockers would prevent, misleading the paramedic into thinking the patient is not shocked.

Blood pressure
- It is important that you try to ascertain the older patient's normal blood pressure history as it is common for the older person to have hypertension, therefore a recording considered normal for a younger person may indicate shock.
- If the patient has very high blood pressure, it may signal an impending stroke or other problem (Snyder, 2016).
- A blood pressure consistently higher than 140/90 mmHg is considered to be hypertensive and patients will often be prescribed medication for this. However, a single blood pressure reading is largely meaningless on its own, as trends give more information on the cardiovascular status of the patient. Obtain at least three readings.
- If the patient presents with a blood pressure of greater than 180/110 mmHg, then considerate immediate referral in discussion with the patient's GP (NICE, 2011).

- If possible, assess the older patient for postural hypotension by taking their blood pressure when supine, semi-recumbent and standing. If the patient's blood pressure drops the more vertical they become, this could indicate a cause for symptoms such as dizziness and syncope.
- Remember to factor in the effects of stress and anxiety on your patient's blood pressure.

ECG recordings
- Arrhythmias in older people are generally a result of age-related changes in the heart, existing cardiac disease, adverse drug effects, or a combination of these factors.
- The most common arrhythmia in the older population is atrial fibrillation (AF) which increases the risk of stroke and heart failure (NICE, 2014).

Neurological system

Glasgow Coma Score (GCS)
- Altered mental status is a common presentation of a number of underlying causes in the older patient which may be due to a malfunction of virtually any body system, therefore it is important to investigate it thoroughly (see Neurological Assessment, Chapter 5).
- It is worth noting that the causes of an altered mental status are the same across the life span but have a higher frequency for older patients (Snyder, 2016).
- When assessing an older patient with an altered mental status, differentiate between delirium and dementia, which are the most common causes of 'confusion' in the older population (Kane et al., 2013).
- Delirium is a symptom with a rapid onset (hours to days) that resolves once the underlying cause has been treated (NICE, 2010). Use the mnemonic 'DELIRIUMS' as a guide to possible causes:

    D – drugs or toxins
    E – emotional (psychiatric)
    L – low pO_2
    I – infection
    R – retention (stool/urine)
    I – ictal (seizures)
    U – under-nutrition/dehydration
    M – metabolism
    S – subdural haematoma

- Dementia is a disease that produces irreversible brain damage. The two most common degenerative dementias are 'multi-infarct' or 'vascular dementia' and Alzheimer's disease which is one of the fastest growing health care issues (NICE, 2007). Research suggests that there are approximately 820,000 people in the UK suffering from dementia and that the estimated cost of dementia to society is approximately £23 billion a year (Luengo-Fernandez et al., 2010).

Blood glucose levels

- Approximately 10% of over-65-year-olds have **Type 2 diabetes**, which is frequently diet or tablet-controlled. These patients are at risk of hypoglycaemia due to such factors as medication, irregular or inadequate dietary intake, failure to recognize the warning signs or blunted warning signs.
- Delirium may be the only indication of hypoglycaemia in the older patient. If the patient is hyperglycaemic, the presentation is likely to be acute confusion with dehydration.

Urine dipstick testing

- Can be used to screen for serious renal, urological and liver disease as well as metabolic disorders such as diabetes.
- Positive result is not sufficient to make a clinical diagnosis.
- Urine constituents that are detectable by commercial dipstick testing include glucose, bilirubin, urobilionogen, ketones, blood, leucocyte esterase, nitrite, protein, albumin, creatinine, trypsinogen, pH and specific gravity.

Pupils

- Decreases in visual acuity are common in older people without underlying diseases.
- Assess pupils – PERRLA. Remember the two most common visual disturbances are cataracts (*hardening lenses that eventually become opaque*) and glaucoma (*increased intra-ocular pressure that damages the optic nerve*).

Temperature

- Thermoregulation in the older patient is impaired due to a slowed endocrine system and can be adversely affected by chronic disease, medications and alcohol use.
- Older people account for half of all deaths and most indoor deaths from hypothermia which can develop in temperatures above freezing from prolonged exposure.
- Hypothermia death rates are more than double for older people with those over 85 years old most at risk (Pilbery, 2014).

Pain score

- Older patients may not perceive pain normally due to a number of factors such as neuropathy caused by diseases (e.g. diabetes) and the ageing process.
- Remember medications or living with chronic pain (*e.g. arthritis*) can give the patient a higher pain tolerance. It is important to note any changes to the level or location of the pain (NAEMT, 2014).
- The standard pain score is still a useful assessment tool with the older patient as it monitors pain levels from a subjective patient viewpoint.

Trauma

- Injuries to the older person should be considered to be more serious than their outward appearance, to have a more profound systemic influence and to have a greater potential for producing rapid decompensation (NAEMT, 2014).
- Medication, such as beta-blockers, can prevent the normal homeostatic responses to shock.
- Osteoporosis can make the older patient more prone to fractures even from low energy impacts and they can even suffer pathological fractures from sudden movements.
- When assessing the older patient, careful questioning about past falls as well as the current incident could highlight an underlying cause. The incidence of falls increases with increasing age and is evenly split between extrinsic causes (*slip or trip*) and intrinsic causes (*dizziness or fainting*) (Pilbery, 2014).
- If the older patient takes anti-coagulation medication such as Warfarin, any haemorrhage could be more severe and last longer due to disruption of the clotting process.

Impressions

The key impressions that the paramedic notes when dealing with the older patient should include the impression of the patient and the condition of their surroundings, in addition to the situation:

- What is the state of the patient's living conditions?
- Does the patient have home oxygen?
- Do you think the patient can manage at home?

The paramedic should ensure that if the patient is taken to hospital, they verbally provide their 'impression' when handing over the patient, and record on their documentation to prevent this information from being lost.

OTHER CONSIDERATIONS

Communication

- Do not shout at an older patient who has a hearing impairment.
- Ensure they are wearing their hearing aid if available.
- Move closer to the patient and speak into their ear or use a 'reverse stethoscope' technique (*the ear pieces of the stethoscope are placed in the patient's ears and the paramedic speaks softly into the diaphragm*).
- If the patient has a visual impairment, do not assume they also have a hearing impairment. It is important that you describe the procedures you wish to carry out and the equipment you are going to use.
- Make sure you are facing the patient and allow your facial expressions to reflect your meaning.
- Use short sentences and avoid technical jargon. This is especially true if the patient does not speak English and you are interviewing the patient through an interpreter.
- If the patient has aphasia, which is the partial or total inability to produce and understand speech as a result of brain damage caused by injury or disease, give them time to talk and encourage all modes of communication.
- If the patient has dementia, use simple, clear language conveying only one idea at a time; there is a delayed reaction time in conversation, so if repeating yourself, use the same words to allow for this.
- If the patient still does not understand, then try re-phrasing possibly using gestures to augment your communication.

Social/family/carer/guardian

- When assessing the older patient, listen to any concerns voiced by the patient's caregiver regarding changes in the patient's health or the ability of the patient to cope.
- If you think the history given by the older patient is unreliable or incomplete, ask the caregiver to confirm the history.
- It is worth noting any signs of stress or frustration in the caregiver as they may need help as well (Snyder, 2016).
- Where the patient lives with their spouse, consider the ability of the spouse to cope should you take your patient to hospital and give consideration to conveying the spouse as well.
- If there are any suspicions of abuse of the older person, then these should be reported to the appropriate authority.
- Remember it is not the paramedic's place to conduct an investigation but to report any concerns (Fisher et al., 2013).

Ethical and legal

- As with all adult patients, the older patient has autonomy over their choices in accordance with their own goals and values.
- Where there may be conflict in 'end-of-life care issues' or the patient has a 'do not resuscitate' order and their family disagree, check documentation.
- As far as possible, the patient's wishes must be respected.
- The paramedic should satisfy themselves that the patient can give informed consent for any proposed treatment and that the patient's decision-making capacity is assessed (DH, 2009).
- Use the local guidelines of your service when assessing a patient's capacity and make sure the process is documented fully.
- When dealing with end-of-life issues, consider the patient's beliefs and how they might impact on the care you propose and the needs of the patient and their family. This may involve facilitating the presence of a religious leader.
- It is important not to let your own beliefs influence the treatment of those who hold a different view to yourself but to deliver the most appropriate care in a professional manner.

Destination/receiving specialist units/non-conveyance

- There is an ever-increasing choice of where to refer your patient and local guidelines should be followed.
- Specialist units include acute stroke units for new onset strokes, hospices for palliative care and trauma centres for major trauma.
- A patient may refuse treatment or transportation and a quick assessment of their capacity is required. There can be many reasons for refusal to go to hospital, from a poor past experience to a fear of never getting home again.
- Reassurance and honesty are the best route in these circumstances.
- If the patient is deemed to have capacity, then their wishes must be respected and the appropriate documentation completed.
- If the patient is not deemed to have capacity, then assistance might need to be sought from the patient's doctor or the police in order to treat the patient.

Professional

The Health and Care Professions Council (HCPC) sets out the expected *Standards of Proficiency – Paramedics* (HCPC, 2014), and the *Standards of Conduct, Performance and Ethics* (HCPC, 2012a) for registrant paramedics, and also provides *Guidance on Conduct and Ethics for Students* (HCPC, 2012b) for 'students' on HCPC-approved pre-registration courses.

- These are regularly reviewed and updated and it is the paramedic's responsibility to be fully conversant with the latest version.
- The *National Service Framework for Older People* (DH, 2001) sets out the minimum level of care an older patient should receive.

Facts and figures

- The Office for National Statistics (2013) reports that the population of the UK is growing increasingly older.
- Over the last 25 years the percentage of the population aged 65 and over has increased from 15% in 1983 to 16% in 2008, an increase of 1.5 million people.
- The fastest population increase has been in the number of those aged 80 and over, the 'oldest old', with their numbers more than doubling since 1983, to reach 1.3 million in 2008.
- By 2037, the number of people aged 80 and over is projected to more than double again to reach 6 million.
- As a result of these increases in the number of older people, the median age of the UK population is increasing – from 35 years in 1983 to 39 in 2008. It is projected to continue to increase over the next 25 years rising to 40 by 2033.

Older people in the population

- In 2013, the number of centenarians (people aged 100 and over) in the UK was estimated at 13,780, of these 710 were estimated to be 105 years or older. Of these there were 586 women aged 100 years of age and over per 100 men of that age, this is a fall from 823 women a decade previously in 2003.
- In 2013, there were over half a million (500,000) aged 90 years and over in the UK.
- In 2013, there were 840 people who were aged 90 years and over per 100,000 population in England and Wales, which was higher than in Scotland (707), and in Northern Ireland (620) (ONS, 2014).

Increases in life expectancy

- The increase in the size of the older population has largely been driven by increases in life expectancy.
- Life expectancy at age 65 in the UK increased by 40% to 18.2 years for men and for women by 23% to 20.7 years in the 30 years between 1980–82 and 2010–12.

- A newborn baby boy could expect to live 78.7 years and a newborn baby girl 82.6 years if mortality rates remain the same as they were in 2010–12. Women continue to live longer than men, but the gap is closing.

CHAPTER KEY POINTS

- Older patients will call the ambulance service as a 'last resort', often apologizing for calling the emergency services.
- The older patient should be, as with any patient, treated with respect.
- Ensure consent is obtained appropriate to the older person and the situation.
- Undertake and follow the structured approach to the primary survey DR ABCDE and manage **time critical** conditions accordingly.
- Undertake and follow the structured approach to the secondary survey, and ensure you cover all important aspects. Do not ignore the patient's social and environmental history.
- Take your time with your verbal history taking, physical assessment and social assessment. If older people feel rushed, they may omit an important piece of information, if they sense you are in a hurry.
- Always ascertain the drug/medication history, as many older patients may have added complications due to pharmacokinetics of multiple medications.
- If appropriate, use bystanders, carers and relatives to ascertain important information.
- As older people are subject to abuse, ensure you have a clear understanding of the vulnerable adult policies and procedures, and always document clearly.

REFERENCES

Age Concern (2009) *Social Exclusion in Later Life: An Exploration of Risk Factors*. London: Age UK.

Bickley, L.S. and Szilagyi, P.G. (2012) *Bates' Guide to Physical Examination and History Taking* (11th edn). Philadelphia, PA: Lippincott Williams & Wilkins.

British Thoracic Society (2015) *Emergency Oxygen Use in Adult Patients Guideline*. Available at: https://www.brit-thoracic.org.uk/searchresults/?txtSearch=2015+Oxygen+Guidelines&search= (accessed. 14 February 2015).

Department of Health (2001) *National Service Framework for Older People*. London: The Stationery Office.

Department of Health (2009) *Reference Guide to Consent for Examination or Treatment* (2nd edn). London: Department of Health.

Fisher, J., Brown, S.N. and Cook, M. (eds) (2013) *UK Ambulance Services Clinical Practice Guidelines 2013: Major Pelvic Trauma*. Bridgwater: Class Professional Publishing.

Health and Care Professions Council (2012a) *Standards of Conduct, Performance and Ethics*. London: HCPC.

Health and Care Professions Council (2012b) *Guidance on Conduct and Ethics for Students*. London: HCPC.

Health and Care Professions Council (2014) *Standards of Proficiency: Paramedics*. London: HCPC.

Kane, R.L., Ouslander, J.G. and Abrass, I.B. (2013) *Essentials of Clinical Geriatrics* (6th edn). New York: McGraw-Hill.

Luengo-Fernandez, R., Leal, J. and Graz, A. (2010) *Dementia 2010: The Prevalence, Economic Cost and Research Funding of Dementia Compared with Other Major Diseases*. Oxford: Oxford University Press.

National Association of Emergency Medical Technicians US (NAEMT) (2014) *PHTLS Pre Hospital Trauma Life Support* (8th edn). Missouri: Mosby Elsevier.

National Clinical Guideline Centre (2010) *Chronic Obstructive Pulmonary Disease: Management of Chronic Obstructive Pulmonary Disease in Adults in Primary and Secondary Care*. London: National Clinical Guideline Centre.

National Collaborating Centre for Chronic Conditions (2008) *Stroke: National Clinical Guideline for Diagnosis and Initial Management of Acute Stroke and Transient Ischaemic Attack (TIA)*. London: Royal College of Physicians.

NHS UK (2015) *Stroke – Act F.A.S.T.* Available at: http://www.nhs.uk/actfast/Pages/stroke.aspx (accessed 9 June 2015).

NICE (National Institute for Health and Clinical Excellence) (2007) *Dementia: A NICE–SCIE Guideline on Supporting People with Dementia and Their Carers in Health and Social Care*. NICE clinical guidance 42. London: British Psychological Society and Gaskell.

NICE (National Institute for Health and Clinical Excellence) (2010) *Delirium: Diagnosis, Prevention and Management*. NICE clinical guidance 103. London: National Clinical Guideline Centre.

NICE (National Institute for Health And Clinical Excellence) (2011) *Hypertension: The Clinical Management of Primary Hypertension in Adults*. NICE clinical guidance 127. London: National Clinical Guideline Centre.

NICE (National Institute for Health and Clinical Excellence) (2014) *Atrial Fibrillation: The Management of Atrial Fibrillation*. NICE clinical guidance 180. London: National Clinical Guideline Centre.

ONS (Office for National Statistics) (2013) *National Population Projections, 2012-Based Projections*. Available at: http://www.ons.gov.uk/ons/rel/npp/national-population-projections/2012-based-projections/index.html (accessed 9 May 2015).

ONS (Office for National Statistics) (2014) *Estimates of the Very Old (including Centenarians) for England and Wales, United Kingdom, 2002 to 2013*. Available at: http://www.ons.gov.uk/ons/rel/mortality-ageing/estimates-of-the-very-old–including-centenarians-/2002–2013–england-and-wales–united-kingdom-/index.html (accessed. 9 June 2015).

Pilbery, R. (2014) *Nancy Caroline's Emergency Care in the Streets: United Kingdom* (7th edn). Burlington, VA: Jones & Bartlett Learning.

Snyder, D.R. (2016) *Geriatric Education for Emergency Medical Services (GEMS)* (2nd edn). Sudbury, MA. American Geriatric Society: National Association Emergency Medical Technicians (NAEMT).

13 Obstetric patient assessment
Graham Harris and Rehan Khan

Childbirth is a natural event which in itself is not a medical emergency, and which for millions of years has required little medical assistance (AAOS, 2011). For paramedics, however, this area of practice has always caused feelings of trepidation even for the experienced practitioner. However, by undertaking a systematic and structured approach when completing a **primary and secondary survey** of the *obstetric* patient, the paramedic will remain not only professional, but will ensure they obtain the relevant obstetric history.

The primary survey is extended in this chapter to include: **F – Fundus** and **G – Get to the point quickly**. The aim of this chapter is to provide the paramedic with a systematic approach to the assessment of the patient which will enable them to ascertain the key features of the obstetric history. It will identify whether the patient has any potential life-threatening conditions, which will require the paramedic to implement the appropriate management and transfer immediately to an obstetric unit.

SCENE ASSESSMENT

The assessment of the scene and the patient occurs as you approach the patient; the paramedic should subconsciously undertake a **DR 'C' ABCDEFG** assessment as they scan the scene. D – Danger, R – Response, C – Circulation (obvious external haemorrhage), A – Airway, B – Breathing, C – Circulation, D – Disability, E – Expose/Environment/Evaluate, F – Fundus, and G – Get to the point quickly, undertake a primary survey.

- Are there other children present? (possibly an indication of previous pregnancies, but check to be certain, do not assume)
- Is the environment clean and warm?
- Is there a midwife present?

PRIMARY SURVEY

The paramedic should remember that with the obstetric primary survey there are two patients (sometimes more in multiple pregnancies). If already born, assess the newborn baby (see *Assessment and Care of the Newborn, Chapter 14*). The primary survey provides the paramedic with the first 'hands-on' examination of the pregnant patient. If the patient has sustained significant trauma, either blunt or penetrating to the abdomen, then they should be referred to hospital for assessment. The primary survey should be modified in accordance with the findings of the element, for example, the presence of vaginal bleeding post-trauma is a **red flag** condition and potentially indicates the patient is **time critical**, until proven otherwise (Woollard et al., 2010).

DANGER

While the majority of obstetric emergency calls attended by paramedics will not present any substantial dangers, the need to ensure that an assessment of this element has been undertaken is important.

- Always ensure the safety of yourself, your colleagues, other health care professionals (midwives) and the patient.
- If pets such as dogs are present, politely request they be removed to another room.
- Remember that obstetric situations have a high risk of body fluids, and the appropriate personal protective equipment (gloves, aprons) should be worn.

Possible actions to be taken:

- Ensure safety of self, colleagues, midwives and patient
- Request pets to be removed if present
- Wear appropriate PPE (gloves, aprons).

RESPONSE

The patient who responds clearly to your questions can be deemed to be conscious, however, remember that if the patient's level of consciousness is altered, this can also have an effect on the unborn foetus.

- Assess the patient's response using the AVPU scale and record appropriately.
- Remember that alterations in the patient's level of consciousness (LOC) may be due to hypoxia caused by an airway, breathing or circulation problem.

Obstetric patient assessment

> **Possible actions to be taken:**
> - Assess and record the patient's level of consciousness (AVPU)
> - Remember that obstetric patients have differing oxygen requirements during the pregnancy, which can affect the patient's level of consciousness.

CIRCULATION (OBVIOUS EXTERNAL HAEMORRHAGE)

This extra element of the primary survey occurs not only because pregnant females increase their blood volume, but also because the placenta and gravid uterus are highly vascular and injuries to these can cause profound haemorrhage. Death due to haemorrhage remains a leading cause of death (CMACE, 2011).

- Is there a significant amount of blood visible on the floor?
- Is the patient's clothing visibly wet/saturated with blood?
- Is blood running down the patient's legs?
- Is there evidence of blood-soaked pads? If so, how many?
- Is the haemorrhage compressible?

Bear in mind that some causes of obstetric haemorrhage, e.g. placenta previa (placenta obstructing the birth canal), lead to REVEALED haemorrhage, i.e. visible blood loss in keeping with haemodynamic state, whereas others, e.g. placental abruption, lead to CONCEALED haemorrhage, i.e. visible blood loss less than that suggested by haemodynamic state.

> **Possible actions to be taken:**
> - If compressible, manage immediately (pressure dressing(s))
> - If it is an ante-partum haemorrhage (APH), remove to the nearest obstetric unit for surgery
> - Cannulate and administer IV fluids en route
> - Pre-alert the hospital/obstetric unit.

AIRWAY

While the airway does not change dramatically due to pregnancy, the paramedic needs to be aware of the issues that may affect the airway of the pregnant patient. Obesity remains a significant contributor to maternal death, the prevalence is increasing in both the general population and the pregnant population. Women with a high body mass index remain over-represented in maternal deaths. Obesity = a body mass index of 30 or more (CMACE, 2011). Oedema of the airway may occur in patients with a hypertensive condition, and due to a decrease in peristalsis of the gastro-intestinal tract, they are at risk of regurgitation and aspiration (Salomone and Pons, 2014).

- Is the patient able to talk clearly and does she have an open airway?
- Is she making unusual noises indicating a possible airway obstruction?
- If obstructed, manage accordingly (stepwise airway management, see *Respiratory Assessment, Chapter 2*).
- If unresponsive, manage the airway with positioning (place the patient in a left lateral tilt 15–30° or manually displace the uterus) to prevent compression of the vena cava.

Possible actions to be taken:

- Ensure airway is patent and secure before proceeding to next element
- If obstructed, manage by using stepwise airway management
- If unresponsive, manage the airway (*place the patient in a left lateral tilt 15–30° or manually displace the uterus*).

Breathing

During pregnancy, the shape of the rib cage alters anatomically to accommodate the enlarging uterus, and pushes up on the diaphragm (NAEMT, 2011). Throughout pregnancy both the vital capacity and respiratory rate increase, but the residual volume decreases and during late pregnancy the patient may exhibit dyspnoea (Marieb and Hoehn, 2014). In late pregnancy the tidal volume increases by 40%, however, the tidal increase causes an increase in the minute ventilation by as much as 50%.

- Ascertain the patient's respiratory rate and effort (increased rate without increased work of breathing may be indicative of an attempt to compensate for a circulatory problem) (Woollard et al., 2010).
- Ascertain the patient's oxygen saturation levels.

- Administer oxygen only in relation to the clinical findings (administering oxygen to well-pregnant patients may cause alarm).
- Auscultate for and clarify if there are adventitious sounds.

> **Possible actions to be taken:**
> - Ascertain the patient's oxygen saturation levels
> - Administer oxygen only in relation to the clinical findings (British Thoracic Society, 2015)
> - Manage breathing problems and/or associated hypoxia effectively before moving on to the next element.

Circulation

Physiological changes occur with the circulatory system as the pregnancy develops; these incorporate an increase in heart rate 15/20 bpm by the third trimester. Blood pressure decreases 5/15 mmHg during the second trimester, but returns to normal by term. Cardiac output increases by 1–1.5 l/min by the tenth week, but by term, blood volume increases by approximately 50% (Resuscitation Council (UK), 2011; Salomone and Pons, 2014). The paramedic should remember that a pregnant patient at term can lose 30%–35% of their blood volume before presenting with signs of hypovolaemia.

- Assess the patient's radial pulse to ascertain the rate and rhythm.
- Assess the patient's blood pressure (BP):
    - A systolic BP of 100 mmHg is not uncommon in the healthy pregnant patient.
    - Mild Hypertension 140/90–149/99: Moderate Hypertension 150/100–159/109: Severe Hypertension 160/110 or higher (NICE, 2015a).
    - A systolic BP of 160 mmHg or over requires urgent further medical assessment.
- Ask the patient if they have had problems with their BP during the pregnancy.
- Always read the patient's hand-held records to assess trends in their blood pressure and judge for the presence of pre-eclampsia (hypertension associated with proteinuria occurring after 20 weeks).
- ECG changes occurring in pregnancy include ectopic beats and supraventricular tachycardia (these are often considered normal).

Possible actions to be taken:

- Assess the patient's heart rate
- Assess the patient's BP (note and record, if severely hypertensive 160/110 mmHg or higher, then arrange further assessment)
- Perform urine analysis
- Ask to see the patient's hand-held records and ascertain trends or problems with blood pressure.

DISABILITY

Pre-eclampsia in late pregnancy is characterized by changes in the patient's mental status, and can result in seizures (eclampsia). Eclampsia and pre-eclampsia were identified as the fifth highest cause of death for pregnant patients (CMACE, 2011). Gestational diabetes is increasing with the rise in obesity.

- Assess the patient's level of consciousness (LOC) (*AVPU*).
- Assess the patient's blood glucose levels (*ascertain if the patient has pre-existing diabetes. If so, is it type I or type II?*)
- Any pregnant woman with any form of diabetes should maintain their capillary plasma glucose level below the following target levels (*if achievable without causing problematic hypoglycaemia*):
  - Fasting 5.3 mmol/litre
  - 1-hour post meals: 7.8 mmol/litre or
  - 2-hour post meals: 6.4 mmol/litre (NICE, 2015b).
- Pregnant women with diabetes who are on insulin or glibenclamide should maintain their capillary plasma glucose level above 4 mmol/litre (NICE, 2015b).
- Assess the patient's pupils for both size and reaction (PERRLA).

EXPOSE/ENVIRONMENT/EVALUATE

The paramedic may or may not be experienced in obstetric situations, however, if you have not already done so, briefly expose and examine the intraoitus (*vaginal opening*). Always ensure you obtain consent first from the patient and that it is recorded (Department of Health, 2009). If the patient is contracting and in apparent labour, consider:

- Have the waters broken? (*spontaneous rupture of membranes (SROM)*)
- Can you see any presenting parts of the baby?
- Environment. Is it warm, and as clean as possible? (*especially if considering to deliver on site*)

- Evaluate the findings from the primary survey and if you have identified any **time critical** problems within any of the elements, then consider the need to transport and transfer immediately to an appropriate obstetric unit, if not, then conduct the secondary survey and then transfer the patient to her pre-booked unit.

> **Possible actions to be taken:**
> - Expose patient and examine
> - Ensure consent and patient dignity
> - Evaluate – time critical obstetric emergencies require transfer to an appropriate obstetric unit, pre-alert the hospital/obstetric unit
> - Request midwife/skilled assistance if remaining on scene
> - Non-time critical – move on to the secondary survey.

FUNDUS

When examining make a quick assessment of the fundal height, a fundus at the height of the umbilicus equates approximately to 22 weeks gestation. At full term the fundus is at the xiphoid process.

GET TO THE POINT QUICKLY

The aim of the primary survey is to identify any potential life-threatening conditions, which will require the paramedic to implement the appropriate management and transfer immediately to an obstetric unit.

SECONDARY SURVEY

Obstetric history

Paramedics may be called to obstetric patients who are either due to undertake, or have undertaken, a home delivery; alternatively they may be booked into a midwifery-led or a consultant-led unit, and, in the worst case scenario, attend patients who have not pre-booked obstetric maternity care. The majority of patients will, however, have accessed antenatal care and be in possession of appropriate hand-held maternity notes. Undertaking a complete obstetric history from the patient, in combination with the information provided in the patient's hand-held maternity notes, will enable the paramedic to identify any potential obstetric or related medical problems that may arise, while the patient is in their care. In the first instance ascertain the following information from the patient:

- The patient's name (*is she agreeable for you to address her by this name?*).

- Date of birth (DOB) or age (*this can provide information regarding the possibility of potential obstetric problems*), is she young or maternal age >40 years of age?
- Which hospital is the patient booked in to (*if the patent has previously booked*)?
- Is she booked into an obstetric or midwife-led unit? (*The latter normally dictates low-risk antenatal care.*)
- The gestation of the pregnancy (*how many weeks pregnant is the patient?*):
  - 1st trimester (1–13 weeks)
  - 2nd trimester (14–27 weeks)
  - 3rd trimester (28–40 weeks).
- If the patient does not know how many weeks pregnant she is, or is unsure, then use the estimated date of delivery (EDD) against the last menstrual period (LMP) to ascertain the gestation (*birth normally occurs within 15 days of the EDD, which equates to approximately 280 days from the first day of the patient's LMP*) (Marieb and Hoehn, 2014).
- Remember to look at the patient's hand-held notes (these will provide the paramedic with information regarding both the current and any previous pregnancies).

Previous medical history

Remember as with any secondary survey, the patient's previous medical history will provide evidence that may be relevant, especially with co-morbidity conditions, or if she has any medical problem that may be related to the reason why you are in attendance.

- Does the patient have hypertension? If so, is this pre-existing hypertension? (*hypertension occurring before the 13th week of gestation, a diastolic BP >110 mmHg would be deemed severe*).
- Is it pregnancy-induced hypertension (PIH)? (*raised BP which occurs after 20 weeks gestation, with the absence of proteinuria, it is usually mild, with readings normally 140/90*).
- Does the patient suffer from epilepsy? If so, has the patient remained compliant with medication?
- Is the patient diabetic? (*again is this pre-existing (type I or II) or gestational diabetes?*)
- Is the patient asthmatic? (*ascertain history of medication compliance and previous attacks*).

Past obstetric history

In other chapters this section of the secondary survey relates to 'past medical history', however, in relation to the obstetric patient, this is specific

Obstetric patient assessment

to their 'past obstetric history', therefore the paramedic will need to clarify and differentiate between 'gravity' and 'parity'. Gravity is the total number of pregnancies including the current, whereas parity relates to the number of live births (live or stillborn).

- How many previous pregnancies has the patient had?
- How many previous deliveries has the patient had?
- How were these delivered? (*naturally, or did she have a caesarean section?*)
- Did the patient have any problems in the previous pregnancies? (*bleeding, BP or pre-term delivery?*)

Previous caesarean section is an important risk factor as in labour it carries a 1 in 200 risk of uterine rupture, presenting as constant pain and bleeding.

History of current pregnancy

The information ascertained here is the history that relates to this particular pregnancy, and allows the paramedic the opportunity to elicit appropriate facts:

- How many weeks pregnant is the patient? Define which trimester the patient is in from this, and consider potential problems.
- Does the patient know her EDD? (*is she premature? or overdue?*)
- How many babies is she expecting? (*single, twins or multiple?*)
- Have there been any concerns with the baby? (*scans and ante-natal appointments, check notes for information and attendance*).
- Has the patient had any problems? (*pregnancy-induced hypertension, pre-eclampsia, gestational diabetes*).

History of current problem

The paramedic should use questions that are aimed at clarifying the patient's current problem. Consider the following structure to assist this format of questions: **L**abour, **P**ain, **D**ischarge, **B**leeding, **F**oetal, and **F**its.

Labour
- Is the labour at term (*after 3 weeks*) or preterm?
- At what stage of labour is the patient in? (*first, second or third stage?*)
- How many contractions are there in a 10-minute period? (*three or more contractions in 10 minutes is considered established labour*).
- Are there more than five contractions in a 10 minute period? (*if so, consider abruption*).
- Have the waters broken? If so, when? (*as prolonged rupture of membranes is associated with infection*).

Pain

Abdominal pain is a common complaint during pregnancy, most women suffer from it at some stage. Ascertain if it is physiologically normal (muscle stretching or indigestion), or is due to a severe pathological condition (appendicitis or an ectopic pregnancy) (Marshall and Raynor, 2014). Ascertain from the patient in the first instance the *location* of the pain, and then obtain a description of the pain, by using the SOCRATES framework (AACE, 2013):

> **S** – Site. Where exactly is the pain?
>
> **O** – Onset. What were they doing when the pain started? Ask the patient: When did the pain start? (was it rapid, over minutes or gradual, over hours?)
>
> **C** – Character. What does the pain feel like? Ask the patient to describe the pain:
>
> - Contractions – does the uterus go hard?
> - Is it constant?
> - Is it stabbing?
> - Does it come and go?
> - Is it like an ache?
>
> **R** – Radiate. Does the pain go anywhere else? Ask the patient if the pain moves anywhere, or if it stays in one place.
>
> **A** – Associated symptoms. Is it associated with any other symptoms? For example, nausea and/or vomiting
>
> **T** – Time/duration. How long have they had the pain? Is there any history of trauma it may be related to?
>
> **E** – Exacerbating/relieving factors. Does anything make the pain better or worse?
>
> **S** – Severity. Obtain an initial pain score (*0 = no pain, 10 = worst pain ever*).

Discharge

All women have some vaginal discharge or 'leucorrhoea' (normal discharge is clear, white or creamy and may smell musky but not unpleasant), which normally starts a year or two before puberty and ends after the menopause, and is usually quite harmless. It is quite common for this to increase during pregnancy. In the final weeks of pregnancy the discharge may contain streaks of thick mucus and some blood. This is called a 'show' and happens when the cervical plug (a 'ball' of thick mucus that fills the cervix during pregnancy) comes away. This is a sign that the body is starting to prepare for birth, and the patient may have already had a few small 'shows'. The paramedic should ascertain from the patient if the discharge is normal or has changed,

Obstetric patient assessment

and consider asking the patient about the colour, odour, consistency and quantity of the discharge:

- Colour – ascertain if the discharge is:
  - Clear and odourless
  - Clear and smells of urine
  - Green
  - Yellow
  - Pink
  - Red
- Odour – does the leucorrhoea have an offensive smell?
- Consistency – ascertain if the discharge is:
  - Watery
  - Thick
  - Frothy
  - Jelly-like
- Quantity – ask the patient to clarify if the discharge is:
  - A trickle
  - Gushing
  - Still draining.

Bleeding

While approximately 1 in 10 women experience some bleeding during pregnancy, it is usually a terrifying ordeal at the time for those involved (patient and partner alike). It does not necessarily mean a miscarriage will occur. In early pregnancy the patient may have some light bleeding, called *spotting*, when the foetus implants itself into the wall of the uterus. It is also known as *implantation bleeding* and normally occurs at the time when the patient's first period (post-conception) would have been due. In the first three months of pregnancy, vaginal bleeding may be a sign of miscarriage or ectopic pregnancy, whereas in the later stages of pregnancy, vaginal bleeding may be due to different causes. However, bleeding at any stage of the pregnancy from the genital tract is abnormal and needs to be appropriately assessed by a doctor, irrespective of the amount (Stables and Rankin, 2010).

Ascertain the following information from the patient:

- When did it start?
- How much blood is/was there?
  - Noticed it when wiping self after going to toilet
  - Teaspoon (approximately 5 ml)
  - Soaked pants/trousers
  - Sanitary towel(s) (ascertain how many)
  - Visible on legs.

- Ask the patient if she is still bleeding.
- Ask the patient if there were any clots in the blood (size and quantity).
- Ask the patient if there is any mucus mixed in the blood.

Foetal movements

The first movement of the foetus, also known as *quickening*, usually occurs at 20 weeks in a first pregnancy, with the average time of occurrence being between 16 and 20 plus weeks (Marshall and Raynor, 2014). By week 28, the patient can expect to feel foetal activity every day, this continues throughout the third trimester.

It is crucial to note changes in activity, and any sudden decreases in movements should be addressed accordingly. Ascertain the following from the patient:

- If the baby is moving normally (*after 28 weeks/7 months, 10 movements of any kind in one hour or less are normal*).
- The patient may not feel foetal movement if she is contracting.
- If the baby is moving less.
- When was the last time she felt the baby move?
- If there is no foetal movement, and the patient is presenting with severe pain (*with or without haemorrhage – treat as a placental abruption*).
- Remember 'dead' babies move (*an external movement may cause the baby to move against the uterine wall, and be interpreted as movement*).

Fitting

The paramedic should remember that fitting may occur due to complications of the pregnancy – pre-eclampsia (hypertension and associated proteinuria occurring after 20 weeks gestation) and eclampsia (tonic-clonic, grand mal seizure: associated with signs and symptoms of pre-eclampsia). The incidence of eclampsia in the UK is around 1/2000 pregnancies (Newson, 2012). Epilepsy affects 1 in 200 of all pregnant women (Stables and Rankin, 2010). Ascertain the following information from the patient, partner or bystanders:

- Does the patient have epilepsy? If so, how is this controlled? (NICE, 2012).
  - Valproate (epilim)
  - Lamotrigine
  - Keppra
  - Carbamazepine, oxcarbazepine or others.
- Does the patient have any previous history of fits? When and why did they occur?
- Was the fit witnessed? If so, ask the witness:
  - If there were any tonic-clonic movements
  - How long they lasted.

- Has the patient suffered any associated problems (incontinence, biting tongue/lips)?
- Check the patient's hand-held notes (ascertain any problems with blood pressure, pregnancy-induced hypertension (PIH), pre-eclampsia or eclampsia).

Evaluating the history

On completing the history, the paramedic should evaluate the key components and use the findings of the examination to assist in making a diagnosis. Consideration should be given to the following:

- Did the history identify any risk factors? Such as:
    - previous caesarean section (*increases the risk of uterine rupture*)
    - breech presentation in the transverse lie position (*higher risk of prolapse cord*)
    - twin pregnancy (*increased risk of all obstetric emergencies*).
- Assess and evaluate the severity of symptoms:
    - Systolic blood pressure >160 mmHg or over (*requires further urgent medical assessment*)
    - Hypertension (*increases risk of abruption*)
    - Severe pain
    - Bleeding.

Use all of the information obtained during the secondary survey and the findings of the examination to confirm your diagnosis. If appropriate, pre-alert the obstetric unit.

HANDOVER OF THE OBSTETRIC PATIENT

At some opportune moment, the paramedic will be required to 'hand over' their patient to another health care professional. It should be structured to ensure that important information regarding the patient is not omitted. The initial stage of a handover may have already occurred with a pre-alert communication being forwarded to the maternity/obstetric receiving unit. For the obstetric patient, this should include the following:

- Age
- Signs and symptoms, follow the ABCDEFG framework, include relevant findings (*onset of labour, contractions, SROM, omit categories with atypical findings*)
- History of the current problem
- History of the current pregnancy (*what is the expected date of delivery (EDD), gravidity, number of pregnancies, parity, number of birth events, or any problems identified*)

- Interventions (*describe any management provided, location of IV/IO sites and doses of drugs*)
- Estimated time of arrival (ETA) for those patients with a pre-alert communication.

OTHER CONSIDERATIONS

Communication

Not only does the problem of communicating with patients of different dialects occur to the paramedic (English not being the first language). The paramedic in the worst case scenario may also have to deal with the situation where the baby is born with an unexpected disability, such as cleft lip or clubfoot. In these situations clear, effective and honest communication is considered crucial.

Destination/receiving specialist units/non-conveyance

Depending on the circumstances of the call and the findings of the primary and secondary surveys, the obstetric patient may not even be required to be conveyed. However, if the patient has an obstetric risk factor, then the receiving unit may need to be an obstetric unit. Alternatively the paramedic may need to convey the patient to an emergency department due to the dyspnoea associated with life-threatening asthma.

Social/family/carer

Childbirth in the twentieth century has been transformed from a social, domestic experience into a highly technological medical system. However, evidence clearly shows that there is a link between adverse pregnancy outcomes and vulnerability and social exclusion (CMACE, 2011). Certain groups of patients may be particularly disadvantaged, including women who are asylum seekers, from travelling communities, from black and ethnic minority groups or who have a disability (Marshall and Raynor, 2014). Support from the family network for the new mother may include partner/husband, parents, grandparents etc., while the very young single mother may well have to deal with childbirth entirely alone.

Ethical and legal

As with any patient, the paramedic has a 'duty of care' to their patients, and with obstetric incidents there is the added problem of cultural, religious and gender issues that may affect the ability of conducting a physical examination. Always ask for consent and explain clearly to the patient the need to perform an inspection (document and record this in your notes), maintain the patient's dignity and respect their right to refuse consent.

Obstetric patient assessment

CHAPTER KEY POINTS

- Fully assess each area of the primary survey: DR 'C' ABCDEFG.
- Ensure consent is obtained appropriate to the situation, and is recorded.
- Identify time critical problems within the primary survey.
- Manage time critical problems as they are found, pre-alert the receiving unit.
- Undertake a secondary survey, and evaluate the risks and severity of symptoms.
- Consider cultural, religious and gender issues.
- Provide a structured handover of the patient to other health care professionals.

REFERENCES

American Academy of Orthopaedic Surgeons (AAOS) (2011) *ALS Skills Review*. Burlington, VA: Jones and Bartlett Learning. (DVD).

Association of Ambulance Chief Executives (2013) *UK Ambulance Services Clinical Practice Guidelines 2013 Pocket Book: Pain Assessment Model*. Bridgwater: Class Professional Publishing.

British Thoracic Society (2015) *Emergency Oxygen Use in Adult Patients Guideline*. Available at: https://www.brit-thoracic.org.uk/searchresults/?txtSearch=2015+Oxygen+Guidelines&search= (accessed. 27 Feburary 2015).

CMACE (Centre for Maternal and Child Enquiries) (2011) *Saving Mothers' Lives: Reviewing Maternal Deaths to Make Motherhood Safer: 2006–08*. The Eighth Report on Confidential Enquiries into Maternal Deaths in the United Kingdom. BJOG 2011;118 (Suppl. 1): 1–203.

Department of Health (2009) *Reference Guide to Consent for Examination or Treatment* (2nd edn). London: Department of Health.

Marieb, E.N. and Hoehn, M.D. (2014) *Human Anatomy & Physiology* (9th edn). Harlow. Pearson Education Limited.

Marshall, J. and Raynor, M. (2014) *Myles Textbook for Midwives* (16th edn). Edinburgh: Churchill Livingstone Elsevier.

NAEMT (National Association of Emergency Medical Technicians) (2011) *Advanced Medical Life Support: An Assessment-Based Approach*. St. Louis, MO: Elsevier Mosby.

Newson, L. (2012) Pre-eclampsia and eclampsia. Available at: http://www.patient.co.uk/doctor/Pre-eclampsia-and-Eclampsia (accessed 1 March 2015).

NICE (National Institute for Health and Care Excellence) (2012) *The Epilepsies: The Diagnosis and Management of the Epilepsies in Adults and Children in Primary and Secondary Care*. Available at. https://www.nice.org.uk/guidance/cg137 (accessed 1 March 2015).

NICE (National Institute for Health and Care Excellence) (2015a) *Hypertension in Pregnancy: Pre-Eclampsia*. NICE Guideline. Available at: http://pathways.nice.org.uk/pathways/hypertension-in-pregnancy#path=view%3A/pathways/hypertension-in-pregnancy/pre-eclampsia.xml&content=view-index (accessed 27 February 2015).

NICE (National Institute for Health and Care Excellence) (2015b) *Diabetes in Pregnancy. Management of Diabetes and its Complications from Preconception to the Postnatal Period*. Available at: https://www.nice.org.uk/guidance/ng3 (accessed 27 February 2015).

Resuscitation Council (UK) (2011) *Advanced Life Support* (6th edn). London: Resuscitation Council (UK).

Salomone, J.P. and Pons, P.T. (2014) *Pre-Hospital Trauma Life Support (PHTLS)* (8th edn). Maryland Heights, MO: Mosby Elsevier.

Stables, D. and Rankin, J. (2010) *Physiology in Childbearing: With Anatomy and Related Biosciences* (3rd edn). Edinburgh: Bailliere Tindall, Elsevier.

Woollard, M., Hinshaw, K., Simpson, H. and Wieteska, S. (2010) *Pre-hospital Obstetric Emergency Training: The Practical Approach*. Advanced Life Support Group. Oxford: Wiley-Blackwell.

14 Assessment and care of the newborn
Nandiran Ratnavel

In 2013, there were a total of 778,805 births in the UK (ONS, 2014). Most of these deliveries occurred in hospital. A small number of babies are born as planned home deliveries, a smaller proportion are delivered as unplanned home births. A rather more hazardous situation is the unplanned delivery of a baby in a public place. Recent evidence suggests that unplanned births out of hospital increase the risk of infant mortality (Gunnarsson et al., 2014). This chapter deals with the assessment of the newborn baby and the immediate pre-hospital assessment/management of the newborn baby requiring resuscitation and subsequent transfer to hospital.

SCENE ASSESSMENT

It is important for the paramedic to be aware that attending a delivery potentially involves looking after a minimum of two patients: mother and baby. To that end it may be normal practice for two crews to be dispatched to such events. It may be that a community midwife is in attendance and has called for emergency services for transfer into hospital. Alternatively it may be the case that the paramedic is first to arrive on the scene and is subsequently joined by the midwife. It is recommended that the paramedic take guidance from the birth specialist if they are present.

Actions will be determined depending on whether the baby has delivered or not. If not yet born and a midwife is not in attendance, it may be necessary for the crew to deliver the baby if there is no opportunity to transfer the mother into hospital first. Following delivery, if the baby is well and needs no interventions, the baby can be placed directly onto the mother's chest for skin-to-skin contact and be covered with a blanket. This maintains warmth to the baby, encourages bonding and facilitates breast feeding. The umbilical cord can be clamped and cut after a minute or so. If the infant has already delivered, it is important to make sure that mother and baby are at the same horizontal level so as to avoid feto-maternal or materno-fetal transfusion until the umbilical cord is clamped and cut. Any visible blood at the scene may indicate acute blood loss from either mother or baby.

> **Possible actions to be taken:**
> - If baby has not delivered and birth is imminent, then
>   - Request midwife and second vehicle via control (*if appropriate*)
>   - Prepare for delivery using Maternity and Paediatric Advanced Life Support (PALS) packs
> - If baby is delivered:
>   - Ensure mother and baby are at same horizontal level until cord is clamped and cut
>   - Note the amount of visible blood and ascertain if from mother or baby.

PRIMARY SURVEY

The generic process of conducting the primary survey needs to be modified to a more appropriate approach in accordance with the circumstances surrounding the birth of the baby.

DANGER

Circumstances surrounding the delivery of a baby are not usually hazardous to the paramedic, however, the presence of body fluids mean the paramedic should wear the appropriate personal protective equipment (PPE). Clamping and cutting the cord will require the paramedic to be exposed to these fluids. Newborn babies are extremely susceptible to body temperature loss; to that end it may be necessary to close any windows and doors, as well as increase the environmental temperature if it is possible to do so. In the out-of-hospital setting this will usually occur in a domestic environment although this is not always the case. The newborn baby's size means that it has a relatively large surface area to body weight ratio. For this reason heat loss by convection and radiation will be high. The baby will also be wet which means that heat loss via evaporation will be significant. An unexpected delivery outside of hospital will almost certainly be associated with hypothermia as it is far more difficult to control the environmental temperature. It is well recognized that hypothermic babies have significantly increased morbidity and mortality rates compared to normo-thermic babies (Branco de Almeida, 2014). Thermal stress is exacerbated even further in those who are premature.

With regard to management of the umbilical cord after delivery of the baby, there are currently two approaches:

- *Approach 1: Clamping and cutting the cord* gives the paramedic a clear time point from which adaptation to post-natal life is required and at the beginning of which effective resuscitation must be commenced (if indicated).

This prevents siphoning of blood between the placenta and the infant. There is some evidence to suggest that delayed clamping of the umbilical cord can lead to polycythaemia in the infant if excessive blood passes from mother to baby. Complications associated with hyperviscosity syndrome may then ensue.

- *Approach 2: Not clamping the cord* prior to commencing resuscitation centres around allowing the baby to receive whatever residual support from the maternal circulation there may be for as long a time as there is blood flowing from the placenta to the baby. This is particularly reasonable if the baby is well at birth and does not require active resuscitation.

The converse problem of anaemia in the baby can arise from delayed cord clamping due to flow of blood in the opposite direction.

There is of course the practical problem of attending to mother and baby as separate patients while they are still physically connected.

Possible actions to be taken:
- Ensure that gloves and PPE are worn
- Clamp and cut the cord (*as appropriate to situation*)
- Close windows and doors and increase environmental temperature.

RESPONSE: INITIAL ASSESSMENT AT BIRTH

Following initial introductions and assessment it is vital for the paramedic to establish if any urgent interventions are necessary before ascertaining a complete history. The clinical assessment of the newborn baby immediately after birth allows the paramedic a quick and informative overview that will direct subsequent resuscitative actions (*if required*). The continuing assessment of the newborn will be dependent on the following criteria at birth:

- What is the gestation? Knowing the gestation of the baby will be very helpful both in adjusting the style of respiratory support offered (*if this is needed*) as well as appreciating the higher rates of heat loss

experienced by premature babies. If the mother is unsure, then estimate it, based on the first day of her last menstrual period (LMP), particularly if a dating scan was not performed in the first trimester of the pregnancy.
- Is the amniotic fluid clear? (*if there was meconium present in the amniotic fluid and a greenish tinge to the baby's skin or fingernails, this may indicate foetal distress during labour and the possibility of meconium aspiration syndrome in the newborn*).
- Is the baby breathing or crying?
- Does the baby have good muscle tone?

If the answer to these questions is yes, then routine care should be provided (Resuscitation Council (UK), 2010). To that end, make a note of the time.

Possible actions to be taken:
- Provide warmth
- Dry and wrap the newborn (see Figure 14.1)
- Clear airway if necessary
- Assess colour.

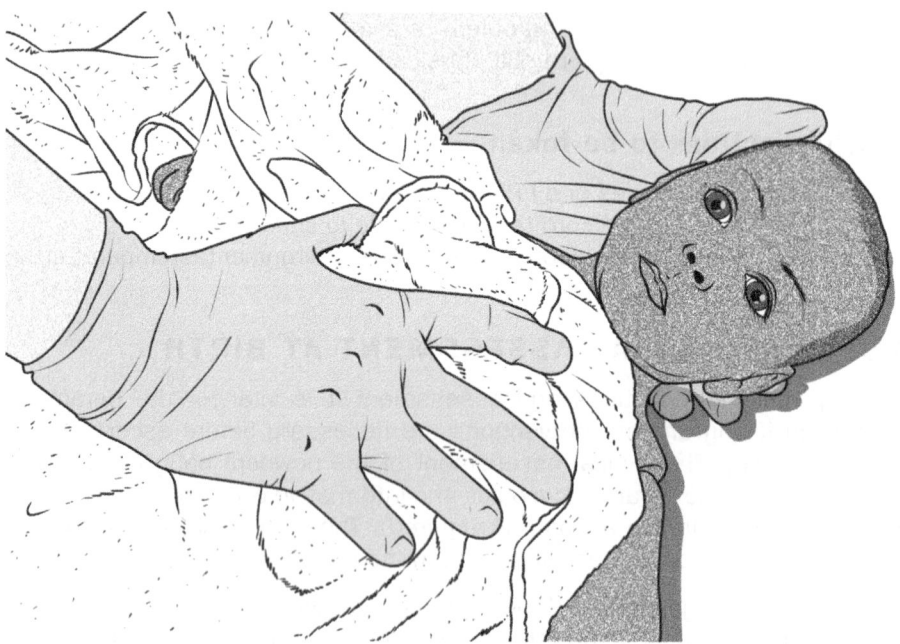

Figure 14.1 Drying a newborn baby

Assessment and care of the newborn

> **Possible actions to be taken:**
> - Dry the baby off thoroughly with a warm dry towel
> - Having done this, discard the wet towel and wrap the newborn up with a new warm dry towel. This will require opening two maternity packs or using domestic towels if in someone's home.

It is important to cover the extremities and the head, which is a source of major heat loss. A small triangle of chest may be left exposed in order to assess respiratory effort, chest movement and to listen to the heart rate with a stethoscope. While undertaking the drying and wrapping process, the paramedic should simultaneously assess and evaluate the following parameters of the newborn: colour, muscle tone, breathing and heart rate.

Colour

Pink	Implies delivery of oxygenated blood to the skin and vital organs
Blue	Implies delivery of deoxygenated blood to the skin and vital organs
White	Implies reduced blood supply to the skin and vital organs

Muscle tone

Normal	Vigorous infant
Abnormal	Some tone but reduced
Absent	Completely floppy and lifeless

Breathing

Normal	Crying infant with regular respirations
Abnormal	Shallow, irregular respirations or gasping
None	No respiratory effort at all

Heart rate

Fast	Above 100 beats per minute
Slow	Between 60 and 100 beats per minute
Very slow	Less than 60 beats per minute
Absent	No audible heart rate

The heart rate should be estimated rather than actually counted so as not to lose time. The paramedic will more often than not estimate within the correct category and act accordingly with the appropriate action. The most accurate method is ascertained by listening to the left side of the praecordium with a stethoscope. It is difficult in the compromised neonate to palpate the brachial, femoral or carotid pulses, particularly in an emergency situation. Experienced midwives may be used to feeling the newborn baby pulse by palpating the base of the umbilical cord, but most paramedics will not have this level of expertise. However, not all cardiac pulsations are transmitted to the cord and particularly if the umbilical vessels have gone into spasm, these pulsations may not be felt, leading to inaccuracies in heart rate estimation.

After completing the assessment evaluations, the newborn baby will fall into one of the following categories:

Pink, vigorous, crying, heart rate >100 bpm

- Keep warm. Raise environmental temperature, if feasible.
- Remain wrapped in dry towels, or skin-to-skin with mother.
- Take lead from birthing specialist. If no midwife present, await arrival while maintaining normothermia.

Blue, reduced or absent tone, irregular or absent breathing, heart rate <100 bpm

- The stimulation produced during the process of drying is usually sufficient to induce effective breathing.
- If not, then place the head into the neutral position (see Figures 14.2, 14.3).

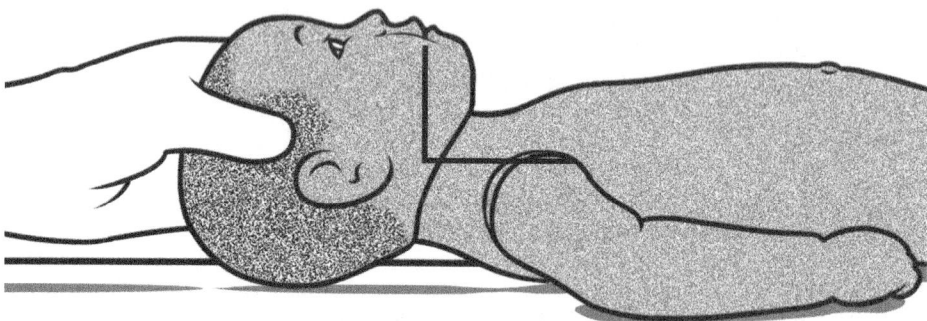

Figure 14.2   Correct neutral head position

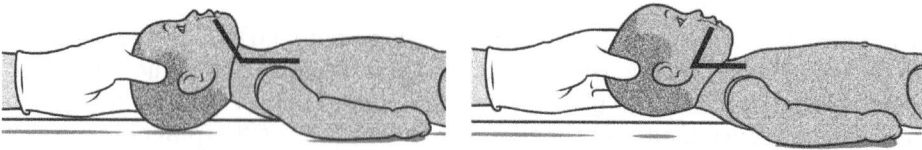

Figure 14.3   Incorrect neutral head positions

The face should be kept horizontal. This position differs from that in children or adults. Avoid hyper-extending or flexing the neck. Either of these positions can result in airway occlusion in a baby due to the shorter and more compressible trachea.

- Open the airway.
- Assess and ascertain if the baby responds. If so, no further resuscitation is needed other than keeping the baby warm.
- If there is no response, then proceed to aerate the baby's lungs (see Breathing).

Blue or pale, reduced or absent tone, irregular or absent breathing, heart rate slow <60 bpm or absent

- Apnoeic babies require resuscitation.
- Place the head into the neutral position.
- Open the airway and aerate the lungs (see Breathing).
- Reassess and ascertain if there is a heart rate response.
- If none, then implement circulatory resuscitation accordingly.
- Reassess heart rate and respiration every 30 seconds.

These depend on the newborn baby's condition at the initial assessment following the drying and wrapping process.

Possible actions to be taken:

- Following assessment implement resuscitation measures accordingly (Newborn Life Support (NLS))
- Airway
- Breathing
- Circulation
- Drugs (*consider adrenaline*) (Resuscitation Council (UK), 2010).

AIRWAY

The appropriate position to achieve an open airway is neutral alignment. The prominent occiput of the baby means that the baby will tend to adopt a flexed position to the neck when lying supine. Equally, extension of the neck will also have a tendency to occlude the airway owing to the newborn's anatomy and the relatively collapsible nature of the trachea. Paramedics may find it useful to place a folded towel under the baby's neck and shoulders to assist in maintaining the airway in a neutral position (Woollard et al., 2010).

> **Possible actions to be taken:**
> - Place the baby supine on a flat surface, with a folded towel beneath the baby's neck and shoulders
> - Position the head in neutral position
> - Open the airway (*if the baby is floppy, consider applying chin lift*)
> - Inspect the oral cavity
> - Do not attempt blind finger sweeps.

BREATHING

The purpose of the initial five breaths is to provide aeration. This is due to the lungs initially being full of fluid. By giving these slow, sustained breaths, the majority of the fluid in the lungs will be driven into the lymphatic system and the alveoli will be inflated and readied for gas exchange with the lung capillaries. These should last 2 to 3 seconds each. The aim of these is to inflate the lungs and establish a resting lung volume. It is imperative to visualize the chest to look for chest rise. The aim is to achieve this by the fifth breath. It is not unusual for the initial one or two attempts to fail to give rise to chest expansion. These can be administered with the infant mask carried in the standard paediatric bag which is suitable for the full-term baby. It should be sized to cover the nose and mouth without pressing on the eyes or overlapping the chin and sufficient pressure applied to provide a good seal. Having done this it should be connected to a bag-valve system, which should have a 500 ml capacity or more to allow for delivery of a 2- or 3-second inflation breath.

The entire capacity of the bag may not need to be used. Smaller bags may not contain the necessary volume to achieve this. Attach the face mask to the bag-valve device away from the baby's face. Check the pressure release valve is working on the bag-valve device. The bag-valve – mask apparatus can be connected to a source of supplemental oxygen but there should be no delay incurred in doing this because achieving lung inflation is far more important than the concentration of inspired oxygen. A newborn baby can be effectively resuscitated with room air. Apply the system over the baby's nose and mouth and give five inflation breaths. The paramedic should simultaneously check for rise of the chest to assess effectiveness. The baby should then be reassessed in terms of colour, tone, breathing and heart rate.

Possible actions to be taken:

- Size mask and attach to 500 ml bag-valve device
- Attach supplemental oxygen if available (*do not delay resuscitation if not available*)
- Administer five aerating 'inflation breaths', each of 2–3 seconds duration
- Check for chest rise (*remember the initial 1–2 breaths may fail to expand the chest*)
- Reassess heart rate and action accordingly.

If chest rise has been seen and the heart rate responds lung inflation has been successful. If the baby's colour becomes pink, the tone improves, the infant starts to cry or breathe regularly and the heart rate remains fast, he/she must be kept warm. Liaise with the midwife/control regarding transferring the baby into hospital while constant reassessment continues.

Should the baby fail to commence spontaneous breathing

If the baby's colour becomes pink, the tone improves, the heart rate increases but the baby fails to establish regular, effective respirations, then ventilation breaths should be administered until he/she is breathing regularly. Reassessment should be performed every 30 seconds to establish whether this has occurred. Ventilation breaths should last 1–2 seconds, a resting lung volume having already been established. The purpose is to maintain continuous alveolar ventilation thus facilitating gas exchange.

The paramedic should ensure that the chest is rising and falling with the assisted ventilation. If the heart rate increases, one can assume that gas has entered the lungs.

Possible actions to be taken:

- Continue to administer regular breaths at a rate of 30–40 per minute (Resuscitation Council (UK), 2010)
- Reassess every 30 seconds.

If the chest does not rise and the heart rate does not improve

NB: If the mother has received morphine or any other opiate during the past four hours and the newborn is not breathing adequately, then administer naloxone intramuscularly and maintain respiratory support (Fisher et al., 2013).

- *Naloxone:* 400 micrograms/1 ml. Initial dose 200 micrograms. Single dose only (AACE, 2013).
- Paramedics must assume that the lungs have not been inflated and an alternative airway manoeuvre must be employed.
- Re-aligning the airway and checking that the neutral position is being maintained may be an appropriate first step with a view to trying the inflation breaths again. If this does not work, then applying jaw thrust, either as a single or two-person manoeuvre is often effective. There are three major tasks to be achieved while performing the jaw thrust:
    - Maintain neutral alignment of the airway (see Figure 14.2).
    - Ensure a good seal of the mask edge over the baby's mouth and nose (see Figure 14.4).
    - Bring the mandible forward.
- When performing the single person manoeuvre, the mask is held around the firm stem between thumb and index finger such that equal pressure is applied to the face all around the mask edge. This prevents deformation of the soft part of the mask and maintains a good seal. The ring finger can be used to bring the mandible forward by applying pressure along the line of the jaw just proximal to the angle of the mandible. The palm of the same hand can be rested gently on the baby's forehead to keep the airway in a neutral position and to prevent flexion or hypertension of the neck.
- In the two-person manoeuvre the mask can be held onto the face by holding the stem of the mask with the thumb and index fingers of each hand on either side with ring fingers on each side providing the jaw thrust and the palms of the hands keeping the neutral position. If the paramedic's hands are small, then the mask can be held on by both thumbs placed over the soft part of the mask on each side while the jaw thrust is achieved with the third finger on each side.
- Insertion of an appropriately sized oropharyngeal airway under direct vision may help to open the airway. Such airways come in different sizes and it is vital that the paramedic correctly sizes the airway prior to insertion. This is done by aligning one end with the angle of the mandible and the other with the middle of the lower lip. The airway that most closely spans these two landmarks is the one that should be used. Insertion should never be performed blind and should always be done under direct vision. This minimizes the risk of the tongue or foreign material being lodged further down the airway. Insertion is carried out with the convex surface of the airway

Assessment and care of the newborn

adjacent to the palate throughout the process. There is no twisting of the airway through 180 degrees as in adult insertion. Direct vision can be achieved using a laryngoscope or a tongue depressor or little finger along with a pen torch. The latter may need a second person to assist. At the time of inspection of the oropharynx, if any physical obstruction of the airway is seen, e.g. a blood clot, vernix or meconium, then suction can be applied using a wide bore catheter and low setting suction.
- Five further inflation breaths can then be administered followed by a reassessment of the baby's colour, tone, breathing and heart rate.

Possible actions to be taken:

- Realign the airway and ensure the head is in the neutral position
- Apply a jaw thrust (*ensure effective seal, neutral alignment and bring mandible forward*)
- Ensure that the aspirator is set to the lowest setting
- Remove visible obstructions/secretions using suction under direct vision
- Insert correctly sized oropharyngeal airway under direct vision
- Administer five further 'inflation breaths', each of 2–3 seconds duration
- Check for chest rise (*remember the initial 1–2 breaths may fail to expand the chest*)
- Reassess heart rate and action accordingly.

If the heart rate remains slow <60 bpm or absent despite good chest movement during the 5 inflation breaths, commence chest compression.

CIRCULATION

If there has been chest movement, then it is likely that the myocardium has become compromised due to hypoxia and needs help to start. This help is provided by giving chest compressions in combination with ventilation breaths at a ratio of three compressions to one ventilation (*3:1 ratio*). The purpose of the chest compressions is to push oxygenated blood from the lungs forward to the heart to perfuse the oxygen-starved myocardium via the coronary arteries. The coronary arteries are branches of the ascending aorta and are perfused during diastole. The relaxation phase of the chest compressions is therefore equally important. The encircling technique is the most efficient method of chest compression on a baby.

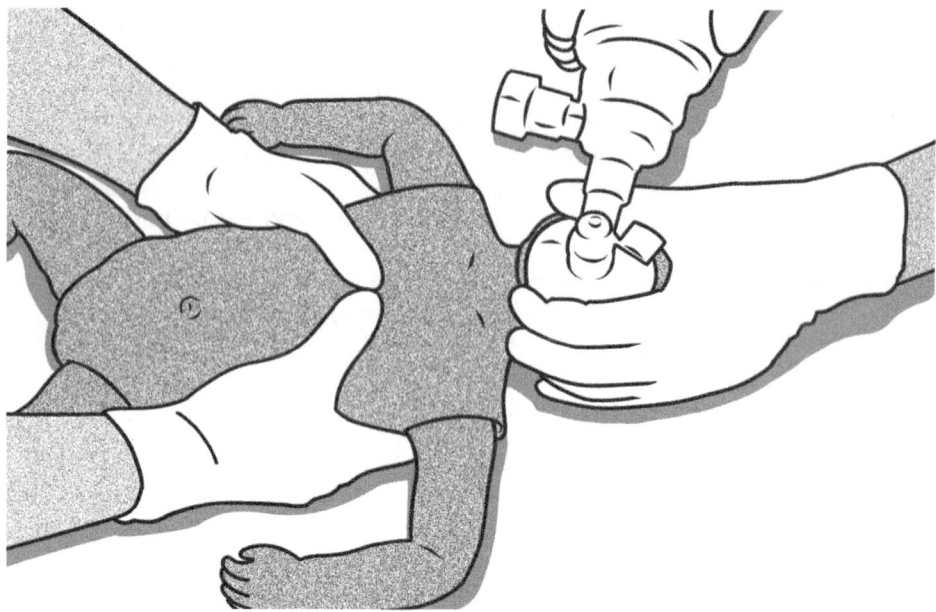

Figure 14.4 Compression technique to be used on a neonate

Chest compression technique (see Figure 14.4):

- The preferred method is to encircle the chest with both hands and press on the sternum with both thumbs.
- The thumbs can be placed either side by side or on top of one another.
- The point of application of pressure for the compressions should be on the lower third of the sternum, just below an imaginary line joining the nipples (Richmond, 2006).

Sufficient pressure should be applied to compress the sternum to one third of the depth of the chest. The speed with which this sequence should be carried out is to achieve a rate of 120 events per minute (i.e. 90 compressions to 30 ventilations per minute). This should actually be carried out for 30 seconds following which the baby should be reassessed. This will therefore allow time for 45 compressions and 15 ventilations to be delivered.

Possible actions to be taken:

- Only commence chest compressions when the lungs have been aerated successfully
- Grip the baby's chest in both hands, position thumbs on sternum and ensure fingers support the spine

Assessment and care of the newborn

- Compress the chest and ventilate the lungs at a ratio of 3:1
- Reassess after 30 seconds
- Once the heart rate is >60 bpm and increasing, then chest compressions can be stopped. Continue ventilation breaths if not breathing.
- Consider drugs if the heart rate does not respond despite effective inflation of the lungs and effective chest compressions.

DRUGS

These are usually unnecessary in the pre-hospital scenario, because effective management of the airway, breathing and circulation is usually sufficient to resuscitate the newborn baby. However, if there is no significant improvement of the baby's cardiac output despite effective lung inflation and chest compressions, then the following drugs are needed:

- Adrenaline 1:10,000
- Dextrose 10%
- Sodium bicarbonate 4.2%.

The doses are weight dependent and are ideally administered centrally via either an umbilical venous catheter or an infant intra-osseous needle. Paramedics will be proficient in the latter. Recommended doses are:

- *Adrenaline:* 10 microgram/kg (0.1 ml/kg, 1:10,000). If ineffective, then a dose of up to 30 microgram/kg (0.3 ml/kg, 1:10,000) may be administered on repeat after 5 minutes.
- *Sodium bicarbonate:* 1–2 mmol/kg (2–4 ml/kg, 4.2% bicarbonate solution). (This drug is not routinely available to paramedics in the pre-hospital environment and needs to be administered intravenously.)
- *Dextrose:* 250 ml/kg (2.5 ml/kg, 10% dextrose). Energy in the form of glucose may be depleted during a prolonged resuscitation.
- *Saline 0.9%:* On rare occasions the heart rate may not be able to increase due to loss of blood volume. On such occasions the use of an isotonic crystalloid for emergency volume replacement is preferred. 10 ml/kg of 0.9% saline bolus administered over 10–20 seconds (may be safely repeated if required after 5 minutes).

Possible actions to be taken:

- Obtain intra-osseous access and administer drugs accordingly
- Consider hypovolaemia
- Consider when to move to hospital
- Notify receiving unit via control with appropriate history/information.

OTHER CONSIDERATIONS

Premature babies

Fortunately, the same principles apply to the resuscitation of pre-term infants as to full-term babies. The important additional considerations are that both inflation and ventilation breaths may need to be done more gently. However, it is vital that the chest is seen to move with these insufflations. Second, thermal control is even more important. The premature baby's skin is often thin with a reduced epidermal layer and less subcutaneous fat. The practice of delivering babies at 28 weeks gestation or less into plastic bags is only indicated if they are simultaneously placed under a radiant heat source which is not usually available outside of hospital. Therefore for premature babies who are born outside of hospitals they should be dried off and wrapped in a fresh towel, as described above for the full-term infant.

Departure to hospital

Most neonates will respond to simple measures during resuscitation at birth. It is important to institute these promptly and effectively on scene rather than simply transfer a compromised baby into hospital without the proper initial actions. Unnecessary hypoxic injury can then be avoided which may not have been sustained if the correct manoeuvres were employed in the first place. It is, however, also important to recognize the window to move the patient. If regular spontaneous respirations and a fast heart rate have been found on reassessment, then the baby can be transferred with close monitoring. If the baby's condition has improved but not to normality, then another cycle of resuscitation appropriate to the infant's current condition can be employed followed by the reassessment. If the baby's condition is approaching normality, then he/she can be transferred. If the clinical condition remains the same or is worsening despite effective technical manoeuvres, then this plateau phase should be recognized and the patient moved into hospital without further delay. Whatever the level of resuscitation, this should be continued until arrival and handover in the hospital setting. A decision will need to be made regarding transfer of the mother into hospital either with the baby if he/she has stabilized or separately if ongoing resuscitation of either patient is necessary. Once the baby is in hospital an experienced paediatrician or neonatologist can make the decision to discontinue resuscitation armed with the appropriate facts and background if the baby shows no response to good quality ongoing resuscitation in the hospital setting.

Calling ahead via ambulance control to the local accident and emergency department or labour ward to inform them of the imminent arrival of a potentially critically unwell baby will allow the appropriate staff (i.e. paediatrician or

Assessment and care of the newborn

neonatologist and neonatal nurse) to attend the baby on arrival at the hospital as well as the accident and emergency staff.

Apgar score

Four of the clinical parameters assessed above during the resuscitation are also found in the Apgar score (see Table 14.1). This score was devised to evaluate a newborn baby's adaptation to extra-uterine life. It was created by Virginia Apgar, Professor of Anaesthetics at Columbia University, USA, in 1949. While a useful tool in describing a baby's condition shortly after birth, it is best used as a retrospective scoring system rather than being used to guide the resuscitation.

Table 14.1 Apgar scoring

Sign	Score 0	Score 1	Score 2
Heart rate	Absent	<100 per minute	>100 per minute
Breathing	Absent	Weak cry or hypoventilation	Good
Colour	Pale/blue	Body pink, limbs blue	Pink
Tone	Limp	Some flexion	Normal
Reflex response	None/nil	Some movement	Cries

Communication

Remember that the birth of a child is an important event for parents, and in situations involving the resuscitation of the newborn, this can be an extremely anxious time for them; paramedics should be objective with the information they give regarding possible outcomes. In situations where communication with the parents is a problem, the paramedic should request an interpreter via language line; remember the use of friends or relatives as an interpreter is considered poor practice (Richmond, 2006).

Handover of the patient in the accident and emergency department or on the labour ward of the local hospital is very important. A succinct description of the time of birth and condition of the baby as well as details of the resuscitation will be key to ongoing management. The timing of the infant's responses to resuscitation and the retrospective Apgar scores applied will help to guide the subsequent management of the baby. It will also help the paediatrician in making later decisions regarding prognosis which will of course be central to any discussions with the parents. A **S**ituation **B**ackground **A**ssessment **R**ecommendations (SBAR) format can be used for this transfer of crucial information (NHS, 2008).

CHAPTER KEY POINTS

- Control the environmental temperature.
- Minimize heat loss by drying the baby off and wrapping in a fresh dry towel.
- Most babies will respond well to basic manoeuvres performed effectively.
- Reassess the baby's condition at intervals described above.
- Decide on the opportune time to move the patient into hospital.
- Communicate with parents, control and other health care professionals.
- Give a good quality handover that accurately describes the timeline of events, particularly treatments given and the baby's response to these.

REFERENCES

Association of Ambulance Chief Executives (2013) *UK Ambulance Services Clinical Practice Guidelines 2013 Pocket Book: Naloxone*. Bridgwater: Class Professional Publishing.

Branco de Almeida, M.F., Guinsburg, R., Sancho, G.A., Rosa, I.R.M., Lamy, Z.C., Martinez, F.E. et al. (2014) Hypothermia and early neonatal mortality in preterm infants. *The Journal of Pediatrics* 164(2): 271–5. Available at: http://www.sciencedirect.com/science/article/pii/S0022347613012201 (accessed 19 May 2015).

Fisher, J., Brown, S.N. and Cooke, M. (eds) (2013) *UK Ambulance Services Clinical Practice Guidelines 2013: Newborn Life Support*. Bridgwater: Class Professional Publishing.

Gunnarsson, B., Smàrason, A.K., Skogvoll, E. and Fasting, S. (2014) Unplanned births out of hospital increases risk of infant mortality. *Acta Obstetricia et Gynecologica Scandinavica*. Available at: http://medicalxpress.com/news/2014-09-unplanned-births-out-of-hospital-infant-mortality.html (accessed 19 May 2015).

National Health Service (NHS) Institute for Innovation and Improvement (2008) *Quality and Service Improvement Tools: SBAR Situation-Background-Assessment-Recommendation*. http://www.institute.nhs.uk/quality_and_service_improvement_tools/quality (accessed 25 June 2015).

ONS (Office for National Statistics) (2014) *Births in England and Wales 2013*. Available at: http://www.ons.gov.uk/ons/rel/vsob1/birth-summary-tables--england-and-wales/2013/stb-births-in-england-and-wales-2013.html (accessed 19 May 2015).

Resuscitation Council (UK) (2010) *Resuscitation Guidelines 2010*. Available at: http://www.resus.org.uk/pages/guide.htm (accessed 19 May 2015).

Richmond, S. (2006) *Newborn Life Support: Resuscitation at Birth* (2nd edn). London: Resuscitation Council (UK).

Woollard, M., Hinshaw, K., Simpson, H. and Wieteska, S. (2010) *Pre-hospital Obstetric Emergency Training: The Practical Approach*. Advanced Life Support Group. Oxford: Wiley-Blackwell.

15 Mental health assessment
Graham Harris and Ursula Rolfe

Health and well-being include the physical and 'mental' aspect of each individual, as both our mental health and psychological well-being are an integral part of our ability to lead fulfilling lives, including studying, forming and maintaining relationships, our work and leisure interests, and the capacity to make decisions on a daily basis. Any disruption to the individual's mental well-being (albeit on a temporary or permanent basis) can and will compromise these decisions, which affect not only them as individuals, but sometimes at the wider family and societal level.

Since 1948, the World Health Organization (WHO) have provided an intrinsic significance of positive mental health in their definition of health, which it describes as 'a state of complete physical, mental, and social well-being and not merely the absence of disease or infirmity' (WHO, 1948: 100; 2006).

Paramedics have seen an increase in calls relating to mental health issues in the out-of-hospital environment (College of Paramedics, 2015), and evidence indicates that one in four people experience a mental health problem at some point in their life and one in six adults has a mental health problem at any one time (ONS, 2011). The problem is not restricted to adults, with one in ten children aged between 5 and 16 years also having a mental health problem, and many of these continue to have mental health problems into adulthood (Department of Health, 2011).

The Department of Health, the National Collaborating Centre for Mental Health (NCCfMH), and the National Institute for Health and Care Excellence (NICE) provide considerable evidence and guidance regarding the recognition, assessment and treatment of common mental health disorders which paramedics may meet in practice (Department of Health 1999, 2001a, 2001b, 2002a, 2002b, 2004, 2005, 2011; NCCfMH 2006, 2009, 2011a, 2011b, 2011c, 2013, 2014a, 2014b: NICE 2004, 2005, 2007, 2009, 2011, 2013, 2015):

- Depression, general anxiety disorder (GAD), panic disorder, phobias, ante and post-natal depression (PND)

- Obsessive compulsive disorders (OCD), post-traumatic stress disorder (PTSD), social anxiety disorder
- Psychosis and schizophrenia
- Self-harming, attempted suicide
- Bipolar disease
- Alcohol and drug misuse.

More often than not, prior information is provided before arrival at a scene; however, the incidental occurrence requires paramedics to be fully versed with the necessary tools for the correct assessment of each patient. The aim of this chapter is to illustrate relevant key issues the paramedic may find helpful when dealing with patients with mental health issues, and a list of useful mental health organizations is provided at the end of the chapter which can be referred to for further information.

SCENE ASSESSMENT

The scene itself may provide information to the paramedic. When approaching any scene where the patient has (or potentially may have) a mental health issue, consider the following aspects of the scene:

Physical environment

- Type of micro environment – domestic two-storey house, multi-storey apartments, industrial garage space, assisted living facilities (chaotic living conditions)
- Access and egress routes – narrow passageways, stairs, open spaces
- Potential hazards – poor lighting, obvious obstructions, the patient
- Paraphernalia like spoons, tin foil, matches, syringes and makeshift tourniquets
- Smells (particularly alcohol, cannabis or smoked cocaine).

Personnel already in attendance

- Police
- Relatives/friends
- Social service personnel
- GPs
- Ambulance personnel.

Patient presentation

- Stance – sitting, withdrawn posture, standing, incessant pacing, rocking
- Verbal communication – silence, inappropriate language, aggression, shouting

- Alcohol – visible evidence, smell
- Drug usage – both prescription and illicit
- Appearance – dishevelled, unwashed, state of undress.

PRIMARY SURVEY

The purpose of any primary survey is to ascertain if the patient has any **time critical** conditions which require immediate life-saving attention. The primary survey of the patient with a mental health issue continues the ethos of the **DR ABCDE** framework; however, in incidents that involve self-harm or attempted suicide, the paramedic may need to consider catastrophic haemorrhage. Paramedics should also understand that a distressed patient may react extremely to being hurried. Consider and use the following approach:

- Do not rush.
- Take your time (*explain your actions, to patient and relatives*).
- Make every attempt to be honest.
- Explain what is likely to happen (*obtain consent, ensure patient has capacity, GP, assessment, hospital, potential admission*) (Fisher et al., 2013).

Information regarding the patient may have to be obtained from concerned family, partners and/or friends, and in certain instances an Approved Mental Health Professional (AMHP) and the police. The presentation of the patient will vary considerably depending on the condition and the severity of their symptoms. A common symptom, psychosis, affects the patient's mind and causes them to change the way that they think, feel and behave, resulting in them being unable to distinguish between reality and their imagination. The symptoms may be due to:

- Mental health conditions, such as schizophrenia, bipolar disorder (*manic depression*)
- Physical conditions (*Parkinson's disease, meningitis*)
- Drug or alcohol misuse.

About 1 in every 200 adults experience a 'probable psychotic disorder' in the course of a year (Singleton et al., 2001).

Psychosis due to drug or alcohol misuse may only last for a few days. However, the psychosis that results from schizophrenia or bipolar disorder may last indefinitely unless it is treated, hence the importance of obtaining the appropriate care. Ascertain if the patient presents with or has suffered from either:

- Hallucinations – the patient may see or hear things that are not there.
- Delusions – the patient believes things that are untrue.

DANGER

Most people who suffer from mental illnesses are vulnerable and present no threat to anyone but themselves. Patients with schizophrenia and related disorders may be intensely distressed, especially during the acute phases, which may manifest as fear, agitation, suspicion or anger. Consider the patient's needs but always ensure the safety of self, colleagues, bystanders and the patient at all times. Never place yourself in a situation where you cannot readily exit. Remember the value of an open, non-judgemental approach and the use of a calming voice to assist in easing the situation and in achieving a conversation with the patient and then explaining that you are there to help.

Possible actions to be taken:

- Always ensure safety of yourself, your colleagues and the patient – in that order
- Ensure a viable escape route
- Obtain consent, and ensure patient has capacity (Department of Health, 2005)
- Speak in a calming tone and use an open, non-judgemental approach
- Remember the value of good verbal and non-verbal communication
- If applicable, ensure that appropriate personal protective equipment (PPE) is worn.

Be particularly aware that performing any assessment may have the opposite effect of creating more worry and anxiety for the patient, so describe all of your intended actions.

RESPONSE

Remember to exclude all probable medical or drug-related reasons for any patient presenting with altered mental status (hypoglycaemia, head injuries, alcohol or drugs) before considering psychological causes. Obtain the patient's level of consciousness (LOC) using the AVPU scale and remember that schizophrenic patients often appear emotionless, flat and apathetic.

- If possible, ascertain the patient's LOC (AVPU).
- Ascertain if the patient responds to a calm reassuring voice.
- Does the patient present with incessant pacing (akathisia – a movement disorder characterized by a feeling of restlessness and the need to be in constant motion) (NCCfMH 2013, 2014b)?

Mental health assessment

- Ascertain if the patient has a history of long-term use of antipsychotic drugs (akathisia is a side-effect).
- Have they used cannabis or cocaine? The latter is associated with a variety of movement disorders, including akathisia (*crack dancers*).

Possible actions to be taken:

- Ascertain and record the patient's AVPU scale
- Ascertain if the patient responds to a calm reassuring voice
- Ascertain the cause, if present, of 'incessant pacing' (*antipsychotic or cocaine use*) (NCCfMH, 2013, 2014b).

AIRWAY

A patient who is talking incessantly may initially appear to have a patent airway, however, remember that the patient who has misused alcohol or drugs may have an airway problem. Alternatively, the patient may present with tardive dyskinesia, another effect of long-term use of antipsychotic drugs. The patient may present with involuntary movements which normally commence with the face: mouth, lips and tongue, and include grimacing, lip-smacking, tongue and chewing movements (MIND, 2015).

- Does the patient appear to have excess salivation (*likely to occur with second generation antipsychotics* (SGAs))?
- Is the airway patent?
- Is the patient able to maintain their own airway?
- Correct any airway deficits immediately by stepwise airway management (*see Respiratory Assessment, Chapter 2*).

Possible actions to be taken:

- Ensure the patient has a patent airway
- Use stepwise airway management as appropriate (*see Respiratory Assessment, Chapter 2*)
- Identify if the patient has any involuntary movements of mouth, lips and tongue (*ascertain the use of first generation or second generation antipsychotic drugs*)
- Ensure airway is secure before moving to the next element.

BREATHING

The patient may be intensely distressed and agitated, and their emotional responses and/or medications may potentially have a direct influence on the respiratory system. These elevated anxiety levels may be the cause of an adrenergic response, resulting in an increase in respiration and other symptoms. Remember that a considerable number of individuals with mental health problems also misuse substances (*cocaine 'smoked or snorted', cannabis*) (Department of Health, 2002a; 2011). Patients using these substances may present with:

- Shortness of breath
- Productive cough
- Chronic rhinitis (*intra-nasal use of cocaine – snorting*)
- Oropharyngeal ulcers
- Wheezing
- Chest pain
- Haemoptysis
- Exacerbation of asthma.

Assess and manage any of the above conditions appropriately.

Listen to the patient talking and assess if their speech is:

- Disorganized (frequent derailment or incoherent, also known as *word salad*).
- Disjointed or rambling monologues (patient appears to be talking to themselves or imagined people or voices).
- Alogia – lessening of fluent speech and productivity (*patient may either speak very little or with a lack of spontaneous content*). This is also known as poverty of speech.
- Identify the presence of either normal or abnormal breathing patterns.
- If possible, obtain a SpO_2 reading, manage accordingly.
- Note any particular odour that may lead you to identify differential complications (*alcohol, sweet or pear drop odour*).
- Ascertain if the patient has asthma and treat accordingly.

Possible actions to be taken:

- Ascertain the patient's breathing pattern (*normal or abnormal*)
- Identify acute respiratory symptoms (*manage accordingly; ensure the patient is not hypoxic*)
- Obtain an SpO_2 reading
- If **time critical** conditions are identified, manage and transfer in relation to condition
- Note abnormal odours
- Identify if their speech is disorganized, disjointed or if they have alogia.

CIRCULATION

Patients with schizophrenia have an increased risk of cardiovascular disease, including myocardial infarction (NCCfMH, 2014b). Some antipsychotic medications have been shown to induce cardiovascular side effects (lengthening of the QT interval on ECG) (NCCfMH, 2014b), whilst tricyclic drugs may cause postural hypotension, tachycardia and ECG changes (BNF, 2015).

Remember that patients who use cocaine are also at risk of cocaine-induced myocardial infarction/cardiac arrest (Burnett, 2015). Various pharmacologically active substances have reportedly been used with cocaine, alcohol and nicotine being the most common.

Alternatively, the effects of the patient's medication or the fact that they are agitated and distressed may have resulted in elevated anxiety levels and be the cause of an adrenergic response, directly causing an increased pulse rate and blood pressure. The patient, however, may present with injury as a result of self-harm or a failed suicide attempt. Assess the following aspects of circulation:

- Ensure the immediate control of obvious external bleeding.
- Assess and record the patient's pulse (*bradycardic, normal or tachycardic*).
- Assess and record the patient's blood pressure (BP) (*hypotension or hypertension may occur as a side effect of the patient's medication*).
- Does the patient appear diaphoretic?
- Ask the patient if they smoke (including cannabis and cocaine) or use other illicit drugs. If so, ascertain frequency and quantity.
- Obtain a 12-lead ECG trace and ascertain if there is lengthening of the QT interval (*measured from the beginning of the QRS to the end of the 'T' wave*) (Figure 15.1).

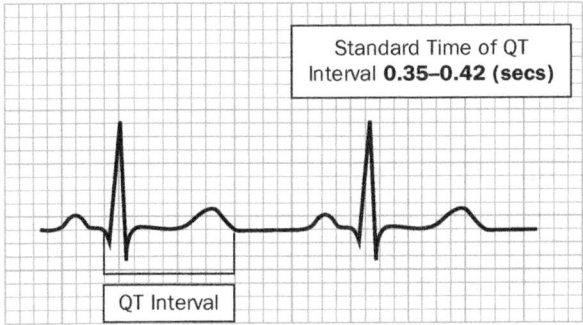

Figure 15.1 QT Internal Measurement

Possible actions to be taken:

- Ensure the immediate control of obvious external haemorrhage (see *Trauma Assessment, Chapter 7*)
- Assess and record the patient's pulse and BP
- Obtain a 12-lead ECG trace and assess for lengthening of the QT interval
- Ascertain if they use illicit drugs
- If a 'time critical' condition is identified, manage and transfer as appropriate

DISABILITY

As with any patient, the assessment of disability includes checking their neurological function and their level of consciousness. It also includes assessing and recording their blood glucose levels and conducting an examination of their pupils. In a patient with mental health issues, these may all potentially be affected. A patient who has catatonic schizophrenia may present with:

- Bizarre posture
- Muscle immobility
- Stupor (*semi-consciousness due to mental illness, wherein the patient does not move or speak, and does not respond to stimuli*).

Alternatively, the patient may present with other effects of tardive dyskinesia (MIND, 2015). These include involuntary movements which affect other parts of the body, resulting in gestures, tics and writhing movements. It may include the fingers making it look as if the patient is playing an invisible guitar or piano. It can also cause rapid blinking, making the assessment of the patient's pupils more difficult for the attending paramedic. Unfortunately for the patient, another side effect of antipsychotic medication is the onset of diabetes. Assess and record the patient's level of consciousness, blood glucose level and pupils (Pilbery, 2014).

Possible actions to be taken:

- Assess and record the patient's level of consciousness (AVPU)
- Record any abnormal postures
- Do they present with any other involuntary movements? (*note and record*)

- Assess and record the patient's blood glucose level (*manage accordingly*)
- Assess the patient's pupils (PERRLA)
- If a **time critical** condition is identified, manage and transfer as appropriate.

EXPOSE/EXAMINE/EVALUATE

All reasonable steps should be taken to engage individual patients in meaningful discussion about issues relating to consent, remembering that examining any patient will require their consent. Ensure that the patient has capacity; specific guidance is provided regarding the patient with mental health problems (Department of Constitutional Affairs 2007; Department of Health, 2009). Due consideration must be given to the results of a physical examination of any patient with mental health issues as their emotional responses and/or medication may have a direct influence. The paramedic will have evaluated all of the information obtained from the elements of the primary survey and the patient's environment (Pilbery, 2014), and linked this to their presenting disorder. This should be appraised and the need to remove the patient (time critical conditions) from the scene considered and, if appropriate, a secondary survey should be completed.

Possible actions to be taken:

- Consider the effects of the patient's emotional response and/or medication
- Expose patient and examine (*remember appropriate consent, and ensure the patient has capacity*)
- Evaluate the findings of the primary survey
- If time critical, transfer to the appropriate treatment unit or centre
- Undertake a secondary survey.

SECONDARY SURVEY

Presenting complaint

In relation to attending emergency calls involving mental health issues, the paramedic may be called to patients who present for various reasons. While the call may have been received as *'person having hallucinations'* or *'hearing voices'*, there are specific mental disorders which paramedics will be called to attend, which include:

- Mood, stress-related and anxiety disorders
- Psychosis
- Mania/hypomania
- Schizophrenia
- Paranoia.

A patient who is in the initial phase of schizophrenia may present with symptoms of unusual and uncharacteristic behaviour, disturbed communication, bizarre ideas, poor personal hygiene, and reduced interest in and motivation for day-to-day activities, and may explain that they feel that their world has changed. However, their family and friends may advise that the patient has changed *in themselves*. Alternatively, the presenting complaint may be due to either a self-harm or suicide attempt. Continue the ethos commenced in the primary survey (*not rushing, being open and non-judgemental*), as misinterpretation due to the paramedic's view of the events or perceived problems may lead to an incorrect starting point. This can affect the history obtained and potentially have consequences for the patient's care.

- Ascertain the exact causes of the presenting complaint (from the patient if possible, alternatively from the family, partner or friends).
- Ascertain if this is the first time the problem has occurred.
- Use the patient's own words when detailing and documenting the presenting complaint.
- Undertake a suicide and self-harm risk assessment (see Table 15.1).

As previously stated, the assessment of patients presenting with mental health problems (once you have excluded any physical cause) requires the paramedic to sometimes adopt a different approach from usual, in that you do not rush, take your time to establish a rapport and are usually on scene for a longer period of time. It may be that you struggle for questions to ask that may reveal more about your patient's mental state. In such cases, the mnemonic GASPIPES may be useful (Whitnell, 2012). Ask yourself and the patient whether they are experiencing any of the following:

- **G** – Guilt and self-reproach
- **A** – Appetite is disturbed
- **S** – Sleep disturbance, suffering insomnia
- **P** – Paying attention to your questions, or not, orientation to time, place and person
- **I** – Interest in things lacking, such as football, music
- **P** – Psychomotor disturbance-slow, agitated, pacing, mood, hallucinations and belief expressed
- **E** – Energy loss, tired, slow, non-stop
- **S** – Suicidal, expressed thoughts

Table 15.1 Suicide and self-harm risk assessment

Item	Value	Patient score
Gender: Female	0	
Gender: Male	1	
Age: <19 years old	1	
Age: >45 years old	1	
Depression/hopelessness	1	
Previous self-harm attempts	1	
Evidence of excess alcohol/use of illicit drugs	1	
Absence of rational thinking	1	
Separated/divorced/widowed	1	
Organized or serious attempt	1	
Absence of close/reliable family or job or active religious affiliation	1	
Determined to repeat attempt or ambivalent	1	
Total patient score		

AACE (2013).

Once you have answers to specific questions, or a general impression of your patient's mood, it needs to be combined with the suicide and self-harm risk assessment tool, detailed in Table 15.1. The answers to specific questions and your impressions of the patient's mood will all be extremely valuable for handover at hospital or referral pathways that may be available to you (*paramedic practitioner, community psychiatric liaison team, crisis team*). Such focused questioning will often provide you with information that will be useful, taken seriously and demonstrates education in the assessment of patients with mental health problems to other allied health professionals and colleagues. It may be the difference between a referral that you are trying to make being accepted or declined.

In emergency situations, it is important to address whether the patient is at immediate risk of self-harm or suicidal intent. The use of the risk assessment scoring system in Table 15.1 can identify key markers regarding the patient's risk of repeating the self-harm/suicide attempt.

- Score <3 indicates low risk.
- Score 3–6 indicates medium risk.
- Score >6 indicates high risk.

> **Possible actions to be taken:**
> - Ascertain the presenting complaint
> - Undertake a suicide and self-harm risk assessment (*record and document low risk as part of history*)
> - Medium/high risk patient should be referred/conveyed to an appropriate unit for further assessment.

History of presenting complaint

The actual history of the presenting complaint will specifically vary depending on the *reason* for the presenting complaint. The history of a patient whose presenting complaint is *self-harm* may be due to the fact that they are depressed due to either child or domestic abuse (NICE, 2004, 2011). Alternatively, another patient may have a history of suffering from schizophrenia for several years and is suffering an acute exacerbation or relapse and requires additional intervention (NCCfMH, 2013, 2014b). Remember that not all patients that present with indicators for mental health illness will have a definitive diagnosis prior to the time of your assessment. Particular consideration should be made to particular demographic groups:

- Current or ex-military personnel (*who may be suffering from post traumatic stress disorder (PTSD)*) (Pedrotti, 2011)
- New mothers (*who may be suffering from post-natal depression (PND)*) (NCCfMH, 2014a)
- Children and adolescents (*who may perform intentional acts of deliberate self-harm (DSH)*). Children as young as 7 have been found to self-harm; the average age for children commencing self-harm is 13 years and it is a common occurrence in the 10–14 year age group. Until the age of 12 years, DSH is more common in boys than girls. After this age, DSH is four times more common among girls (Hawton et al., 2009; Whitnell, 2012).

Endeavour to ascertain any triggering or exacerbating factors that may have led to the patient's present situation. Remember that patients may suffer from more than one mental health problem simultaneously; as well as potentially being drug-/alcohol=dependent, with specific groups being particularly at risk:

- Young people
- Homeless people
- Offenders
- Women
- Ethnic minority groups (Department of Health, 2002a).

Ascertain the history of the presenting complaint:

- Confirm the findings from relatives and friends (*time period, symptoms, etc.*).

- Obtain information regarding vulnerable persons (*record and complete documentation as per local guidelines, refer to the appropriate agency*).
- Depending on the patient's age/gender, consider the need for a chaperone (World Health Organization, 2012a).

Possible actions to be taken:
- Record and document information obtained regarding vulnerable persons (*comply with local guidelines and refer to appropriate agencies*).

Past medical history

A full account of a patient's past medical history is invaluable when deciding on an appropriate course of treatment for the individual; these are not normally decided by the paramedic for patients with mental health problems. However, a patient's past medical history and any pre-existing mental health problems should be obtained by the paramedic. Ascertain the nature of any pre-existing mental health conditions:

- Depression, general anxiety disorder (GAD), panic disorder, phobias, ante and post-natal depression (PND)
- Obsessive compulsive disorder (OCD), post-traumatic stress disorder (PTSD), social anxiety disorder
- Psychosis and schizophrenia
- Self-harming, attempted suicide
- Bipolar disease.

Patients will and do have other co-morbidity conditions that, as with any patient, may be relevant to the existing problem; these can include endocrine (*diabetes*), cardiovascular (*hypertension, lipid levels, heart attack – myocardial infarction*), or respiratory conditions (*asthma*). Evidence suggests that psychiatrists and the patient's GP are particularly poor at recognizing and treating physical conditions in patients who suffer from a mental health problem (Roberts et al., 2007).

Drug/medication history

A precise notation of all the medications taken by the patient should be obtained wherever possible; although the paramedic must always be aware that any underlying mental health issues can preclude an accurate list. Also, drug regime compliance and regular concordance must always be taken into consideration. Be cautious of the accuracy of this information from other parties, as emotion may cloud accuracy issues. The use of illegal, illicit or herbal drugs must also be considered as these can interact with prescription medications.

Specifically check for St. John's wort (*Hypericum perforatum*), which is a popular herbal remedy and available to the public for mild depression. It has drug-metabolizing enzymes, which differ with the strength of the preparation. Care must be taken to avoid toxicity due to drug interactions between prescribed and alternative (e.g. herbal) or over-the-counter remedies (BNF, 2015).

Patients with mental health problems are prescribed anti-depressants, anti-psychotic and anxiolytic medications. Anti-depressant drugs relieve the symptoms of depression and include four main types:

- Monoamine oxidase inhibitors (MAOIs)
- Selective serotonin reuptake inhibitors (SSRIs)
- Serotonin and noradrenaline reuptake inhibitors (SNRIs)
- Noradrenaline and specific serotonergic antidepressants (NASSAs) (Royal College of Psychiatrists, 2015).

Anti-psychotic drugs, also known as neuroleptics, and which affect various chemicals in the brain, tend to be classified into two specific groups:

- Typical – first generation antipsychotics (FGAs) (see Table 15.2)
- Atypical – second generation antipsychotics (2nd GAs) (see Table 15.3).

Table 15.2 Typical anti-psychotics (FGAs)

Medication	Trade name
Chlorpromazine	Largactil
Haloperidol	Haldol
Pimozide	Orap
Trifluoperazine	Stelazine
Sulperide	Dolmatil

Table 15.3 Atypical anti-psychotics (2nd GAs)

Medication	Trade name
Amisulpiride	Solian
Ariprazole	Abilify
Clozapine	Clozaril
Olanzapine	Zyprexa
Quetiapine	Seroquel
Risperidone	Risperdal
Sertindole	Serdolect
Zotepine	Zoleptil

Royal College of Psychiatrists (2015).

Table 15.4 Common anxiolytic drugs

Medication	Trade name
Ativan	Lorazepam
Valium	Diazepam
Librium	Chlordiazepoxide
Serax	Oxazepam
Xanax	Alprazolam
Dalmane	Flurazepam
Halcion	Triazolam
Klonopin/rivotril	Clonazepam

BNF (2015).

Anxiolytics are used for the short-term relief of severe anxiety. Table 15.4 includes some of the common anxiolytics.

Social/family medical history

Consideration needs to be given to a patient's social and family history, which may have an influence upon a patient's state of mind and therefore thought processes. In the out-of-hospital setting, acquiring an accurate and detailed social and family medical history may not always be possible; however, when treating a patient with acute mental health issues, extended on-scene time may allow for a more detailed questioning regimen. Evidence suggests that various factors may cause mental health problems (Rethink, 2015):

- Physical
- Environmental
- Psychological
- Social.

Alternative evidence explains these factors as biological, sociocultural and psychosocial issues (see Table 15.5).

Remember that relatives, families and carers of patients suffering mental health problems may also need support; they may be emotionally and psychologically affected by caring for someone with a mental health problem. They may have been coping with this for days, weeks or even years and be feeling distressed, fearful and isolated, which can have a significant impact on their quality of life.

Table 15.5 Biological, sociocultural and psychosocial factors

Biological	Sociocultural	Psychosocial
Genetic factors	Personal relationships	Childhood trauma
Pre- and postnatal factors	Family stability	Childhood abuse/neglect
Neuro-biochemical imbalance	Economic status	Dysfunctional family structure
	Social cohesion	Biological disorders
	Work environment	
	Personal belief values	

Gregory and Ward (2010).

REVIEW OF SYSTEMS AND VITAL SIGNS

As mentioned earlier, the exclusion of any physical or medical conditions is important when formulating a treatment plan. Therefore, acquiring a set of vital sign observations will not only assist the paramedic, but may also provide the patient with reassurance that they are receiving treatment and thereby help to reduce their anxieties. The vital signs ascertained, if possible, should include:

- Respiratory rate, character and work of breathing (*breathing: rate, depth and efficacy*)
- Heart rate, character (*circulation: rate, depth and efficacy*)
- Blood pressure
- Result of 12-lead ECG
- Blood glucose levels
- AVPU, GCS/neurological status, including pupillary reaction
- Temperature
- SpO_2.

Consideration, however, must be given to the acquisition and results of any physical examination of patients with a mental health problem, as their emotional response and/or medication may have a direct influence. Be particularly aware that performing these assessments may also have the opposite effect of creating more worry and anxiety for a patient, so describe all of your intended actions, and obtain appropriate consent prior to examining.

MENTAL CAPACITY ACT 2005

The Mental Capacity Act 2005 relates to patients over the age of 16 in England and Wales. If the patient has a mental disorder in Scotland or Northern Ireland, the paramedic should note the exceptions in the Mental Health Act 2003 (as amended by the Mental Health Act 2006), the Mental Health (NI) Order 1986, and the Mental Health (Care and Treatment) (Scotland) Act 2003 (General Medical Council, 2015). The paramedic should therefore understand what the Act defines as a lack of *capacity*: 'a person lacks capacity in relation to a matter if at the material time he is unable to make a decision for himself in relation to the matter because of an impairment of, or a disturbance in the functioning of, the mind or brain' (Department of Health, 2005; Mental Capacity Act 2005, 4.3, Section 2(1)).

This means that a person lacks capacity if they cannot do one or more of the following four things, known as *inability to make a decision*:

- Understand information given to them.
- Retain that information long enough to be able to make a decision.
- Use or weigh up the information available to make a decision.
- Communicate their decision.

An assessment of a person's capacity must be based on their ability to make a specific decision at the time it needs to be made, and not their ability to make decisions in general. This incorporates the five statutory principles included within Section 1 of the Act:

- A person must be assumed to have capacity unless it is established that he or she lacks capacity.
- A person is not to be treated as unable to make a decision unless all practicable steps to help him or her to do so have been taken without success.
- A person is not to be treated as unable to make a decision merely because he or she makes an unwise decision.
- An act done, or decision made, under this Act for or on behalf of a person who lacks capacity must be done, or made, in his or her best interests.
- Before the act is done, or the decision is made, regard must be had to whether the purpose for which it is needed can be as effectively achieved in a way that is less restrictive of the person's rights and freedom of action (Department of Health 2005; Mental Capacity Act 2005, Section 1).

MENTAL HEALTH ACT 1983 (AMENDED 2007)

The Mental Health Act of 1983 provides special legal provision for any person displaying any disorder or disability of the mind and who is considered a danger to either themselves or others, and who refuses to accept treatment that they require. They may be detained under the Mental Health Act 1983 (amended 2007) for a limited time, in order to be assessed or treated accordingly. An application for assessment can be made by an Approved Mental Health Professional (AMHP) (*previously known as Approved Social Worker, ASW*), or the patient's nearest relative who has cause for concern over their welfare.

The duration and circumstances of the compulsory admission (commonly termed as *being sectioned*) can be broken down into three main sections that are more pertinent to paramedic out-of-hospital practice (Table 15.6).

Section 135 enables an approved social worker or an Approved Mental Health Professional (AMHP) to seek a warrant from a Justice of the Peace which will allow the police to enter the premises (with force if necessary) if there is reasonable cause to believe a patient has mental health problems and to take this patient to a place of safety. Paramedics need to be aware of this section if they have trouble accessing premises as they can call on the police to invoke this section. Section 135 has a duration period of 72 hours which cannot be renewed. The police who attend and access the premises (with force if necessary) must be accompanied by an (AMHP) and a doctor (Mental Health Act 1983, Section 135).

There may be times when the paramedic comes into contact with patients who are at risk to themselves or others and require to be placed into a place of safety. Section 136 of the Mental Health Act 1983 covers this (see Table 15.7).

The paramedic may also come across patients who have been discharged following a period of compulsory hospital admission (Section 3). Depending on the circumstances they may be discharged with aftercare (Section 117). The local social services authority (LSSA) is required to provide the patient with the aftercare services, which may include: accommodation, psychological, physical health care, daytime activities or employment needs arising from drug, alcohol or substance misuse.

OTHER CONSIDERATIONS

Communication

Consideration should be given to patients whose first language is not English or who have a visual or hearing impairment as misinterpretation and confusion can lead to an escalation of the patient's symptoms. Consider if the information could be explained or presented in a way that is easier for the patient to understand (*visual aids*). Endeavour to use alternative methods (*non-verbal*) or other people to aid communication:

Mental health assessment

Table 15.6 Compulsory admission to hospital

Mental Health Act	Purpose	Duration	Decision direction
Section 2	Compulsory admission for assessment or assessment followed by treatment	Up to 28 days	Application must be made by AMHP, or nearest relative who has seen the patient in the past 14 days. Also seen (examined) by two separate doctors (one of which must be approved under the Mental Health Act) within 5 days of each other. Admission must be within 14 days of last examination.
Section 3	Compulsory admission for treatment	Up to 6 months (may be renewed for further 6 months, and after that 12 monthly)	Application must be made by AMHP, or nearest relative who has seen the patient in the past 14 days. Also seen (examined) by two separate doctors (one of which must be approved under the Mental Health Act) within 5 days of each other. Admission must be within 14 days of last examination.
Section 4	Enables admission in an emergency	Up to 72 hours (can be converted to another section (usually 2) if required)	Application must be made by AMHP, or nearest relative. Must be seen by a doctor (preferably one that knows the patient or one that has been approved under the Mental Health Act). The doctor and the applicant must have seen the patient within the previous 24 hours and the patient must be admitted to hospital within 24 hours of being examined by the doctor or from when the application was made.

Mental Health Act (2007).

Table 15.7 Section 136: Mentally disordered people found in public places

Mental Health Act Code of Practice	Section 136: Mentally disordered people found in public places
Chapter 10 Section 10.12	Section 136 allows for the removal to a place of safety of any person found in a place to which the public have access (by payment or otherwise) who appears to a police officer to be suffering from mental disorder and to be in immediate need of care or control.
Chapter 10 Section 10.13	Removal to a place of safety may take place if the police officer believes it necessary in the interests of that person, or for the protection of others.
Chapter 10 Section 10.14	The purpose of removing a person to a place of safety in these circumstances is only to enable the person to be examined by a doctor and interviewed by an AMHP, so that the necessary arrangements can be made for the person's care and treatment. It is not a substitute for an application for detention under the Act, even if it is thought that the person will need to be detained in hospital only for a short time. It is also not intended to substitute for or affect the use of other police powers.
Chapter 10 Section 10.15	The maximum period a person may be detained under Section 136 is 72 hours. The imposition of consecutive periods of detention under Section 136 is unlawful.

Department of Health (2008)

- Interpreter (*language line*)
- Family member
- Support worker
- Speech and language therapists
- Advocate.

Social/family/carer/guardian

Never forget the distress and emotional pressure that can be experienced by relatives or carers of any patient suffering a mental health illness, especially if they have had to instigate a compulsory admission. Remember to fully explain any actions or interventions undertaken in the patient's best interest to any

Mental health assessment

family members present to help avoid misunderstanding and therefore undue distress.

Ethical and legal

Mental illness is not a condition affecting adults alone. Patients under 18 years of age can be subject to acute episodes of mental illness and therefore due consideration must be given to how to manage a young patient accordingly. Compliance with The Children Act 1989 (amended 2010) must be maintained wherever possible. The Act's starting point is to confirm in legislation that it should be assumed that an adult (aged 18 or over) has full legal capacity to make decisions for themselves (the right to autonomy) unless it can be shown that they lack capacity to make a decision for themselves at the time the decision needs to be made. This is known as the presumption of capacity.

Destination/receiving specialist

Always ensure that all documentation appertaining to any patient's compulsory admission to hospital under the Mental Health Act 2007 is transferred to an appropriate receiving professional (Approved Mental Health Professional, nurse or doctor) on their arrival.

Mental health: facts/figures

The World Health Organization advised that over 350 million people in 2012 suffered from depression globally (WHO, 2012b). In the United Kingdom one in four people experience a mental health problem at some point in their life and one in six adults has a mental health problem at any one time (ONS, 2011).

Mental health problems – 2011 statistics:
- At least one in four people will experience a mental health problem at some point in their life and one in six adults have a mental health problem at any one time.
- One in ten children aged between 5 and 16 years has a mental health problem, and many continue to have mental health problems into adulthood.
- Half of those with lifetime mental health problems first experience symptoms by the age of 14, and three-quarters before their mid-twenties.
- Self-harming in young people is not uncommon (10–13% of 15–16-year olds have self-harmed).
- Almost half of all adults will experience at least one episode of depression during their lifetime.

- One in ten new mothers experiences postnatal depression.
- About one in 100 people has a severe mental health problem.
- Some 60% of adults living in hostels have a personality disorder.
- Some 90% of all prisoners are estimated to have a diagnosable mental health problem (*including personality disorder*) and/or a substance misuse problem (Department of Health, 2011).

CHAPTER KEY POINTS

- The safety of both yourself and your colleagues is paramount when managing any situation involving patients with mental health illness.
- Where possible and safe, allow any patient suffering from a mental health illness to be involved in their assessment and management.
- Ensure consent is obtained, and, if required/appropriate, assess the patient's capacity.
- Remember the value of effective verbal and non-verbal communication.
- Be careful to exclude any physical and medical causes of altered mental status before considering psychological causes.
- If the patient is being compulsorily admitted to hospital, ensure that the appropriate documentation has been completed.
- Current legislation must always be complied with when dealing with any patient with a mental health issue, especially regarding consent and capacity.

REFERENCES

Association of Ambulance Chief Executives (2013) *UK Ambulance Services Clinical Practice Guidelines 2013 Pocket Book: Suicide and Self-Harm Risk Assessment Form*. Bridgwater: Class Professional Publishing.

BNF (British National Formulary) (2015) *BNF Online*. Available at: http://www.bnf.org/bnf/index.htm (accessed 20 May 2015).

Burnett, L.B. (2015) *Cocaine Toxicity in Emergency Medicine*. Available at: hhttp://emedicine.medscape.com/article/813959-overview (accessed 20 May 2015).

College of Paramedics (2015) *Paramedic Curriculum Guidance* (3rd edn) (Revised). Bridgwater: College of Paramedics.

Department of Constitutional Affairs (2007) *Mental Capacity Act 2005: Code of Practice*. London: The Stationery Office.

Department of Health (1999) *The National Service Framework for Mental Health*. London: Department of Health Publications.

Department of Health (2001a) *Consent – What You Have a Right to Expect. A Guide for Adults*. London: Department of Health Publications.

Department of Health (2001b) *National Service Framework for Older People*. London: The Stationery Office.

Department of Health (2002a) *The Mental Health Policy Implementation Guide: Dual Diagnosis Good Practice Guide*. London: Department of Health Publications.

Department of Health (2002b) *National Suicide Prevention Strategy for England*. London: Department of Health Publications.
Department of Health (2004) *The National Service Framework for Mental Health – Five Years On*. London: Department of Health Publications.
Department of Health (2005) *Mental Capacity Act*. London: The Stationery Office.
Department of Health (2008) *Code of Practice. Mental Health Act 1983*. London: The Stationery Office.
Department of Health (2009) *Reference Guide to Consent for Examination of Treatment* (2nd edn). London: Department of Health.
Department of Health (2011) *No Health Without Mental Health: A Cross-Government Mental Health Outcomes Strategy for People of All Ages. Mental Health and Disability*. London: Department of Health Publications.
Fisher, J., Brown, S.N. and Cooke, M. (eds) (2013) *UK Ambulance Services Clinical Practice Guidelines 2013. Mental Disorder*. Bridgwater: Class Professional Publishing.
GMC (General Medical Council) (2015) *Consent Guidance: Endnotes*. Available at: http://www.gmc-uk.org/guidance/ethical_guidance/consent_guidance_endnotes.asp (accessed 22 May 2015).
Gregory, P. and Ward, A. (eds) (2010) *Sanders' Paramedic Textbook*. London: Elsevier Health Sciences.
Hawton, K., Rodham, K., Evans, E. and Harris, L. (2009) Adolescents who self harm: a comparison of those who go to hospital and those who do not. *Child and Adolescent Mental Health* 14(1): 24–30.
Mental Health Act (2007) Chapter 12: Amendments to the Mental Health Act 1983. Legislation.gov.uk. Available at: http://www.legislation.gov.uk/ukpga/2007/12/contents (accessed 22 May 2015).
MIND For better mental health (2015) *Tardive Dyskinesia (TD)*. Available at: http://www.mind.org.uk/help/diagnoses_and_conditions/tardive_dyskinesia (accessed 20 May 2015).
National Collaborating Centre for Mental Health – Commissioned by NICE (2006) *Post Traumatic Stress Disorder: The Management of PTSD in Adults and Children in Primary and Secondary Care*. NICE clinical guideline 26. London: Gaskell and the British Psychological Society.
National Collaborating Centre for Mental Health – Commissioned by NICE (2009) *Depression in Adults with a Chronic Physical Health Problem: The NICE Guideline on the Treatment and Management*. NICE clinical guideline 91. London: The British Psychological Society and The Royal College of Psychiatrists.
National Collaborating Centre for Mental Health – Commissioned by NICE (2011a) *Common Mental Health Disorders: Identification and Pathways to Care*. NICE clinical guideline 123. London: The British Psychological Society and The Royal College of Psychiatrists.
National Collaborating Centre for Mental Health – Commissioned by NICE (2011b) *Generalised Anxiety Disorder in Adults. Management in Primary, Secondary and Community Care*. NICE clinical guideline 133. London: The British Psychological Society and The Royal College of Psychiatrists.
National Collaborating Centre for Mental Health – Commissioned by NICE (2011c) *Psychosis with Coexisting Substance Misuse: Assessment and Management in Adults*

and Young People. NICE clinical guideline 120. London: The British Psychological Society and The Royal College of Psychiatrists.

National Collaborating Centre for Mental Health – Commissioned by NICE (2013) *Psychosis and Schizophrenia in Children and Young People. Recognition and Management*. NICE clinical guideline 155. London: The British Psychological Society and The Royal College of Psychiatrists.

National Collaborating Centre for Mental Health – Commissioned by NICE (2014a) *Antenatal and Postnatal Mental Health: The NICE Guideline on Clinical Management and Service Guidance*. (Updated edn). NICE clinical guideline 192. London: The British Psychological Society and The Royal College of Psychiatrists.

National Collaborating Centre for Mental Health – Commissioned by NICE (2014b) *Psychosis and Schizophrenia in Adults. Treatment and Management*. (Updated edn). NICE clinical guideline No. 178. London: National Collaborating Centre for Mental Health.

NICE (National Institute for Health and Clinical Excellence) (2004) *Self-harm: The Short-Term Physical and Psychological Management and Secondary Prevention of Self-Harm in Primary and Secondary Care*. NICE clinical guideline 16. London: The British Psychological Society.

NICE (National Institute for Health and Clinical Excellence) (2005) *Core Interventions in the Treatment of Obsessive Compulsive Disorder and Body Dysmorphic Disorder*. NICE clinical guideline 31. London: The British Psychological Society and The Royal College of Psychiatrists.

NICE (National Institute for Health and Clinical Excellence) (2007) *Drug Misuse: Psychosocial Interventions*. National Clinical Guideline No. 51. London: The British Psychological Society and The Royal College of Psychiatrists.

NICE (National Institute for Health and Clinical Excellence) (2009) *Depression: The NICE Guideline on the Treatment and Management of Depression in Adults* (Updated edn). NICE clinical guideline 90. London: The British Psychological Society and The Royal College of Psychiatrists.

NICE (National Institute for Health and Clinical Excellence) (2011) *Self-Harm: Longer-Term Management. Baseline Assessment – Implementing Nice Guidance*. NICE clinical guideline133. London: The British Psychological Society and The Royal College of Psychiatrists.

NICE (National Institute for Health and Clinical Excellence) (2013) *Social Anxiety Disorder: Recognition, Assessment and Treatment*. NICE clinical guideline 159. London: The British Psychological Society and The Royal College of Psychiatrists.

NICE (National Institute for Health and Clinical Excellence) (2015) *Addendum to Clinical Guideline 28. Depression in Children and Young People. Clinical guideline addendum28.1. Methods, evidence and recommendations*. NICE clinical guideline 28.1. London: National Institute for Health and Clinical Excellence.

ONS (Office for National Statistics) (2011) *General Lifestyle Survey 2009 Data*. Available at: www.statistics.gov.uk/StatBase/Product.asp?vlnk=5756&Pos=&ColRank=1&Rank=256 (accessed 19 May 2015).

Pedrotti, D. (2011) Heroes to hometown: when veterans come home. *Journal of Emergency Medical Services* 36(3): 64–72.

Pilbery, R. (2014) *Nancy Caroline's Emergency Care in the Streets: United Kingdom* (7th edn). Burlington, VA: Jones & Bartlett Learning.

Rethink (2015) *Living with Mental Illness?* Available at: http://www.rethink.org/living-with-mental-illness (accessed 22 May 2015).
Roberts, L., Roalfe, A. and Wilson, S. (2007) Physical health care of patients with schizophrenia in primary care: a comparative study. *Family Practice* 24: 34–40.
Royal College of Psychiatrists (2015) *Antipsychotic Medication.* Available at: http://www.rcpsych.ac.uk/mentalhealthinfo/treatments/antipsychoticmedication.aspx (accessed 22 May 2015).
Singleton, N., Bumpstead, R., O'Brien, M., Lee, A. and Meltzer, H. (2001) *Psychiatric Morbidity Among Adults Living in Private Households, 2000.* London: The Stationery Office.
The Children Act (1989) Online. Available at: http://www.legislation.gov.uk/ukpga/1989/41/introduction (accessed 22 May 2015).
Whitnell, J. (2012) Abnormal Psychology: an introduction. In A.Y. Blaber (ed.) *Foundations for Paramedic Practice: A Theoretical Perspective* (2nd edn). Maidenhead: OU Press.
World Health Organization (1948) *Preamble to the Constitution of the World Health Organization,* as adopted by the International Health Conference, New York, 19–22 June, 1946; signed on 22 July 1946 by the representatives of 61 States (Official Records of the World Health Organization, no. 2, p. 100) and entered into force on 7 April 1948.
World Health Organization (2006) *Constitution of the World Health Organization. Basic Documents* (45th edn). Supplement. October.
World Health Organization (2012a) *Risks to Mental Health: An Overview of Vulnerabilities and Risk Factors.* Available at: http://www.who.int/mental_health/mhgap/risks_to_mental_health_EN_27_08_12.pdf (accessed 21 May 2015).
World Health Organization (2012b) *Depression: Fact Sheet No. 369.* Available at: http://www.who.int/mediacentre/factsheets/fs369/en/ (accessed 22 May 2015).

Useful organizations

Hearing Voices Network: Providing help and assistance to those who hear voices. Contact. Sheffield Hearing Voices Network, Limbrick Day Service, Limbrick Road, Sheffield, S6 2PE. Email: nhvn@hotmail.co.uk | Phone: 0114 271 8210.
Mind and Mind Cymru: Mindinfoline: 0845 766 0163. Mind provides information and advice, training programmes, 'Mind in your area', grants and more.
National Schizophrenia Fellowship (Scotland): Works to improve the well-being and quality of life of those affected by schizophrenia and other mental illness, including families and carers.
Rethink: National voluntary organization that helps people with any severe mental illness, their families and carers.
Saneline: Helpline: 0845 767 8000. A national mental health helpline offering emotional support and practical information for people with mental illness, families, carers and professionals.
Shine: Supporting people with mental ill health.
Young Minds: www.youngminds.org.uk. A UK charity committed to the emotional well-being and mental health of children and young people. Website has sections for young people, parents, parent helpline and training services for professionals.

Conclusion
Amanda Blaber and Graham Harris

As a paramedic, your skills of assessment are crucial to the outcome of your patient. It is hoped this text has provided you with an easy-to-read, structured approach and ultimately an educational 'starting point' to assessment skills. This will aid you when you are beginning to develop these skills under the supervision of your practice educator. As you progress and develop your expertise, this text will remain useful as an aide-mémoire for the skill of assessing certain patient groups, for example, neonates, whom you may not encounter on a daily basis.

Those who have compiled this text are passionate about their skills of assessment. The book has been written to equip new and existing paramedic professionals with the knowledge they need to carry out assessment to the best of their ability.

Glossary of terms

Accessory muscles – any neck, back and abdominal muscles that may assist the internal and external intercostals and diaphragm in respiration. Can be observed in people during periods of exercise and/or people during exacerbation of breathing disorders, such as asthma.

Adventitious sounds – when listening (auscultating) to a person's chest using a stethoscope, the sounds you hear (breath sounds) can either be normal or abnormal (adventitious). These adventitious sounds may be heard when listening over the lungs. They may include rales or crackles and rhonchi (a coarse rattling sound).

Angina – is caused by ischaemia (insufficient blood supply to heart muscle). A person with angina will generally complain of chest pain, discomfort and/or a feeling of pressure in the chest.

Apnoea – the absence of breathing.

Asthma – is an inflammatory disease of the airways. Narrowing of the bronchi (two main branches of the trachea that go into the lungs) is caused by chronic inflammation, making them narrower. Surrounding muscles of the respiratory system become irritated and contract (become tighter) causing a worsening of the symptoms. Mucus glands also produce excessive sputum, due to the inflammation, which further obstructs the airways. Has varying levels of severity from mild/moderate, severe, life-threatening and near fatal.

Auscultate – to auscultate is to listen. Auscultation is a procedure that involves listening to sounds within the body, usually using a stethoscope, as part of a physical assessment, e.g. chest or abdomen.

Bradycardia – refers to a slow heart rate, usually defined as less than 60 beats per minute. Be aware that this may be 'normal' for people who are very fit.

Bradypnoea – slow breathing <10 per minute in adults.

Bronchiectasis – abnormal dilation of the bronchi, commonly seen in young children and infants, rare in adults.

Bronchiolitis – is an acute viral infection of the small air passages of the lungs called the bronchioles.

Bronchospasm – narrowing of the airway caused by the contraction of smooth muscles in the walls of bronchioles within the lungs.

Capacity – refers to the 'mental capacity' of the person to use and understand information in order to make a decision. Refer to the Mental Capacity Act (2005).

Capnometry (EtCO$_2$) – monitoring device that measures the concentration of carbon dioxide in exhaled respiratory gases. Usually presented as a waveform on the monitoring device.

Glossary

Catastrophic haemorrhage – a sudden, hard-to-control haemorrhage affecting all body physiology. A major haemorrhage is defined as the loss of 100% of total blood volume within 24 hours, loss of 50% within four hours, or the loss of 150 mL per minute. Catastrophic haemorrhage is more sudden and significantly threatens life.

Cerebral insult – an abnormal condition of the brain characterized by occlusion by an embolus, thrombus, or cerebrovascular haemorrhage or vasospasm, resulting in ischemia of the brain tissues normally perfused by the damaged vessels.

Chronic bronchitis – inflammation of the bronchi. Chronic is usually caused by smoking, although allergies in some people may be a cause. Symptoms include chest pain, difficulty breathing and a hoarse cough with sputum production.

Chronic obstructive pulmonary disease (COPD) – an obstruction of air flow to and from the lungs. Is a consequence of several forms of pulmonary disease, including chronic bronchitis, cystic fibrosis and emphysema.

Complementary therapy medicines – otherwise known as Complementary and alternative medicines (CAMs). These are treatments that fall outside of mainstream healthcare, such as acupuncture, homeopathy.

Consent – NHS Choices (2010) defines consent as: 'the principle that a person must give their permission before they receive any type of medical treatment. Consent is required from a patient regardless of the type of treatment being undertaken, from a blood test to an organ donation', it must be valid and the person must have capacity.

Conveyed – transported to another place. This term is likely to be used in situations where a patient/service user is taken to a health care facility, such as a hospital; specialist unit; or minor injury unit, etc.

Croup – laryngo-tracheo-bronchiolitis is a viral infectious disease that is quite common among infants and young children. Produces a hoarse cough with a sound resembling the bark of a dog, resulting from the acute obstruction of the larynx.

Cyanosis – a blue/grey discoloration of the skin, usually more noticeable around the lips. Resulting from abnormally low levels of oxygen and high levels of carbon dioxide in the tissues.

Decerebrate posturing – the position of a patient, who is usually comatose, in which the arms are extended and internally rotated and the legs are extended with the feet in forced plantar flexion. It is usually observed in patients afflicted by compression of the brain stem at a low level.

Decorticate posturing – the position of a comatose patient in which the upper extremities are rigidly flexed at the elbows and at the wrists. The legs also may be flexed. The decorticate posture indicates a lesion in a mesencephalic region of the brain. In some instances the posture may be produced by applying a painful stimulus to a comatose patient. Also called decorticate rigidity.

DR 'C' ABCDE – Danger, Response, Catastrophic Haemorrhage, Airway, Breathing, Circulation, Danger, Expose-Examine-Evaluate.

Dyspnoea – the symptom of difficulty in breathing.

Electrocardiogram (ECG) – a graphic tracing of the variations in electrical potential caused by the excitation of the heart muscle and detected at the body surface. Usually performed in either 3-lead or 12-lead ECG context.

Emphysema – chronic lung disease. Patients will have dyspnoea, chronic cough, formation of barrel chest due to laboured breathing and a gradual deterioration caused by chronic hypoxemia and hypercapnia.

Endotracheal tube (ETT) – a non-collapsible breathing tube inserted into the trachea through the mouth. Performed to open the airway or if the patient is unconscious/comatose, to keep the airway open.

Epipen – an auto-injector containing adrenaline (epinephrine), used to treat severe allergic reactions (anaphylaxis). Dose is fast-acting and can be self-administered. Epipen is a trade name.

Ethical – relating to ethics. Conforming with the rules governing personal and professional conduct.

Extension – the act of straightening or extending a flexed limb.

Flaccid – limp or without muscle tone.

Flail segments – usually refers to chest trauma, where the term 'flail chest' is used. This refers to loss of stability of the chest wall due to three or more ribs that are broken in two or more places as a result of a crushing chest injury. The loose chest segment moves in a direction in the reverse of normal; that is, the segment moves inward during inhalation and outward during exhalation (paradoxical respiration). Other signs and symptoms may include shortness of breath, cyanosis, and extreme pain in the area of trauma.

Flared nostril – may also be termed nasal flaring and refers to an increase in the size of the nostrils associated with work of breathing, for example, in patients with severe asthma.

Flexion – bending of a joint to decrease the angle between two bones or two body parts. Is the opposite of extension.

Fundus – a larger part, base or body of a hollow organ, such as the dome-shaped top of the bladder, uterus above the Fallopian tubes, or rounded, most superior part of the stomach.

Glasgow Coma Score or Scale (GCS) – a quick, standardized tool for measure consciousness. Used especially after a head injury, in which scoring is determined by three factors: amount of eye opening, verbal responsiveness, and motor responsiveness.

Glyceryl tri-nitrate spray (GTN) – a potent smooth muscle relaxant and vasodilator used in transdermal patches and in a paste as well as in oral and sublingual tablets. Used for prevention and treatment of angina pectoris and severe cardiac origin chest pain.

Haemoptysis – symptom of coughing up and spitting out blood.

Haemorrhage – the escape of blood from any part of the vascular system.

Haemothorax – the pooling of blood within the pleural cavity surrounding the lungs, may be caused by trauma or underlying pathology, e.g. cancer.

Handover – the term used to describe the communication process between health professionals, usually involving explaining patient symptoms, condition, treatment to date and personal details. Confidentiality of patient details is important to consider during handover.

Hypercapnia – excessive levels of carbon dioxide in the blood.

Glossary

Hyperglycaemia – an abnormally high concentration of glucose in the blood, a feature of diabetes mellitus.

Hyperpnoea – abnormally deep breathing or an abnormally high rate of breathing.

Hypertension – high blood pressure.

Hyperventilation – a fast breathing rate.

Hypocapnia – low levels of carbon dioxide in the blood.

Hypoglycaemia – an abnormally low concentration of glucose in the blood.

Hypotension – low blood pressure.

Hypothermia – a potentially fatal condition, occurs when body temperature falls below 35°C (95°F).

Hypoxaemia – abnormally low levels of oxygen in the blood.

Hypoxia – deficiency in the amount of oxygen reaching the tissues

Intercostal recession – a clinical sign of respiratory distress which occurs as increasingly negative intra-thoracic pressures cause in-drawing of part of the chest.

Jaundice – a medical condition with yellowing of the skin or whites of the eyes, arising from excess of the pigment bilirubin and typically caused by obstruction of the bile duct, by liver disease, or by excessive breakdown of red blood cells.

Left ventricular failure (LVF) – heart failure in which the left ventricle fails to contract forcefully enough to maintain a normal cardiac output and peripheral perfusion. Pulmonary congestion and oedema develop from back pressure of accumulated blood in the left ventricle. Signs include breathlessness, crackles, dyspnoea, orthopnoea, pallor, sweating, and peripheral vasoconstriction.

Lucid interval – is a temporary improvement in a patient's condition after a traumatic brain injury, after which the condition deteriorates. A lucid interval is especially indicative of an epidural haematoma.

Mechanism of injury (MOI) – the circumstance in which an injury occurs, for example, sudden deceleration, crushing by a heavy object.

Meninges – membranes that protect the brain and spinal cord. There are three: the dura mater, arachnoid and pia mater.

Meningitis – inflammation of the meninges of the brain or spinal cord by a bacterial or viral infection.

Obstetrics – the branch of medicine that deals with the care of women during pregnancy, childbirth, and the recuperative period following delivery.

Orthopnoea – describes the limited ability to breathe when lying down. Is relieved by sitting upright.

Oximetry (Oxygen saturation SpO$_2$) – procedure that measures oxygen levels in the blood using an instrument called an oximeter. Is non-invasive and usually only involves physical contact with a patient's finger, although it may be measured elsewhere on the body, such as an earlobe.

Paradoxical breathing – breathing in which all or part of the chest wall moves in during inhalation and out during exhalation. Lack of symmetry between rib cage and abdomen, causing a 'seesaw' type motion.

Peak expiratory flow (PEF) – also called peak expiratory flow rate (PEFR) is a person's maximum speed of expiration, as measured with a peak flow meter, a small, hand-held device used to monitor a person's ability to breathe out air.

Perfusion – blood flow to a particular part/region of the body.

Personal protective equipment (PPE) – includes items, such as gloves, face shields, high visibility jacket, footwear and helmet.

Pneumothorax – large volume of air that forms in the pleural space and, as progresses, separates the two pleural membranes. Can be spontaneous (occurs for no obvious reason) or caused by trauma.

Primary angioplasty – is the emergency treatment for a myocardial infarction (MI) or, in lay terms, a 'heart attack'. The aim of any heart attack treatment is to clear the blockage in the artery as quickly as possible. Primary angioplasty is one way of doing this.

Primary survey – a structured format to ascertain if someone has any injuries or conditions which are life-threatening. Each element needs to be followed methodically, in order to identify each life-threatening condition and deal with it in the order of priority.

Productive cough – produces phlegm or mucus (sputum). The mucus may have drained down the back of the throat from the nose or sinuses or may have come up from the lungs.

Pursed lips/pursed lip breathing – one of the simplest ways to control shortness of breath. It provides a quick and easy way to slow your pace of breathing, making each breath more effective. Commonly seen in patients with chronic obstructive pulmonary disease (COPD).

Reflex – involuntary muscle reaction that is controlled by the spinal cord.

Secondary survey – follows the primary survey and constitutes a focused history, vital signs and physical examination.

Stethoscope – a medical instrument for listening (auscultate) to the action of someone's heart or breathing, typically having a small disc-shaped resonator that is placed against the chest, and two tubes connected to earpieces.

Stridor – a harsh vibrating noise when breathing, caused by obstruction of the windpipe or larynx.

Sucking chest wound – an open pneumothorax caused by a penetrating injury to the chest wall, causing air to enter the pleural space. The negative pressure created in the thoracic cavity can draw air through the hole in the chest wall.

Tachycardia – rapid heart/pulse rate >100 per minute in adults.

Tachypnoea – rapid breathing >20 per minute in adults.

Time critical – a life-threatening condition that requires immediate pre-hospital intervention and treatment followed by immediate transfer to an appropriate hospital or specialist facility.

Tracheostomy – surgical creation of an opening into the trachea, usually for the insertion of a breathing tube. The incision is called a tracheotomy.

Turgor – an skin assessment used by health professionals to assess dehydration in patients.

Glossary

Type Diabetes 1 – Type 1 diabetes develops when the insulin-producing cells in the body have been destroyed and the body is unable to produce any insulin. Type 1 diabetes can develop at any age, but usually appears before the age of 40, and especially in childhood. It is the most common type of diabetes found in childhood.

Type Diabetes 2 – Type 2 diabetes develops when the insulin-producing cells in the body are unable to produce enough insulin, or when the insulin that is produced does not work properly (known as insulin resistance). Usually develops in people over the age of 40 years.

Unconsciousness – a state of impaired consciousness in which the patient shows no responsiveness to environmental stimuli but may respond to deep pain with involuntary movements. Assessed in primary survey by AVPU and in more detail by using GCS.

Vagus nerve – (X (10th) cranial nerve). Sensation and movement of the throat. Sensory and motor for thoracic and abdominal organs.

Ventilation – bulk movement of gas into and out of the lungs.

Virus – parasitic micro-organism that depends on other cells for its metabolic and reproductive needs.

Vital signs – medical procedure during a physical examination in which the temperature, pulse, respirations (T, P, R) and blood pressure (B/P) are measured to establish a baseline, prior to treatment being instigated.

Index

abdomen
    abdominal sounds 98, 101
    distension and swelling of
        45, 69, 108, 170, 198
    examination in
        cardiovascular
        assessment 66
    examination in trauma
        assessment 169-70
    quadrants of 89, 97-8, 99,
        101, 103, 105, 106-7,
        108
abdominal and gastro-
    intestinal assessment
    abdominal conditions 105-9
    airway of patient 84-5
    avoidance of professional
        misconduct 105
    breathing of patient 85-6
    circulatory system of
        patient 86-8
    disability of patient 88
    ethical and legal
        considerations 103-4
    exposure, examination and
        evaluation of patient
        89-91, 95-103
    patient destination
        decisions 104-5
    patient history 91-5
    patient responses 84
    primary survey 83-4
    review of systems and vital
        signs 103
    risk of danger 84
    scene assessment 82-3
    secondary survey 91
    trauma and 108-9
abuse, child 202, 207, 215,
    258, 259, 262, 266

accessory nerves 125
active movements
    musculoskeletal
        assessment 182
activities of daily living
    (ADLs) 10, 88, 184-5,
    186, 187, 199, 202,
    223, 281
acute cholecystitis 106-7
acute myocardial infraction
    (AMI) 58, 68
acute torticollis 208-9
admission, hospital
    newborns care and
        assessment 322-3
adrenaline in care of newborn
    315, 324
aeration in care of newborn
    316
ailments, minor
    of ear, nose and throat
        227-33
    of gastrointestinal and
        urinary system
        238-42
    of joints 237-9
    of skin 233-5
    see also injuries, minor
airways, patient
    abdominal and
        gastro-intestinal
        assessment 84-5
    alignment of in neonate
        care 315-16, 318
    cardiovascular assessment
        48
    child assessment 248-9
    incident assessment of 4
    mental health assessment
        329

    musculoskeletal
        assessment 180
    neonate care and
        assessment 315-16
    neurological assessment
        113-14
    obstetric patient
        assessment 295-6
    older person assessment
        275
    principles of assessment 4
    respiratory assessment 17
    spinal injuries assessment
        141–2
    trauma assessment 154-5
    see also noises,
        respiratory
alimentary canal 82
allergies, history of
    in respiratory assessment
        21-2
alternating movements 126-7
Alzheimer's disease 285-6
amniotic fluid 36, 310
anaphylaxis
    epidemiology 38
    pathophysiology 38
    patient specific questions
        39
    respiratory assessment
        38-9
    signs and symptoms 38-9
anatomy, patient
    musculoskeletal system
        176-7
aneurysm, aortic 49-50, 66,
    96, 106
angina 67
ankles and feet, patient
    minor injuries of 214-16

Index

musculoskeletal
  assessment 200-201
Simmonds' calf squeeze
  200
ankylosing spondylitis 148
anterior chest auscultation 31
antidepressant drugs 338
antiphospholipid syndrome
  119
antipsychotics 329, 338
anxiolytic drugs 338-9
aorta
  coarctation of aorta 71
  pain in 54
apex beat 61-2, 64
Apgar score 323
apnoetic babies 315
appearance, patient
  of joints in musculoskeletal
    assessment 195,
    197, 198
  of patient in cardiovascular
    assessment 58
appendicitis 105-6
Approved Mental Health
  Professional (AMHP)
  327, 342, 343, 344
arms, patient
  examination in trauma
    assessment 171
  musculoskeletal
    assessment of
    forearms 196-7
  patterns of injury in
    forearms 196
  see also hands, patient;
    wrists, patient
arrhythmias, cardiac, cardiovascular assessment
  70
arrhythmogenic right
  ventricular
  cardiomyopathy
  (ARVC) 72
arthritis
  in older people 278
  see also gout; rheumatoid
    arthritis; septic
    arthritis
ascites 45, 66, 69, 97
assessment, patient

danger at incident 2-3
dementia 207
ethical and legal considerations 12
exposure/examination/
  evaluation of patient
  7-8
importance of
  communication 12
importance of patient
  destination 12
importance of social
  implications 12
incident situation 2
of airway and breathing
  4-5
of circulation 5-6
of disability 6-7
patient responses as
  element of 3
primary survey of incident
  2
safety considerations 1, 2
scene assessment 1, 2
secondary survey 8-11
significance of first
  impressions 12
see also situation e.g.
  development, child;
  respiratory system
  assessment
asthma
  acute severe asthma 34
  child assessment 267
  epidemiology 33
  life threatening asthma 34
  pathophysiology 33-4
  patient specific questions
    34
  prevalence and incidence
    33
  respiratory assessment
    33-5
  signs and symptoms 34
assessment, muscle strength
  126
ataxia
  neurological assessment
    of 126
ATMIST acronym 161
atrial fibrillation (AF) 67

auscultation
  as element of abdominal
    examination 98-101
  in cardiovascular
    assessment 62-5
  in chest trauma
    assessment 168, 169
  in respiratory assessment
    31-3
  principles of assessment
    11
  see also IPPA
AVPU framework
  abdominal and gastro-
    intestinal assessment
    84, 88
  cardiovascular assessment
    48, 51, 76
  child assessment 247,
    255
  mental health assessment
    328, 329, 340
  neurological assessment
    113
  obstetric patient
    assessment 294
  older person assessment
    275
  principles of assessment
    3, 4, 7
  respiratory assessment
    16, 19, 27
  trauma assessment 153

babies
  blue babies 315
  history of presenting
    complaint 260
  masks for 316
  see also child assessment
backs, patient
  child assessment 263
  trauma assessment
    170-71
barking cough 20, 248, 259,
  267-8
BECHS framework 258
biological factors, mental
  health assessment
  339-40
back, patient

Index

in child assessment 263
birth
  criteria of 311-12
  history of in child
    assessment 260-61
blood and bleeding
  catastrophic 2, 154
  gastro-intestinal
    assessment 105
  mental health assessment
    333
  obstetric assessment 293,
    295, 303-4
  potential blood loss from
    fractures 157-8
blood glucose level (BGL)
  abdominal and gastro-
    intestinal assessment
    88
  cardiovascular assessment
    51, 66
  child assessment 255,
    256
  neurological assessment
    117, 133
  older person assessment
    286
  principles of assessment
    7, 11
  respiratory assessment 27
  spinal injuries assessment
    144, 145
blood pressure (BP), patient
  cardiovascular assessment
    60-61
  child assessment 252-3
  older person assessment
    284-5
  respiratory assessment 26
  trauma assessment 164
blood vessels
  examination of 194, 196,
    197, 198, 199, 201
blue babies 315
blunt trauma 42, 108, 152,
  158, 168, 172-3,
  193, 206
bowel
  obstruction 97, 100, 107-8
  sounds 96, 97, 98, 99-
    100, 101, 108

bradycardia 254
bradypnoea 128, 130
breathing, patient
  abdominal and gastro-
    intestinal assessment
    85-6
  cardiovascular assessment
    49
  child assessment 249-52
  incident assessment of 4-5
  mental health assessment
    330
  musculoskeletal
    assessment 180-81
  neurological assessment
    114
  newborn care and
    assessment 316-19
  obstetric patient
    assessment 296-7
  older person assessment
    276
  principles of assessment
    4–5
  respiratory assessment
    17-18
  shortness of breath 22,
    38, 40, 49, 209, 276,
    279, 283, 330
  spinal injuries assessment
    142-3
  trauma assessment
    154-5
  see also efficacy, of
    breathing; effort,
    of breathing;
    spontaneous
    breathing
bronchiolitis, child
  assessment 268-9
bronchospasm 5
Brugada syndrome 71-2
bruising, child assessment
  258
burns, trauma assessment
  161, 173

'C' cervical spine injury 139,
  167
'C' spine manoeuvre 4, 154
capillary bed refill (CBR)

musculoskeletal
  assessment 181, 201
principles of assessment 6
respiratory assessment
  26-7
spinal injuries assessment
  144
trauma assessment 164,
  171
capnometry (ETCO2)
  respiratory assessment
    24-6
  trauma assessment 164-5
cardiac tamponade 60, 61,
  155, 158, 167, 181
cardiovascular assessment
  airway of patient 49
  breathing of patient 49
  circulation of patient 49-50
  danger of patient in 48
  disability of patient 50
  ethical and legal
    considerations 78
  examination processes
    58-66
  importance of patient
    appearance 58
  need to expose/examine/
    evaluate patient 51-2
  patient destination
    decisions 78
  patient history 52-8
  patient responses 48
  primary survey 48
  scene assessment 47-8
  secondary survey 52
  importance of
    communication 78
  significance of ethnicity 77
  significance of family and
    carers 78
  significance of sepsis 73-7
  see also conditions
    e.g. asthma; atrial
    fibrillation; congenital
    heart disease;
    congestive cardiac
    failure; heart attack;
    ischaemic heart
    disease
cardiovascular systems

Index

review in older person
    assessment 284-5
review in respiratory
    assessment 22-3
carpal tunnel syndrome 186
Carter, S. 227
cellulitis 235
central capillary refill (CCR)
    253
central pulses, in child
    assessment 253
cerebral depression 251
Charcot joint 187
chest, patient
    auscultation of 11
    child assessment 250,
        263
    compression in newborns
        319-20, 321
    examination in trauma
        assessment 168
    pain in 49, 53-4, 55-6,
        57, 66-8, 70, 71, 76,
        77, 78
    trauma assessment 42
child assessment
    airway of patient 248-9
    breathing of patient
        249-52
    circulation 252-5
    consent to treatment
        263-4
    danger of patient 246-7
    destination decisions 266
    disability of patient 255-6
    ethical and legal
        considerations 267
    exposure, examination and
        evaluation of 257-9
    importance of
        communication 266
    patient responses 247-8
    primary survey 246
    safeguarding of 264-6
    scene assessment 245-6
    secondary survey 259-62
    social considerations 266
    'top to toe' assessment
        262-3
    see also conditions
        affecting e.g. asthma;

bronchiolitis; croup;
    gastroenteritis;
    measles
childbirth
    criteria of 311-12
    history of in child
        assessment 260-61
Children Act (1989, amended
    2004) 264, 345
cholecystitis, acute 106-7
chronic cough 20, 49
chronic obstructive
    pulmonary disease
    (COPD)
    epidemiology 35
    older person assessment
        278
    pathophysiology 35
    patient specific questions
        36
    respiratory assessment 35-6
    signs and symptoms 35-6
circulation
    abdominal and gastro-
        intestinal assessment
        86-8
    cardiovascular assessment
        49-50
    child assessment 252-5
    incident assessment of
        patient 5–6
    mental health assessment
        331-2
    musculoskeletal
        assessment 176, 179,
        181-2
    newborn care and
        assessment 319-21
    neurological assessment
        114-15
    obstetric patient
        assessment 295,
        297-8
    older person assessment
        276-7
    respiratory assessment 18
    spinal injuries assessment
        143-4
    trauma assessment 163
    see also blood and
        bleeding

classification, wounds 217
coarctation of aorta 71
communication
    cardiovascular assessment
        78
    child assessment 266
    mental health assessment
        342-4
    musculoskeletal
        assessment 181-2,
        202
    newborn care and
        assessment 323
    neurological assessment
        134
    obstetric patient
        assessment 306
    older person assessment
        288
    principles of assessment
        12
    spinal injuries assessment
        148
compartment syndrome
    171-2
compression, chest 319-20,
    321
congenital heart disease
    70-71
congestive cardiac failure
    (CCF) 69-70
consciousness
    child assessment 255
    level of 2, 6, 14, 48, 84,
        88, 113, 116, 121,
        128, 129, 130, 131,
        133, 141, 144, 146,
        154, 156, 159, 166,
        167, 180, 183, 239,
        247, 248, 255, 275,
        283, 294-5, 298,
        328, 332
    neurological assessment
        121
    principles of assessment
        6
    spinal injuries assessment
        141, 144
    trauma assessment 154
consent, patient
    child assessment 264-5

Index

musculoskeletal
   assessment 183,
   187, 202
respiratory assessment
   28
trauma assessment 166
constipation
   characteristics, causes and
   treatment 241-2
*Constipation in Children and
   Young People* (2010)
   266
Control of Industrial Major
   Accident Hazards
   (CIMAH) 140
coordination, point-to-point
   neurological assessment
   127
cough, patient
   cardiovascular assessment
   49
   'Cough Test' assessment
   97, 98
   in general principles of
   assessment 8, 9
   respiratory assessment
   20, 23, 34, 35, 36,
   37, 39
   see also chronic cough;
   productive cough
cranial nerves
   need to review in
   neurological
   assessment 122–6
croup 20, 248, 259, 267-8
cultural considerations *see*
   social and cultural
   considerations
current pregnancy, history of
   as element of secondary
   survey 301
Cushing's triad
   child assessment 254
cuts, patient
   pre-tibial 219
   see also blood and
   bleeding
cyanosis 15, 18, 34, 36, 38,
   71, 133, 208, 251,
   258
cystitis 240

danger
   abdominal and gastro-
   intestinal assessment
   84
   assessment of incident
   2–3
   cardiovascular assessment
   48
   child assessment 246-7
   mental health assessment
   328
   musculoskeletal
   assessment 179
   neurological assessment
   113
   newborn care and
   assessment 310-11
   obstetric patient
   assessment 294
   older person assessment
   274-5
   respiratory assessment 16
   spinal injuries assessment
   140
   trauma assessment 153
Deakin, C.D. 6
decerebrate positioning
   child assessment 256
   neurological assessment
   225
   spinal injuries assessment
   144
decisions, making of
   mental health assessment
   341
decorticate positioning
   child assessment 256
   neurological assessment
   115
   spinal injuries assessment
   144-5
deep vein thrombosis (DVT)
   37, 55
defibrillators 28, 51, 56, 72,
   278
dehydration, patient 88
delirium 275, 285, 286
dementia 148, 207, 275,
   285, 288
depression, cerebral 251
destination, patient

abdominal and
   gastro-intestinal
   assessment 104-5
cardiovascular assessment
   78
child assessment 266
mental health assessment
   345
musculoskeletal
   assessment 202-3
neurological assessment
   135
obstetric patient
   assessment 306
older person assessment
   289
principles of assessment
   12
spinal injuries assessment
   148-9
development, child 261-2
dextrose in care of newborns
   321
diabetes
   child assessment 259
   mental health assessment
   332, 337
   minor injuries assessment
   214, 221, 237, 238
   musculoskeletal
   assessment 186-7
   obstetric patient
   assessment 298,
   300, 301
   older person assessment
   280, 286, 287
Diabetes UK 186
diaphragmatic paralysis
   142-3
diarrhoea, acute
   characteristics, causes
   and treatment
   239-40
   see also gastroenteritis
*Diarrhoea and Vomiting in
   Children under 5*
   (2009) 266
diets, regimens of 281
dilated cardiomyopathy
   (DCM) 72
disability, patient

Index

abdominal and gastro-
intestinal assessment
88
cardiovascular assessment
50
child assessment 255-7
incident assessment of 6-7
mental health assessment
332-3
musculoskeletal
assessment 182-3
neurological assessment
115-17
obstetric patient
assessment 298
older person assessment
277
respiratory assessment
19
spinal injuries assessment
144-5
trauma assessment 159
discharge, vaginal 302-3
diseases, infectious 262
dislocation, shoulder 211
dissection, aortic 155-6
distension and swelling,
abdominal 45, 69,
108, 170, 198
dizziness, patient 121
documentation, wound
injuries 221-2
'do not resuscitate' 289
DR ABCDE framework 2, 45,
153, 173, 245, 246,
291, 293, 305, 307,
327
drop arm test 194
drug/medication history
(DMH)
abdominal and gastro-
intestinal assessment
94-5
cardiovascular assessment
56-7
child assessment 262
element of patient
assessment 9-10
element of secondary
survey assessment
9-10

mental health assessment
337-9
musculoskeletal
assessment 185-6
neurological assessment
119
older person assessment
280-81
premature baby
considerations 322
respiratory assessment
19-22
spinal injuries assessment
148
trauma assessment 162
drugs
in newborns care 321
medication patches 28,
48, 52, 118, 278
drying (body drying) of newborn babies 312-13
Dupuytren's contracture 186
dyspnoea 8, 9, 22, 23, 35,
38, 39

ears, patient
anatomy, examination and
problems 227-8
examination and minor
ailment history 228-9
examination in child
assessment 263
minor ailments affecting
229-30
neurological assessment
123
vestibocochlear nerve 123
eclampsia and pre-eclampsia
119, 132, 297-8,
301, 304-5
ectopic pregnancy 107, 195,
211
efficacy, of breathing
in children 250-51
effort, of breathing
in children 249-50
elbow
examination in
musculoskeletal
assessment 195-6
minor injuries of 211-12

elderly patients, assessment
of see older person
assessment
electrocardiogram (ECG)
cardiovascular assessment
49, 66
recordings in older person
assessment 285
respiratory assessment
26
endotracheal tube (ET) intubation 17, 115, 155
English, B.176, 190
environment
mental health assessment
325, 326
older person assessment
273, 278, 279
principles of assessment 7
regard for 1
respiratory assessment
14, 28
trauma assessment 165-6
epidemiology
anaphylaxis 38
asthma 33, 34
blunt trauma 172
child assessment 267
chronic obstructive
pulmonary disease 35
epistaxis 230-31
erythema, child 257
ethics and law
abdominal and gastro-
intestinal assessment
103-4
cardiovascular assessment
78
child assessment 267
mental health assessment
345
musculoskeletal
assessment 202
neurological assessment
134-5
obstetric patient
assessment 306
older person assessment
289
principles of assessment
12

Index

spinal injuries assessment 148
ethnicity 77
evaluation, patient *see* exposure, examination and evaluation, patient
exclusion, social
  obstetric patient assessment 306
  older person assessment 282
exposure, examination and evaluation, patient
  abdominal and gastrointestinal assessment 89-91
  cardiovascular assessment 51-2, 58-66
  child assessment 257-9, 262-3
  cranial nerve in child assessment 263
  mental health assessment 333
  musculoskeletal assessment 183-4
  neurological assessment 117-18
  obstetric patient assessment 298-9, 305
  older person assessment 277-8
  patient injury at assessment 7-8
  respiratory assessment 19
  spinal injuries assessment 145
  trauma assessment 160
  see also primary survey; secondary survey
extraocular movements, assessment of 123
extremities
  examination in child assessment 263
  examination in trauma assessment 171
eyes
  child assessment 263

neurological assessment 122-3
  see also pupils (eye pupils)

face, neurological assessment 123
FACES pain rating scale 255
fainting, patient
  need to review in neurological assessment 121
families, history of
  in child assessment 262
Feverish Illness in Children Guidelines (2007) 266
falls from height 161
feet and ankles, patient
  minor injuries of 214-16
  musculoskeletal assessment 200-201
  Simmonds' calf squeeze 200
fingers, patient
  wound treatment 218-19
fitting, significance for obstetric assessment 304-5
FLACC rating scale 255
flaccidity, neurological assessment 113
flail segment
  respiratory assessment 42-3
  signs and symptoms 42-3, 158
  trauma assessment 158
flexion, assessment of 115-16, 195
foetal movements, significance for obstetric assessment 303-4
fontanelles, abnormality in 254, 263
forced expiratory volume (FEV) 24
forearms, patient
  musculoskeletal assessment 196-7
  patterns of injury in 196

'four plus 4 more' mnemonic 254
Fraser competence guidelines 264
frozen shoulder 186
function, in musculoskeletal assessment 190, 196, 197, 198, 199, 200
fundus 299

gait, neurological assessment of 126
Galioto, N.J. 233
GASPIPES mnemonic 334
gastroenteritis
  characteristics, causes and treatment 238-9
  child assessment 269
  see also constipation; diarrhoea, acute
gastrointestinal system
  minor injuries affecting 238-42
Gastro-Oesophageal Reflux Disease (2015) 266
General Medical Council (GMC) 264
gestation
  child assessment 260-61
  newborn assessment 311-12, 322
  obstetric assessment 299-300, 304
Gillick competence measure 264
Glasgow Coma Score (GCS) 6-7, 19, 27, 121, 130, 165, 255, 285-6
glossopharyngeal and vagus nerves 123-4
glucose, level of *see* blood glucose level
glycerol trinitrate (GTN) patches 28, 48, 52, 278
gout 237
Gregory, P. 340
grunting, in infants 250

Index

Guidance on Conduct and
 Ethics for Students
 (HPC, 2009) 290
gurgling 4, 27, 99

haematemesis 86-7
haematuria 87
haemoptysis 54
haemorrhage see blood and
 bleeding
haemothorax 44
handover, patient
 obstetric patients 305-6
hands, patient
 condition of in
  cardiovascular
  assessment 59
 examination in
  musculoskeletal
  assessment 196-7
 minor injuries of 212-13
 wound treatment 218-19
 see also fingers, patient;
  wrists, patient
Hazardous Area Response
 Team (HART) 1, 2, 16,
 24, 140
head, patient
 examination in child
  assessment 263
 examination in
  musculoskeletal
  assessment 192-201
 examination in trauma
  assessment 166-7
 neurological assessment
  of injury to 130-31
 neutral position in neonate
  care 314
 see also stroke
headache 130
Head Injury: Triage (2014)
 266
healing and recovery
 compromised wound
  220-21
 factors influencing wound
  221
Health and Care Professions
 Council (HPC) 105,
 166, 289-90

Health and Safety Executive
 176
heart, patient
 disease of 70-71
 failure of 68-70
 myocardial infraction 37,
  42, 52, 53-4, 55, 58,
  60, 67, 68, 70, 71,
  73, 195, 211, 331,
  337
 rate of 313-14, 315, 316-
  17, 319, 321, 322,
  323
Helicopter Emergency
 Medical Services
 (HEMS) 2, 153
herbal drugs 337
hernia 85, 89, 96-7, 104,
 106, 130-31
histories, patient
 abdominal and gastro-
  intestinal assessment
  91-5
 cardiovascular assessment
  52-8
 child assessment 259-62
 element of patient
  assessment 8-10
 minor injury wounds
  217-18
 musculoskeletal
  assessment 184-6
 obstetric patient
  assessment 299-301
 older person assessment
  279-82
 respiratory assessment
  19-22
 spinal injuries assessment
  146-8
 trauma assessment
  160-62
hives 38, 257
hospitals
 admission of newborns
  322-3
 compulsory admission
  343
Hughes Syndrome 119
hyper- and hypoactive bowel
 sounds 100

hyper- and hypothermia 7,
 8, 19, 27, 117, 145,
 179, 183, 220, 270,
 283, 310
hyper-tension 130
hypertrophic cardiomyopathy
 (HCM) 57, 72
hypertropic obstructive
 cardiomyopathy
 (HOCM) 72
hyperventilation syndrome
 41-2
hypo- and hyperactive bowel
 sounds 100
hypo- and hyperthermia 7,
 8, 19, 27, 117, 145,
 179, 183, 220, 270,
 283, 310
hypoglossal nerve 124
hypoglycaemia 116
hypothalmus 258
hypoventilation 85, 323
hypovolaemia 144
hypovolaemic shock
 cardiovascular assessment
  49-50, 66
 child assessment 253-4
 musculoskeletal
  assessment 184
 respiratory assessment 44
 trauma assessment 157-8,
  159
hypoxia 114

immediacy of action
 obstetric assessment 299
immunizations, history of
 in child assessment 262
implantable cardiovascular
 defibrillator 28, 51,
 56, 72, 278
impressions (IMP)
 at incident assessment 12
 neurological assessment
  134
 older person assessment
  287
inadequacy, respiratory
 251-2
infants
 blue babies 315

history of presenting
  complaint 260
masks for 316
infectious diseases
history of in child
  assessment 262
inflation, lung 316-17, 321
inherited cardiac conditions
  (ICCs) 71-2
injuries, minor
  documentation of wound
    injuries 221-2
  examination of and
    common causes of
    neck pain 208-10
  framework for assessing
    pain in 208
  head wounds and bruising
    207-8
  lower limb 213-16
  mechanisms of head injury
    206
  red flag situations for head
    207
  referral of wound injuries
    222-3
  upper limb 210-13
  wound classification,
    types and treatment
    216-21
inspection
  abdomen in trauma
    assessment 169-70
  abdominal and gastro-
    intestinal assessment
    96-8, 108-9
  chest in trauma
    assessment 168
  musculoskeletal
    assessment 194,
    195, 197, 199, 200
  respiratory assessment 28
inspection, palpitation,
  percussion, ausculta-
  tion (IPPA) 28-33, 168
intestines
  obstruction 97, 100, 107-8
  sounds 96, 97, 98, 99-100,
    101, 108
intubation, endotracheal tube
  17, 115, 155

ischaemic heart disease
  (IHD) 67-8

jaw
  examination in
    musculoskeletal
    assessment 192
jaw thrust manoeuvre 318-19,
  141, 142, 155
joints
  classification of 191
  crepitus 182, 189, 192,
    197, 199
  inspection in
    musculoskeletal
    assessment 237-9
  mobility of 186
  see also name and limb
    e.g. Charcot joint;
    feet and ankles; knee
    joints; wrists
jugular venous pressure (JVP)
  62

Kauffman, M. 230
key features, emergency
  abdominal and gastro-
    intestinal assessment
    109
  cardiovascular assessment
    78
  child assessment 269
  mental health assessment
    346
  minor injuries assessment
    224
  minor ailments
    assessment 242-3
  musculoskeletal
    assessment 203
  newborn care and
    assessment 304
  neurological assessment
    136
  obstetric patient
    assessment 307
  older person assessment
    309
  respiratory assessment 45
  spinal injuries assessment
    149

trauma assessment 173
knee joints
  minor injuries of 213-14
  musculoskeletal
    assessment 199-200
knuckles, wound treatment
  218-19
Kussmaul's sign 27, 28,
  62, 85
kyphosis 148, 193, 209,
  275, 283

lacerations
  pre-tibial 219
  see also blood and
    bleeding
Laird, C. 227
large bowel obstruction
  107-8
laryngotracheobronchitis 20,
  248, 259, 267-8
left ventricular failure (LVF)
  9, 22, 40, 49, 52,
  65, 69
legal considerations see
  ethics and law
legs, patient
  examination in trauma
    assessment 171
leucorrhoea 302-3
level of consciousness (LOC)
  2, 6, 14, 48, 84, 88,
  113, 116, 121, 128,
  129, 130, 131, 133,
  141, 144, 146, 154,
  156, 159, 166, 167,
  180, 183, 239, 247,
  248, 255, 275, 283,
  294-5, 298, 328,
  332
life expectancy and
  demography 290-91
light-headedness, patient
  need to review in
    neurological
    assessment 121
listening
  need for in
    musculoskeletal
    assessment 200
long QT syndrome (LQTS) 71

Index

looking *see* inspection
Lowe, J.L. 6
lungs, inflation of
   in neonate assessment
      and care 316-17, 321

masks, for babies 315
massive haemothorax/
   haemorrhage 157-8
measles 268
mechanism of injury (MOI)
   abdominal and
      gastrointestinal
      assessment 82, 86,
      109
   child assessment 259
   minor injuries assessment
      206-7, 209, 213,
      215, 216, 223
   musculoskeletal
      assessment 178-9,
      184, 185, 188, 193
   older person assessment
      280
   principles of assessment
      2, 4, 8
   respiratory assessment 44
   spinal injury assessment
      139-40, 146, 147,
      148
   trauma assessment 151-2,
      158, 160, 161, 167,
      170, 172
medication
   in newborns care 321
   medication patches 28,
      48, 52, 118, 278
melaena
   in abdominal assessment
      87
meningitis
   neurological assessment
      114-15, 131-2
   signs and symptoms 131
meningococcal septicaemia
   117, 128, 132, 254,
   257
Mental Capacity Act (2005)
   134-5, 264, 340-41
Mental Health (Care and
   Treatment) (Scotland)
   Act (2003) 341

Mental Health (NI) Order
   (1986) 341
Mental Health Act (1983,
   amended 2007)
   341-2, 342-4
mental health assessment
   airway of patient 329
   breathing of patient 330
   circulation 331-2
   danger of patient 328
   destination decision 345
   disability of patient 332-3
   ethical and legal
      considerations 345
   exposure, examination and
      evaluation 333
   facts and figures about
      345-6
   importance of
      communication 342-4
   patient responses 328-9
   primary survey 327
   review of systems and vital
      signs 340
   scene assessment 326-7
   secondary survey 333-40
   social considerations
      344-5
mental status
   neurological assessment
      121-2
misconduct, professional
   avoidance in abdominal
      assessment 105
   see also standards,
      professional
mitral regurgitation 72
mitral stenosis 72
motor skills
   neurological assessment
      126-7
mouth, examination of
   child assessment 263
   glossopharyngeal and
      vagus nerves 123-4
movement and positioning
   abdominal and gastro-
      intestinal assessment
      88
   child airway openness 248
   in foetuses 303-4
   neutral head position 314

   of joints in musculoskeletal
      assessment 194,
      195-6, 197, 198,
      199, 200
   see also active
      movements;
      alternating
      movements; passive
      movements; resisted
      movements
murmur, aortic 284
muscles, patient
   assessment of strength
      126
   tone of in neonate care
      312
musculoskeletal assessment
   airway of patient 180
   breathing of patient
      180-81
   danger of patient 179
   destination decisions
      202-3
   disability of patient 182-3
   ethical and legal
      considerations 202
   expose/examine/evaluate
      183-4
   importance of
      communication 181-2,
      202
   patient history 184-6
   patient responses 179-80
   physical assessment
      187-92
   physiological aspects 177
   primary survey 178-9
   review of patient systems
      186
   scene assessment 178
   secondary survey 184
   social considerations in
      202
   *see also particular joints
      and conditions
      e.g. carpal tunnel
      syndrome; knee joint;
      pelvis; tenosynovitis;
      wrist joint*
musculoskeletal systems
   review in respiratory
      assessment 23

Index

review in trauma
  assessment 163
myocardial infraction
  abdominal and gastro-
    intestinal assessment
    195
  cardiovascular assessment
    52, 53-4, 55, 58, 60,
    67, 68, 70, 71, 73
  mental health assessment
    331, 337
  minor injuries assessment
    211
  respiratory assessment
    37, 42

naloxone 318
National Audit Office (NAO)
  151
*National Service Framework
  for Older People* (DoH,
  2001) 290
National Society for Prevention of Cruelty to
  Children (NSPCC)
  264
neck, examination of
  in child assessment 263
  musculoskeletal
    assessment 192
  trauma assessment 167
Neonatal Jaundice (2010)
  266
nerves
  examination in
    musculoskeletal
    assessment 194,
    196, 197, 198, 199,
    201
  see also name e.g.
    accessory nerves;
    cranial nerves;
    glossopharyngeal
    and vagus nerves;
    hypoglossal nerve;
    olfactory nerve; optic
    nerve
neurological assessment
  airway of patient 113-14
  body systems review
    119-27
  breathing of patient 114

considerations for
  successful 134-6
danger of scene 113
disability of patient 115-17
ethical and legal
  considerations 134-5
exposure/examination/
  evaluation 117-18
facts and figures 135-6
impressions 134
of common neurological
  conditions 127-34
patient circulatory system
  114-15
patient responses 113
primary survey 112
scene assessment 112
secondary survey 118-19
vital signs review 119-27
neurological systems
  review in older person
    assessment 285-6
  review in respiratory
    assessment 23
  review in trauma
    assessment 163
newborns, assessment of
  airway of patient 315-16
  breathing of patient
    316-19
  circulation 319-21
  danger of patient 310-11
  departure to hospital
    322-3
  drugs 321
  importance of
    communication 323
  premature baby
    considerations 322
  primary survey 310
  responses of 311-15
  scene assessment 309-10
NHS Choices, 226
NHS England 151
noises, respiratory
  in children 250
non-accidental injury (NAI)
  202, 207, 215, 258,
  259, 262, 266
non-blanching rash 257
non-cardiac pain 54
non-conveyance, patient

abdominal and
  gastro-intestinal
  assessment 104-5
cardiovascular assessment
  78
child assessment 266
musculoskeletal
  assessment 202-3
neurological assessment
  135
obstetric patient
  assessment 306
older person assessment
  289
principles of assessment
  12
non-steroidal anti-
  inflammatory drugs
  (NSAIDs) 94-5, 229,
  237
nose, patient
  examination in child
    assessment 263
  minor ailments affecting
    230-31

obesity 45, 97, 237, 296,
  298
obstetric patient assessment
  airway of patient 295-6
  breathing of patient 296-7
  circulation 295, 297-8
  danger of patient 294
  destination decisions 306
  disability of patient 298
  ethical and legal
    considerations 306
  expose/examine/evaluate
    298-9, 305
  fundus 299
  handover of patients in
    305-6
  history 299-301
  immediacy of action 299
  importance of
    communication 306
  patient responses 294-5
  primary survey 293-4
  scene assessment 293
  secondary survey 299-305
  social, family and carer
    considerations 306

Index

obstruction, bowel 97, 100, 107-8
oedema
  in cardiovascular assessment 65
Office of National Statistics (ONS) 290
older person assessment
  airway of patient 275
  breathing of patient 276
  circulation 276-7
  danger of patient 274-5
  dementia 275
  demography and life expectancy 290-91
  destination decisions 289
  disability of patient 277
  ethical and legal considerations 289
  expose/examine/evaluate 277-8
  importance of communication 288
  patient responses 275
  primary survey 274
  professional standards requirements 289-90
  review of systems and vital signs 283-7
  scene assessment 273-4
  secondary survey 278-82
  social considerations 288
  spinal injuries assessment 173
  trauma assessment of 173
olfactory nerve 122
onset of pain 120
open pneumothorax 43-4, 156
opisthotonus positioning 116
optic nerve 122-3
oropharyngeal airway 142, 249, 318, 319, 330
orthopnoea 54
orthostatic hypotension 61
osteoporosis
  older person assessment 287
  spinal injuries assessment 148
Ottawa ankle rule 201

otitis externa 230
otitis media 229-30
over the counter (OTC) medicines 9-10, 56, 261
oxygen saturation (SpO2)
  abdominal and gastro-intestinal assessment 85
  cardiovascular assessment 48, 49, 66, 73
  child assessment 245, 252
  mental health assessment 330, 340
  neurological assessment 133
  older person assessment 276, 283
  principles of assessment 5, 11, 14, 18
  respiratory assessment 34, 46
  spinal injuries assessment 142
  trauma assessment 155, 156

pain, patient
  abdominal and gastro-intestinal assessment 82, 83, 84, 85, 91-3, 95-6, 97, 98-9, 101-2, 103
  frameworks for assessment 21-2, 255
  neurological assessment 120-21
  non-cardiac and pericardial 53, 54
  palliation of 120
  provocation of 120
  significance in obstetric assessment 302
  see also sources e.g. acute cholecystitis; aorta; chest, patient
  see also type e.g. radiating pain
pain scores

abdominal and gastro-intestinal assessment 93
cardiovascular assessment 66
minor injury assessment 208, 222, 228, 235
neurological assessment 121
obstetric patient assessment 203
older person assessment 287
principles of assessment 22
respiratory assessment 21
trauma assessment 162
palliation, pain 120
palpation, body
  child assessment 253
  element of abdominal examination 96-7, 98, 99, 101-2, 108
  minor ailment assessment 230, 232
  musculoskeletal assessment 182, 189, 192, 194, 195, 196, 197, 198, 199, 200
  of abdominal quadrants 170
  respiratory assessment 23, 28-9
  spinal injuries assessment 146
  trauma assessment 166-7, 169, 170, 171
pancreatitis 108
paralysis and weakness, patient
  need to review in neurological assessment 121
paroxysmal nocturnal dyspnoea (PND) 22, 49, 54, 325, 336, 337
passive movements
  musculoskeletal assessment 182
past medical history (PMH)

Index

abdominal and gastro-
   intestinal assessment
   94
 as element of patient
   assessment 9
 cardiovascular assessment
   56
 child assessment 20
 element of secondary
   survey assessment 9
 mental health assessment
   337
 musculoskeletal
   assessment 185
 neurological assessment
   119
 obstetric patient
   assessment 300
 older person assessment
   280
 respiratory assessment 22
 spinal injuries assessment
   147
 trauma assessment 162
past obstetric history
 significance for obstetric
   assessment 300-301
patches, glycerol trinitrate
   28, 48, 52, 278
peak expiratory flow (PEF) 24
pelvis, examination
 child assessment 254
 musculoskeletal
   assessment 197-8
 trauma assessment 170
percussion
 abdominal and gastro-
   intestinal assessment
   101-3
 chest injuries 168-9
 respiratory assessment
   29-30
periorbital ecchymosis 131,
   167
peripheral pulses
 cardiovascular assessment
   66
 child assessment 253
peri-tonsillar abscess 233
PERRLA (Pupils Equal and
   Round; React to Light

and Accommodation)
   Framework 7, 19,
   51, 88, 116-17, 144,
   145, 159, 165, 255,
   256, 263, 277, 286,
   298, 333
petechiae 257
photophobia 117
physiology, patient
 musculoskeletal system
   176-7
pink and vigourous babies
   313, 314
pins and needles, patient
 need to review in
   neurological
   assessment 121
pleural space of lungs 43-4,
   156-7
pneumonia 39-40
pneumothorax 43-4
point-to-point coordination
 neurological assessment
   127
positioning see movement
   and positioning
possible actions
 abdominal and gastro-
   intestinal assessment
   85, 86, 88, 91, 98,
   101, 103
 assessment general
   principles 3, 4, 5, 6,
   7, 8, 10
 cardiovascular assessment
   49, 50, 51, 52, 58,
   59, 62, 65, 68, 70,
   76
 child assessment 247,
   248, 249, 252, 255,
   256, 258-9
 mental health assessment
   328, 329, 330, 332-3,
   336, 337
 minor ailments
   assessment 231
 minor injuries assessment
   218
 musculoskeletal
   assessment 179,
   180, 181, 183, 184

neurological assessment
   114, 117, 129, 132,
   133
 newborn assessment
   310, 311, 312, 313,
   315, 316, 317, 319,
   320-21
 obstetric assessment 294,
   295, 296, 297, 298,
   299
 older person assessment
   275, 276, 277, 278
 respiratory assessment
   14, 16, 17, 18, 19,
   35, 36, 37, 39, 40,
   41, 42, 43, 44
 spinal injuries assessment
   140, 141, 142, 143,
   144, 145, 147
 trauma assessment 153,
   154, 155, 158, 159,
   160
posterior chest auscultation
   31
posture, patient
 in child assessment 255-5
 pupillary responses and 7
praecordium
 cardiovascular assessment
   61-2
pre-eclampsia and eclampsia
   119, 132, 297-8,
   301, 304-5
pregnancy
 abdominal and gastro-
   intestinal assessment
   83, 96, 97, 103, 106,
   107
 current pregnancy as
   element of secondary
   survey 301
 minor injury assessment
   240
 neurological assessment
   119
 newborns assessment
   312
 obstetric patient
   assessment 293-4,
   295-6, 297-8, 300,
   301, 302-3, 304-5

Index

respiratory assessment
37, 45
see also ectopic pregnancy
premature babies 322
presentation, patient
significance for mental
health assessment
326-7
presenting complaint (PC)
abdominal and gastro-
intestinal assessment
92-3
as element of patient
assessment 8
as element of secondary
assessment 8-9
cardiovascular assessment
53-5
child assessment 259-60
mental health assessment
333-6
musculoskeletal
assessment 185
neurological assessment
118
older person assessment
279
respiratory assessment
19-20
spinal injuries assessment
146
trauma assessment
160-61
presenting complaint history
(HPC)
abdominal and gastro-
intestinal assessment
92-3
as element of patient
assessment 9
as element of secondary
survey 9, 301-5
cardiovascular assessment
55
child assessment 259-60
mental health assessment
336-7
musculoskeletal
assessment 184
neurological assessment
118-19

older person assessment
279-80
respiratory assessment
20-21
spinal injuries assessment
146-7
trauma assessment 161-2
PRICE 212
primary survey
abdominal and gastro-
intestinal assessment
83-4
cardiovascular assessment
48
child assessment 246
mental health assessment
327
musculoskeletal
assessment 178-9
neurological assessment
112
newborns care and
assessment 310
obstetric patient
assessment 293-4
of incidents 2
older person assessment
274
respiratory assessment 16
spinal injuries assessment
139
trauma assessment 152-3
productive cough 20, 49
professionalism
importance in neurological
assessment 135
see also standards,
professional
professional misconduct,
avoidance of 105
pronator drift 126
provocation, pain 120
psychosocial factors in mental health assessment
339-40
pulmonary embolism (PE)
36-7
pulmonary oedema 40-41
pulse, patient
in cardiovascular
assessment 60

see also central pulses
pulse oximetry
respiratory assessment 24
trauma assessment 163
pulse rate
cardiovascular assessment
60
in child assessment 252
older person assessment
284
respiratory assessment
26
trauma assessment 164
pupils (eye pupils)
assessment in trauma
cases 165
cardiovascular assessment
51, 66
child assessment 255-6
examination in neurological
assessment 116-17
head injury 130
older person assessment
286
pupillary responses 7,
128, 256-6, 340
radiating pain 120
purpura 257
pyelonephritis 240-41

QT internal measurement
331
*Quality Standards for Asthma
(2013)* 266
quickening 303-4
quinsy 233

radial pulse, assessment of
5, 18, 50, 60, 159,
164, 297
radiating pain 190, 191-2,
194, 195, 197, 198,
199
rashes and marks
abdominal and
gastro-intestinal
assessment 96
cardiovascular assessment
76-7
child assessment 257,
263, 268

Index

minor injuries and ailments assessment 209, 234
neurological assessment 117, 131-2
respiratory assessment 28
recovery and healing
compromised wound 220-21
factors influencing wound 221
Reference Guide to Consent for Examination and Treatment (DoH, 2009) 264
referral
of wound injuries 222-3
regimens, diet 281
regurgitation, aortic 73
rescue, patient
general considerations 1
resisted movements 182
respiratory assessment
airway of patients in 17
breathing of patient in 17-18
circulation in 18
danger of patient in 16
disability of patient 19
exposure/examination/evaluation of patients in 19
global overview in scene assessment 14
injuries to respiratory system 42-4
mechanical factors affecting the respiratory system 45
patient history in 19-22
patient responses 16-17
physical assessment 27-8
primary survey 16
process of 28-33
review of systems (ROS) 22-3
scene assessment 14-15
secondary survey of 19-22
vital signs in 23-7
see also inadequacy, respiratory; noises, respiratory

see also conditions e.g. asthma; chronic obstructive pulmonary disease; pulmonary embolism
respiratory rate
abdominal and gastro-intestinal assessment 85, 86, 103
cardiovascular assessment 66, 73, 74, 77
child assessment 245-6, 248, 249
inadequacy of in children 250, 251-2
mental health assessment 340
neurological assessment 132
obstetric assessment 296-7
older person assessment 283
principles of assessment 5, 11
respiratory assessment 17, 23
trauma assessment 156, 163
respiratory system
older person assessment 283
trauma assessment 163
response, process of
abdominal and gastro-intestinal assessment 84
as element of incident assessment 3
at initial assessment at birth 311-15
cardiovascular assessment 48
child assessment 247-8
mental health assessment 328-9
musculoskeletal assessment 179-80
neurological assessment 113

obstetric patient assessment 294-5
older person assessment 275
respiratory assessment 16-17
spinal injuries assessment 140-41
trauma assessment 153-4
responses, pupillary 7, 128, 256-6, 340
resuscitation
newborn assessment and care 311-12, 315, 316, 317, 321-2, 323
older person assessment 289
trauma assessment 154-5
Resuscitation Council (UK) 68
reverse stethoscope technique 288
review of systems (ROS)
abdominal and gastro-intestinal assessment 103
as element of assessment secondary service 10-11
mental health assessment 340
musculoskeletal assessment 186-7
neurological assessment 119-27
older person assessment 283-7
respiratory assessment 22-3
trauma assessment 162-5
rheumatoid arthritis 9, 56, 96, 148, 176, 185, 195, 209, 211, 212
RICE acronym 215
right ventricular failure (RVF) 68-9
road traffic collisions (RTC) 2, 3, 82, 89, 98, 139, 149, 151, 153, 161, 173, 179, 206, 245, 274

Index

Romberg test 127
rotation, external arm 195
rubeola 268

safeguarding
  child assessment 264-6
  see also abuse, child
safety, incident
  importance and
    considerations 1, 2
saline
  in neonate care 321
SAMPLE framework
  child assessment 261
  older person assessment
    279
  principles of assessment
    11
  respiratory assessment 21
SCENE acronym 151-2
scene assessment
  abdominal and gastro-
    intestinal assessment
    82-3
  cardiovascular assessment
    47-8
  child assessment 245-6
  mental health assessment
    326-7
  musculoskeletal
    assessment 178
  newborns care and
    assessment 309-10
  neurological assessment
    112
  obstetric patient
    assessment 293
  older person assessment
    273-4
  principles of assessment 1
  respiratory assessment
    14-15
  spinal injuries assessment
    139
  trauma assessment 151-2
  see also primary surveys;
    secondary surveys
schizophrenia 326, 327,
  328, 331, 332, 334,
  336, 337
secondary surveys

abdominal and gastro-
  intestinal assessment
  91
  at incident assessment
    8-11
  cardiovascular assessment
    52
  child assessment 259-62
  mental health assessment
    333-40
  musculoskeletal
    assessment 184
  neurological assessment
    118-19
  obstetric patient
    assessment 299-305
  older person assessment
    278-82
  respiratory assessment
    19-22
  spinal injuries assessment
    146-8
  trauma assessment
    160-62
seizures
  neurological assessment
    121, 132-3
  vital signs 133
self-harm and suicide, risk of
  mental health assessment
    335
senses, patient
  need to review in
    neurological
    assessment 126
septic arthritis 236-7
shock, hypovolaemic see
  hypovolaemic shock
shortness of breath (SOB)
  22, 38, 40, 49, 209,
  276, 279, 283, 330
shoulders (glenohumeral)
  joint
  accessory nerve and 125
  examination in
    musculoskeletal
    assessment 193-5
  minor injuries of 210-11
Simmonds' calf squeeze
  200
skin, patient

child assessment 253,
  263
  minor ailments affecting
    233-5
  neonate care and
    assessment 309,
    312, 313, 314, 322
  respiratory assessment
    18
  significance for general
    assessment 6
  spinal injuries assessment
    143
SLIPDUCT framework 182,
  188-9
small bowel obstruction,
  107-8
smell
  neurological assessment
    122
  olfactory nerve and 122
smoking
  significance for abdominal
    and gastro-intestinal
    assessment 83, 95
  significance for
    cardiovascular
    assessment 57-8
  significance for general
    assessment 22
  significance for minor
    injuries 221
  see also chronic
    obstructive pulmonary
    disease 35
snoring 4, 17, 250
social and cultural considerations
  cardiovascular assessment
    57
  child assessment 263
  mental health assessment
    339-40, 344-5
  musculoskeletal
    assessment 18
  neurological assessment
    134
  obstetric patient
    assessment 306
  older person assessment
    281-2

principles of assessment 10
see also particular e.g. exclusion, social
social/family medical history (S/FMH)
  abdominal and gastro-intestinal assessment 95
  as element of patient assessment 10
  cardiovascular assessment 57-8
  child assessment 266
  mental health assessment 339-40
  musculoskeletal assessment 186
  neurological assessment 119
  older person assessment 288
  respiratory assessment 22
SOCRATES framework 11, 21, 55, 92, 109, 120, 146, 162, 208, 209, 215, 228, 235, 260, 279-80, 302
sodium bicarbonate
  in neonate care 321
sore throat 231-2
  see also tonsillitis
sounds
  abdominal and gastrointestinal assessment 98, 101
  auscultation respiratory assessment 31-3
  bowel 96, 97, 98, 99-100, 101, 107-8
  trauma assessment 156, 158, 168-9
Special Operations Response Team (SORT) 1, 2, 3, 16, 24, 140, 153
spinal column
  examination in musculoskeletal assessment 193
spinal injuries assessment
  airway 141-2

breathing of patient 142–3
circulation in 143-4
danger of patient 140
dementia 148
destination considerations 148-9
disability of patient 144-5
ethical and legal considerations 148
exposure/examination/evaluation in 145
importance of communication 148
patient history 146-8
patient responses 140-41
prevalence of 149
primary survey 139
scene assessment 139
secondary survey 146-8
thorax and spinal injuries 143, 155
spontaneous breathing
  failure of newborn to commence 317
sprains and strains, lower limb 215-16
stable angina 53, 68
standards, professional
  older person assessment 289-90
  see also professionalism
stenosis, aortic 60-61, 64, 65, 70, 72-3
stepwise approach
  child assessment 249
  musculoskeletal assessment 180, 183, 187-8
striae 89
stridor 4, 11, 17, 38, 169, 231, 250, 263, 268
stroke
  neurological assessment 127-8
  vital signs 128
sub-arachnoid haemorrhage 129
suicide and self-harm, risk of
  mental health assessment 335

support for older people, forms of 273-4
swelling and distension, abdominal 45, 69, 108, 170, 198
sympathetic autonomic control 143
syncope, patient 121
systolic blood pressure 6, 26, 41, 75, 253, 305
systolic murmur 71, 284

tachycardia 252
tactile fremitus 29
temperature
  cardiovascular assessment 66, 74
  child assessment 258
  loss of in newborns 310, 314
  minor injuries assessment 220, 232, 233
  musculoskeletal assessment 187, 194, 197, 199
  neurological assessment 117, 129, 132
  older person assessment 286
  respiratory assessment 27
spinal injuries assessment 144, 152
tenosynovitis 186
tension pneumothorax 43, 156
term gestation 311, 322
thorax and spinal injuries 143, 155
throat, patient
  minor injuries affecting 231-3
tonic clonic seizure 132-3
tonsillitis 232-3
'toxic trio' 265
tracheal deviation 18, 167
transient ischaemic attack 128-9
transient loss of conscious-ness 51, 53, 107
trauma assessment

Index

abdomen and gastro-
intestinal system
108-9
airway of patient in 154-5
AVPU framework 153
breathing of patient in
155- 8
catastrophic haemorrhage
in 154
circulation and 159
danger of patient 153
definition and
characteristics 151
disability of patient 159-60
exposure/examination/
evaluation in 160
head to toe assessment in
166-73
patient history 160-62
patient response 153-4
physical assessment in
165-6
primary survey 152-3
review of systems related
to trauma 162-3
scene assessment
151-2
secondary survey 160-62
vital signs and 163-5
see also recipients and
focus of e.g. airways,
patient; older person
assessment
Trauma Audit and Research
Network (TARN) 151
trigeminal nerve 123
TWELVE framework 167-9

umbilical cord management
309-10, 311, 314
unconsciousness 113
unstable angina 53, 60, 68
urinary system
minor injuries affecting
240-41
urinary tract infection (UTI)
240
urine dipstick testing 286
urticaria 38, 257

vagus nerve 123
valvular heart disease 72-3
ventilation
principles of assessment 4
respiratory assessment
24, 42
spinal injuries assessment
142-3
ventricular septal defect
(VSD) 71
vertigo, patient 121
vestibocochlear nerve 123
vision, optic nerve and 122-3
vital signs
abdominal and gastro-
intestinal assessment
103
cardiovascular assessment
66
mental health assessment
340
neurological assessment
128
older person assessment
283-7

respiratory assessment
23-7
trauma assessment 163-5
vulnerability, patient
abdominal and gastro-
intestinal assessment
95
minor injuries assessment
207, 219
musculoskeletal
assessment 202
neurological assessment
135
older person assessment
273, 282
obstetric patient
assessment 306
mental health assessment
328, 337

Ward, A. 340
Wardrope, J. 176, 190
weakness and paralysis,
patient 121
Wong-Baker FACES pain
rating scale 255
World Health Organisation
(WHO) 325, 345
wounds
classification, types and
treatment 216-23
wrists, patient
examination in
musculoskeletal
assessment 196-7
minor injuries of 212-13
wry neck 208-9

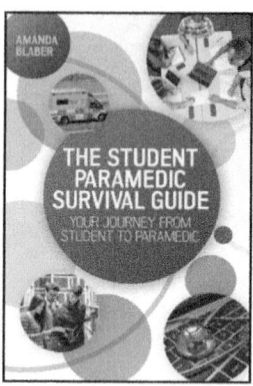

The Student Paramedic Survival Guide

Blaber

ISBN: 9780335262366 (Paperback)
eBook: 978033526373
2015

The Student Paramedic Survival Guide gives information and advice to help you succeed in your education and become a registered paramedic. The book supports you from the start of your journey as you choose a programme, through study and practice placements, to the final stages of registration and applying for work. Finally, the book prepares you to make the transition into your first paramedic job.

To equip you with insights into what studying to be a paramedic is really like, the book is packed full of comments from students, paramedics, mentors, paramedic educators and academics. Their expertise and experience will be invaluable as you study and prepare for practice. Other useful tools are included, such as web links for suggested further reading. The book will answer questions such as:

- Is this the right career for me?
- What do I need to consider when choosing a university and programme of study?
- What will I be studying?
- How can I make the most of the simulations that are part of my course?
- Who is there to support me on placements?
- What is it like caring for patients and their families?
- How can I adjust to shift work?
- What can I do to prepare for registration and securing my first job?

www.mheducation.co.uk

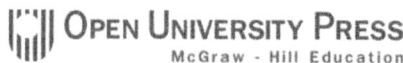

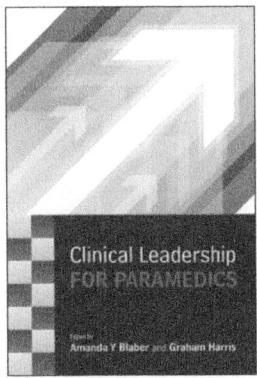

Clinical Leadership for Paramedics

Amanda Blaber and Graham Harris

ISBN: 9780335263127 (Paperback)
eBook: 9780335263134
2014

Clinical Leadership for Paramedics is the first book of its kind to demonstrate just how vital leadership skills are for all paramedics and explore how paramedics can lead in their everyday practice. Divided into two parts the book looks at both the context of contemporary leadership for paramedic practice and then the specific skills of leadership.

Key chapters include:

- What is leadership and who does it?
- Communication skills & leadership
- Working as a team

www.mheducation.co.uk

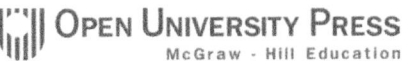